GUIDE TO LIVER TRANSPLANTATION

GUIDE TO LIVER TRANSPLANTATION

THOMAS L. FABRY, M.D., Ph.D.
Associate Clinical Professor of Medicine
Mount Sinai School of Medicine
Associate Attending
Mount Sinai Hospital
New York, New York

FRANKLIN M. KLION, M.D.
Clinical Professor of Medicine
Mount Sinai School of Medicine
Chief, Liver Clinic
Mount Sinai Hospital
New York, New York

IGAKU-SHOIN New York • Tokyo

Published and distributed by

IGAKU-SHOIN Medical Publishers, Inc.
One Madison Avenue, New York, N.Y. 10010

IGAKU-SHOIN Ltd.,
5-24-3 Hongo, Bunkyo-ku, Tokyo

Library of Congress Cataloging-in-Publication Data

Guide to liver transplantation [edited by] Thomas L. Fabry, Franklin M. Klion.
p. cm.
Includes bibliographical references and index.
1. Liver—Transplantation. I. Fabry, Thomas L. II. Klion, Franklin M.
[DNLM: 1. Liver Transplantation. WI 770 G946]
RD546.G85 1992
617.5′56—dc20
DNLM/DLC
for Library of Congress 92-1461
CIP

ISBN: 0-89640-211-8 (New York)
ISBN: 4-260-14211-9 (Tokyo)

Printed and bound in the U.S.A.

10 9 8 7 6 5 4 3 2 1

FOREWORD
An Institutional Perspective on Liver Transplantation

In 1984, The Mount Sinai Medical Center, comprising the Mount Sinai Hospital and the Mount Sinai School of Medicine, decided to develop a liver transplantation program. It was not a decision taken lightly. Rather, it evolved from extensive discussions among the medical staff of many departments, including Surgery, Medicine, Pediatrics, Anaesthesia, Pathology, Psychiatry, the Blood Bank, and Radiology, as well as the hospital Nursing, Social Service, and Pharmacy staffs, administration at many levels, and, ultimately, the separate but overlapping Boards of Trustees of the Hospital, the Medical School, and the Medical Center.

The first liver transplantation operation at Mount Sinai was performed in September 1988. As this is written, in late 1991, we are nearing our 300th recipient. An anticipated 130 patients will receive approximatley 145 new livers in 1991, and current projections are that we will exceed 150 new recipients in 1992. The program has been a striking success in every way that we could possibly have anticipated, and in many unanticipated ways as well.

This *Guide to Liver Transplantation* has evolved out of the Mount Sinai experience. Nevertheless, the Mount Sinai staff brought to the program diverse backgrounds in many disciplines, learned during periods of training in many institutions. Hence, the outlook is not parochial. Moreover, while the practicing transplant physician or surgeon is unlikely to find in these pages any startling revelations, any physician seeing patients with liver disease who are potential candidates for liver transplantation, or whose patients have returned after undergoing successful transplantation, will find in this volume much essential information, based on long and extensive experience. The chapters that follow will assist in guiding appropriate patients to liver transplant centers at appropriate times in the course of their diseases; will provide an appreciation of the medical and surgical technology and the biological and psychosocial stresses that will be focused on these patients as they undergo the transplant experience; and will describe the numerous problems that may occur at various times in the post-transplant period, with emphasis on early recognition and on a rational basis for deciding which can be dealt with by the referring physician and which require the services of the transplant center.

Why did Mount Sinai decide to embark on this complex and costly venture? And why did we succeed where others have not? Both of these questions, and their interrelated answers, may be of interest to those who are considering initiating similar programs.

The answer to the first question is embedded in Mount Sinai's institutional history: for more than 50 years, diseases of the liver have been a central focus of both the patient care activities and research interests of many members of our staff. Hans Popper, the world's premier hepatopathologist, virtual creator of the modern discipline of hepatology, and a founder of the American Association for the Study of Liver Disease and of the International Association for the Study of the Liver, was, sequentially, Chairman of the Department of Pathology, and then President of the Mount Sinai Medical Center and Dean of the Mount Sinai School of Medicine. He was a vital and active component of the hepatologic scene at Mount Sinai until a few weeks before his death in 1988. His close friend and associate, Fenton Schaffner, with whom Hans coauthored the first modern textbook in the English language devoted to liver disease, was for many years Chief of the Division of Liver Diseases within the Department of Medicine. He remains an active member of our program with a vast clinical experience. Thomas Chalmers, well-known for his design, conduct, and critical analysis of numerous valuable clinical trials in the field of hepatology, was Popper's successor as President and Dean. Before coming to Mount Sinai in a move orchestrated by Popper, he had been one of my mentors at the National Institutes of Health, where he had been instrumental in creating the first intramural Section on Diseases of the Liver, and in having me named as Section Chief. After moving to Mount Sinai, he was equally instrumental in my recruitment here.

Dr. Popper was particularly proud (as are we all) of the many younger faculty members who trained with us, and who are the backbone of a thriving multidepartmental effort in both the clinical and basic aspects of hepatology. They have contributed many of the chapters in this volume. The programs developed by these individuals brought to Mount Sinai a large population of patients with liver diseases of all types. Adults and children, from diverse socioeconomic backgrounds, they filled the appointment rolls of a busy liver clinic and several separate but cooperating referral practices. The liver and biliary tract were also the focus of extensive activity within the Department of Surgery. Mount Sinai prided itself on its role as the ultimate, tertiary referral center for patients with liver disease.

Once hepatic transplantation became an accepted modality in the treatment of end-stage liver disease, this history, this staff, and these patients became the imperatives that drove the creation of the liver transplant program at Mount Sinai. Not to have done so would have been to concede that Mount Sinai was no longer at the cutting edge of patient care in a field central to the institution's self-image. Mount Sinai was already sending a stream of patients each year to other centers for liver transplantation. The lack of any liver transplant programs within the New York metropolitan area of more than 15 million people meant that these were long-distance referrals, which were often a particular hardship on our patients and their families. At the same time, this lack of other local programs also assured an adequate patient base to support a program, were we to embark on one.

Because the interest in liver disease pervaded so many departments at Mount Sinai, support for the program was broadbased. And because of the size and visibility of the hepatologic activities at the institution, even administrative enthusiam was readily achieved, despite a period of particular financial stringency throughout the health-care system of New York State which has, if anything, worsened with the subsequent passage of time. In short, the decision to seek state approval to launch a liver transplant program represented a consensus at many levels. No arm twisting was necessary at any point.

A critical decision was taken by Dr. Arthur Aufses, Chairman of the Department of Surgery and a highly enthusiastic proponent of a liver transplant program at Mount Sinai. Rather than attempt to recruit a liver transplant surgeon with experience, but with no ties to or familiarity with our complex institution, he selected a young member of his staff, Dr. Charles Miller, already fully trained in vascular and renal transplant surgery, to head the new program. Two facets of the person selected have been crucial to the success of the program: his skills as a surgeon and as a team player. The operative words are "we" and "our," rather than "I" and "my." Credit is widely and generously shared, making this everyone's program, not merely the transplant surgeon's. The sense of being a participant, even a partner, is what brings 75 people with various skills from many departments to our regular, two-hour recipient review meetings, and what brings them in, as well, with enthusiasm and good will, at whatever hour of the day or night their skills are needed. In my view, a liver transplant program can succeed or fail on the personality, no less than on the technical skills, of its surgeon.

Dr. Miller spent a year in Pittsburgh training with Dr. Thomas Starzl. He had done more than 30 transplant operations there himself, with excellent results, before doing his first case at Mount Sinai. Mount Sinai physicians from anaesthesia and the surgical recovery room, as well as nurses and coordinators, also received special training in Pittsburgh, which proved invaluable when our own program was finally launched. Dr. Aufses, himself, went to Pittsburgh for hands-on training, and actively participated in the early operations at Mount Sinai.

This training was expensive. The liver transplant program had an annual budget of more than $1,000,000 before seeing its first patient. However, the magnitude of the undertaking was clearly recognized by administration, as well as by the medical staff, and there was an unequivocal commitment to do everything possible to ensure the success of the program from the outset by minimizing the "learning curve." The generosity and support of our own administration were matched by those of Dr. Starzl and the University of Pittsburgh in welcoming our staff and providing them with the training they needed.

While the surgical, anaesthesia, and nursing staffs were honing their skills, the medical and pediatric subspecialties were also preparing. In addition to the obvious involvement of adult and pediatric hepatologists and gastroenterologists, other specialists, such as cardiologists, hematologists, immunologists, infectious disease specialists, nephrologists, pharmacists, pulmonary physicians, and psychiatrists, were identified by their respective division chiefs as liaison to the liver transplant program. They familiarized themselves with the problems to be anticipated, and have provided invaluable consultative support in the pre-, inter-, and postoperative settings. It is important to note that enthusiasm, rather than the nature of an academic appointment, has been the driving force for the participation of these individuals. Many, not surprisingly, are full-time academics. Probably unique to our program, however, are the many members of the voluntary faculty who have contributed an enormous amount of time and effort. Notable members of this group are Tom Fabry and Frank Klion, who, along with many other contributions, have provided the impetus for this book.

In short, our liver transplant program is truly institutional, and not merely a program of the Department of Surgery. It was enthusiastically supported from the outset at all levels, including administration and trustee levels, and this support and enthusiasm, substantial from the outset, have been maintained and have grown with the program. The program was a natural outgrowth of extensive clinical and research activities related to the liver in many departments, at an institution situated in a community with a large population base that cried out for such a program. These are the factors that, along with the technical, intellectual, and interpersonal skills of our surgeon, have ensured the program's success.

What are the benefits? The obvious ones are the sense of personal and institutional satisfaction that derive from a complex job well done. These are magnified by the realization that, in doing well, we are also doing good. No one who visits our pretransplant clinics and then witnesses the annual volleyball game between our medical staff and liver transpant recipients, held in Central Park, just across Fifth Avenue from the hospital, will question the rationale for this program. Giving a transplanted liver to a patient with end-stage liver disease is the ultimate gift of life.

An increasing tide of referred patients and favorable recognition in the media are tangible benefits to the institution of a successful liver transplant program. Less tangible but no less real are the benefits that derive from the enthusiasm of the staff, an enthusiam that expresses itself in a constant, self-driven effort to learn more and do better on the part of many individual physicians; in the fostering of productive interactions between divisions and departments with respect to patient care, clinical research, and teaching; and in the involvement of wives, friends, and members of the community in many activities that support the program. These benefits, while fostered initially by the program in liver transplantation, ultimately invigorate the entire institution.

Despite major advances in the understanding, prevention, and medical treatment of liver diseases, the ultimate goal of eradicating end-stage liver disease by medical means remains a distant one. In the interim, which is the entire foreseeable future, liver transpantation is here to stay. Both short- and long-term results, already astonishingly good compared to those of a decade ago, will improve further, and costs will also decrease, in parallel with such parameters as blood utilization and length of hospital stay. Virtually all physicians who treat patients, no matter what their specialty, will have contact with those who need, or have undergone, liver transplantation. Much of what such physicians need to know about this procedure will be found in the pages that follow.

Paul D. Berk, M.D.
Lillian and Henry M. Stratton Professor of Molecular Medicine
Professor of Medicine and Biochemistry
Chief, Division of Liver Diseases
Mount Sinai School of Medicine
New York, New York

This book is dedicated to our children, Jeannie, Susan, Stephen and Amy and Mark for all of the time we did not spend with them.

PREFACE

Liver transplantation, the ultimate treatment for end-stage liver disease, has developed so quickly over the last few years that its clinical application is still not well defined.

After initiation of our transplant program, it became obvious to us that information was not readily available in textbooks or even journal articles to evaluate patients for possible liver transplantation and care for them before and after transplantation. Knowledge of end-stage liver disease and its pathogenesis is not enough. It is necessary to know the interaction of organ systems and be familiar with other disciplines such as infectious disease, immunology, nephrology, cardiology, and pulmonary disease. Sensitivity to psychosocial issues also plays a central role in a successful transplant program.

We address this book to internists, surgeons, gastroenterologists, house officers, transplant coordinators and all health care providers. We felt that a concise and up-to-date book reflecting the experience of a single transplant team would serve as a useful guide and introduction to the field of transplantation.

The referring physician, whether internist, gastroenterologist, or other health professional plays a key role and acts as a partner with the transplant team. The referring physician acts as a gatekeeper of the transplant center and cares for the patient in the pre- and posttransplant period. These roles are crucial components in the successful transplantation of these patients.

The book is organized so that each chapter is complete and readable on its own. Chapters are complementary to each other. Different aspects of the same topics are presented by authors from different disciplines to demonstrate the integrated approach for comprehensive care. We have repeated some topics rather than cross-reference to enhance readability.

Each transplant center has its own individuality. By choosing authors from the same team we hope to present a cohesive methodology and show the importance of the team approach and demonstrate interaction of the team members.

It is our hope that this book will provide an outline and guide the internist, gastroenterologist, and health professionals who select and ultimately care for the patient.

Thomas L. Fabry
Franklin M. Klion

CONTRIBUTORS

Keith J. Benkov, M.D.
Assistant Professor of Pediatrics
Division of Pediatric Gastroenterology, Hepatology & Nutrition
Mount Sinai School of Medicine
New York, New York

Paul D. Berk, M.D.
Lillian and Henry M. Stratton Professor of Molecular Medicine
Professor of Medicine and Biochemistry
Chief, Division of Liver Diseases
Mount Sinai School of Medicine
New York, New York

Wayne Dewell
Data Base Coordinator
Division of Liver Transplantation
Department of Surgery
Mount Sinai School of Medicine
New York, New York

Sukru Emre, M.D.
Fellow in Liver Transplantation
Division of Liver Transplantation
Department of Surgery
Mount Sinai School of Medicine
New York, New York

Thomas L. Fabry, M.D., Ph.D.
Associate Clinical Professor of Medicine
Mount Sinai School of Medicine
Associate Attending
Mount Sinai Hospital
New York, New York

Michael A. Gerber, M.D.
Professor of Pathology
Department of Pathology
Tulane University Medical Center
New Orleans, Louisiana

Margaret M. Kadian, R.N., B.S.N., C.C.T.C.
Senior Clinical Coordinator
Division of Liver Transplantation
Department of Surgery and Nursing
Mount Sinai Medical Center
New York, New York

Eliezer Katz, M.D.
Transplant Surgeon
Division of Liver Transplantation
Department of Surgery
Mount Sinai School of Medicine
New York, New York

Barbara Klion
Co-Director
The Transplant Living Center, Inc.
New York, New York

Franklin M. Klion, M.D.
Clinical Professor of Medicine
Mount Sinai School of Medicine
Chief, Liver Clinic
Mount Sinai Hospital
New York, New York

Cosme Manzarbeitia, M.D.
Director of Liver Transplant Program
Fairfax Hospital
Falls Church, Virginia

Lloyd Mayer, M.D.
Professor of Medicine and Microbiology
Chief, Division of Clinical Immunology
Mount Sinai School of Medicine
New York, New York

Charles M. Miller, M.D.
Director of Liver Transplantation
Alfred and Florence Gross Professor of Surgery
Division of Liver Transplantation
Department of Surgery
Mount Sinai School of Medicine
New York, New York

Erica Miller
Co-Director
The Transplant Living Center, Inc.
New York, New York

Juan Prieto, M.S.W.
Social Worker
Liver Transplant Program
Mount Sinai Medical Center
New York, New York

Lynn Rogut, MCRP
Executive Director
New York Center for Liver Transplantation, Inc.
New York, New York

Joel R. Rosh, M.D.
Assistant Professor of Pediatrics
Division of Pediatric Gastroenterology, Hepatology & Nutrition
Mount Sinai School of Medicine
New York, New York

Maureen Rueger, R.N., M.B.A.
Staff Associate
New York Center for Liver Transplantation, Inc.
New York, New York

Fenton Schaffner, M.D.
George Baehr Professor of Medicine Emeritus
The Mount Sinai School of Medicine
Consultant to Mount Sinai Hospital
New York, New York

Myron E. Schwartz, M.D.
Associate Director, Liver Transplant Program
Assistant Professor of Surgery
Department of Surgery
Mount Sinai School of Medicine
New York, New York

Audrey H. Schwersenz, M.D.
Assistant Professor of Pediatrics
Division of Pediatric Gastroenterology, Hepatology & Nutrition
Mount Sinai School of Medicine
New York, New York

Stephen Snyder, M.D.
Clinical Assistant Professor of Psychiatry
Division of Behavioral Medicine and Consultation Psychiatry
Mount Sinai School of Medicine
New York, New York

Kirk Sperber, M.D.
Assistant Professor of Medicine
Division of Clinical Immunology
Mount Sinai School of Medicine
New York, New York

Swan Nio Thung, M.D.
Professor of Pathology
The Lillian and Henry M. Stratton-Hans Popper Department of Pathology
Mount Sinai School of Medicine
New York, New York

Abraham Zifroni, M.D.
Kaplan Hospital, Rehovoth
Tel-Aviv, Israel

Joel M. Zinberg, M.D., J.D.
Assistant Professor of Surgery
Department of Surgery
Mount Sinai School of Medicine
New York, New York

CONTENTS

—1—

AN OVERVIEW OF TRANSPLANTATION OF THE LIVER

Fenton Schaffner

INTRODUCTION

Many spectacular advances have been made in the field of liver diseases in the second half of the twentieth century. One of the most dramatic of these has been the successful transplantation of the human liver, now on a worldwide scale. For this to have occurred and to have reached its present state of expertise, many new developments in diverse areas of medicine were necessary. These include new surgical techniques, understanding the immunologic mechanisms underlying transplant rejection, development of immunosuppressive therapy, providing means of prolonged organ preservation, preventing and combatting infections, attracting an adequate number of donors, and selection of recipients who will benefit most. This chapter presents an overview of these diverse developments in the field of liver transplantation with the details filled in by the subsequent chapters.

Human hepatic transplantation is no longer considered an experimental procedure, and hence third-party reimbursement has been forthcoming. However, the cost of the procedure (about $150,000–$250,000 per transplant in the United States) and the availability of transplantation procedures for other organs is making a major impact on the cost of medical care. Expense is becoming a driving force in promulgation of the concept of rationing of medical care, a basically abhorrent thought but something that our society will have to concern itself with as the twenty-first century approaches.

HISTORY OF SURGICAL TECHNIQUES

Initial attempts at transplanting the liver were made in dogs and involved insertion of a second liver as an auxiliary or heterotopic graft.[1] These grafts atrophied probably as a result of rejection, inadequate blood supply, and lack of trophic factors originating mainly from within the pancreas. However, when the native liver was damaged or a large portion of it was removed, the grafts survived longer. These old observations led to the recent reintroduction of auxiliary grafts as a stopgap measure while waiting for a donor or for the liver to heal in patients too sick to undergo orthotopic transplantation, as mentioned by Miller in Chapter 11.

The first successful experimental orthotopic liver transplants were performed on dogs in the laboratories of Moore[2] in Boston and Starzl[3] in Chicago in 1959–1960. Starzl performed the first human orthotopic liver transplant in March 1963[4] and during the next 4 years did a total of seven.[1] None of these survived for more than 23 days. Many factors were responsible for the short survival, notably the poor condition of the patient to begin with, the poor state of preservation of the graft at the time of transplantation, inadequate immunosuppression, insufficient control of infection, and as yet undeveloped necessary surgical techniques and skills. Many credits are due Tom Starzl, especially for his stubborn perseverance in the face of the early discouraging results. During the 13 months beginning in July 1967 he attempted 14 more transplants, and 11 of these subjects survived longer than a month. While recurrence of malignant disease and difficulties with vascular and biliary anastomoses created most of the postoperative problems, a new entity became apparent: chronic rejection, which was indolent but relentlessly progressive. Steroids, azathioprine, and antilymphocytic globulin were obviously inadequate for immunosuppression. Nevertheless, more transplants were done and by more surgeons in other countries; the first outside the United States was Calne in England.[5] Several technical problems were tackled in order to improve results. The first was trying to ensure an adequate arterial blood supply by trying to prevent kinking, thrombosis, and other anastomotic difficulties. These problems, which involve the hepatic artery, have not yet been thoroughly resolved, but the number of vascular problems has diminished with increasing experience. The problem of thrombosis of the native portal vein has been partially resolved by venous grafting and partly by preoperative vascular studies using ultrasound and Doppler (frequency-modification) techniques to prepare the surgeon for venous grafting by using either a long segment of the donor portal vein or a graft of a recipient leg vein. The problem of biliary anastomosis has undergone changes, and revisions remain necessary but not as often as previously. Originally, preservation of the sphincter of Oddi was thought to be helpful in preventing cholangitis, but the efficacy of this technique has not been proven, and Roux-en-Y reconstructions are done as a primary procedure rather than a duct-to-duct connection. Donor–recipient size mismatches are less frequently encountered as more transplants are being performed, mainly because donor and recipient are being matched for size. Ultrasound estimation of liver mass of the recipient as well as including recipient height and weight in donor searches has minimized this problem. The paucity of small livers for children, discussed by Benkov and Rosch in Chapter 16, has led to trimming the size of the donor liver and even to cutting the donor liver in half and using each half in separate donors.[6] The development of using portions of liver for orthotopic transplantation resulted in the use of living donors.[7] Several centers around the world have used this procedure for small children with close relatives such as parents and even grandparents serving as donors. Whether the close genetic matching this affords is an advantage worth the risk to the donor remains to be established.

REJECTION

The increasingly widespread use of liver transplantation has led to the need for providing a new chapter of hepatic pathology, that of the structural changes caused by graft rejection.[8] Also the immunologic details of rejection are now being elucidated and, most importantly, rejection is now being largely controlled immunologically and pharmacologically.

Morphology of Rejection

Some grafts never function and the patient remains essentially anhepatic postoperatively. This primary-graft failure may have several causes, few of which have been elucidated in any individual case. Causes for this failure may be inadequate preservation or blood supply, trauma, adverse pharmacologic factors in the donor or recipient, and perhaps an immediate immunologic response of (i.e., rejection by) the recipient.[9,10] The last is characterized by gammaglobulin deposition in graft sinusoids immediately after reperfusion, as described by Thung in Chapter 17. Primary nonfunction is more likely to occur in ABO blood group mismatches and when the donor liver is steatotic, as discussed by Miller et al. in Chapter 11. Little can be seen in biopsies of the reperfused liver when examined under the light microscope, but electron-microscopic studies have revealed extensive sinusoidal lining cell damage. Primary nonfunction of a graft probably should not be considered rejection even though it may have an immunologic component in its development. Rather, it is most often a vascular problem stemming from a hypercoagulable state, possibly induced by endothelial damage.[11] Thrombotic vascular lesions did not seem to be related to persistent perivenular necrosis described in almost 20% of posttransplant liver biopsies.[12] A possible cause of this necrotic lesion may be rejection-induced damage to the sinusoidal endothelium since it was often followed by bile duct disappearance.

Acute rejection manifests itself within the first week after transplantation and is mediated by host cells directed against histocompatibility antigens displayed on cell surfaces.[13] Since hepatocytes normally display few, if any, such antigens, the initial attack is against the vascular lining cells. Liver biopsy specimens show damage to hepatic artery, portal vein, and hepatic venule branches with lymphocytes and macrophages and edema accumulating around these vessels. The extent of damage and inflammatory response reflect the intensity of the reaction and may be early indicators of the need for retransplantation. Damage to hepatocytes follows the vascular injury and, in part, is the result of the disturbed circulation. However, some hepatocellular injury is also immunologically mediated because the hepatocytes display MHC (major histocompatibility complex) class I antigens and lymphocytes can be seen adjacent to them.[14,15] The T-cells and, to a lesser extent, natural-killer cells are the primary effector lymphocytes,[16] although macrophages and, within days, fibroblasts and plasma cells are present. The T-cells express interleukin-2[17] and gamma/delta (γ/δ) T-cell receptors on their surface.[18] The changes are reversible with adequate immunosuppression therapy. All patients have some degree of rejection, much of which is not clinically significant. Routine laboratory test results are helpful in indicating the presence of rejection, particularly aminotransferase activity. However, the correlation between laboratory values and histologic appearance is poor. Hence, liver biopsies are needed to determine which medications are needed and what response they should elicit.[19,20] Indeed, since the introduction of our transplant program, the number of liver biopsies performed at The Mount Sinai Hospital has more than doubled. Fine-needle aspiration biopsy has been suggested as a more rapid and safer method for finding and following rejection episodes.[21]

Chronic rejection may begin anytime after the first couple of weeks following transplantation. It is histologically characterized by portal inflammation, consisting mainly of mononuclear cells and associated with changes indicating injury to bile ducts. The biliary epithelial cells show swelling, vacuolization, fraying, or duplication of the basement membrane and periductal edema. Lymphocytes can be found within the basement membrane, and bile duct cells begin to disappear. Eventually the entire duct is gone and is replaced by fibrosis, the "vanishing bile duct syndrome." MHC class II antigens are displayed by the biliary epithelium, notably HLA-DR antigens. As the bile ducts disappear, perivenular cholestasis becomes increasingly predominant. Changes in the hepatic artery branches are also noted with arteritis and thickening of the vessel wall. Clinically the vanishing bile duct syndrome is marked by increasing cholestasis with high alkaline phosphatase activity and rising bilirubin levels in serum. The early bile duct changes are reversible with adequate therapy in many instances, but when the syndrome is fully established, retransplantation is the only recourse. Differential diagnosis of the vanishing bile duct syndrome may be difficult since disturbed biliary drainage, cholestatic hepatitis (especially hepatitis C), drug-induced cholestasis, cholangitis (either bacterial or sclerosing), and recurrence of primary biliary cirrhosis may produce similar pictures. Graft-versus-host (graft–host) disease, which resembles rejection, also rarely occurs when the donor immune cells survive and proliferate.

IMMUNOSUPPRESSIVE THERAPY

The modern era of liver transplantation began in 1980 with the introduction of cyclosporine, as described by Schwartz et al. in Chapter 13. This substance is an antibiotic, the product of two molds, and was prepared by Borel in Switzerland. It could be administered intravenously as well as orally, and it proved to be the most powerful immunosuppressive agent found up to that time. The use of cyclosporine spread rapidly for all organ transplantations, and made possible dramatic increases in survival of grafts and recipients and in the total number of transplants performed throughout the world. Techniques rapidly developed for monitoring blood levels of the drug using chromatographic and radioimmunoassay so that optimal doses were easily achieved and toxicity due to excess dosing could be avoided. Problems caused by the drug, however, were apparent from the outset. The most common side effects are renal dysfunction and hypertension. These are dose-related, but some tubular damage and some rise in blood pressure are unavoidable even with the most careful monitoring of blood levels. The short-term renal and vascular effects are reversible, but long-term use often leads to permanent renal impairment and fixed hypertension that is recalcitrant to antihypertensive medications. Generally, the best drugs to lower blood pressure have been some of the calcium entry blockers and the angiotensin converting enzyme inhibitors. Several drugs interact with cyclosporine that is metabolized in the liver. Some drugs increase blood levels of cyclosporine by blocking its metabolism (some hormones, cimetidine, danazol), while some decrease the blood levels of cyclosporine by increasing its metabolism (barbiturates, phenytoin, some antimicrobials). Some drugs enhance the renal toxicity of cyclosporine (aminoglycosides, alkylating agents, antimicrobials). Some drugs, particularly antibiotics, interfere with absorption of oral cyclosporine. Prior to use, all drugs should be checked for interactions in sources such as *The Medical Letter Handbook of Drug Interactions.* Cyclosporin has a direct effect on hepatocellular mitochondria by inhibiting calcium-ion-induced large-amplitude swelling.[22] Whether this effect is responsible for the mild cholestasis that the drug can produce[23] or the stimulus to regeneration of hepatocytes that has been described[24] is not known. Food and oral bile acid supplements as well enhance the absorption of cyclosporin, thereby enhancing its bioavailability,[25] while bile acid sequestering resins decrease absorption.

Cyclosporine alone may suffice for immunosuppression, but better results are obtained when small doses (10 mg/day) of prednisone are also given. When cyclosporine doses have to be reduced because of toxicity or when immunosuppression appears inadequate, azathioprine (50–100 mg/day) is used in addition to the prednisone. When rejection worsens despite seemingly adequate doses of cyclosporine, prednisone, and azathioprine, large boluses (1.0 g) of hydrocortisone or methylprednisolone are given intravenously. Should these all appear to be failing, monoclonal anti-T-cell antibody (OKT3) is used.[26] When the latter is used alone, prior to cyclosporine, difficulties may be encountered in initiating cyclosporine. Monoclonal antibody to the interleukin-2 receptor has also been suggested as a means of improving immunosuppression early after transplantation.[27]

Oral cyclosporine has been dispensed as a liquid, but recently the manufacturer has introduced a capsule formulation. Analogs of cyclosporine are currently being tested with the hope of finding one with less renovascular toxicity.

The search for other immunosuppressive agents has led to the discovery in Japan of a macrolide antibiotic derived from a streptomyces species. Still unnamed, this substance is designated as FK506. It has been used as rescue therapy when cyclosporine has failed or led to serious toxicity and also as primary therapy.[28] FK506 inhibits the mixed-lymphocyte reaction, blocks cytotoxic T-cell formation, inhibits interleukin-2 release, and diminishes the number of interleukin-2 receptors. It causes a great deal of gastrointestinal distress and headache initially, but this diminishes in a couple of weeks and ultimately disappears.[29] Some renal dysfunction has been noted, but infrequently when compared to cyclosporine.[30] Because synergy was noted in vitro between FK506 and cyclosporine, they were tried together but the renovascular toxicity was worse than with cyclosporine alone, and so combination therapy was abandoned early. The next several years of testing will determine whether FK506 or cyclosporine is to be the first-line drug for immunosuppression.

The search for better immunosuppressive agents continues. Recently 15-deoxyspergualin, a guanidine derivative synthesized in Japan, was used as an adjunct to cyclosporine.[31] It appeared to exert a powerful immunosuppressive effect in patients as well as in experimental animals. It was well tolerated, although it may diminish white blood cell and platelet counts. Its mode of action may involve inhibition of macrophage function and T-lymphocyte proliferation. Ursodeoxycholic acid has also been used as an adjunct to cyclosporine to prevent cholestasis and to create a less toxic bile acid pool.[32] These adjuncts need careful trials to establish their value.

ORGAN PRESERVATION

Initially transplantation had to occur as soon as possible after the donor was declared dead. This restriction resulted from inadequate means of preserving organs on one hand and delays in certifying death with prolonged use of life-support systems. The acceptance of a flat-line electroencephalogram as evidence of death and the identification of potential donors long before death have shortened the delay in organ harvesting. The greater number of physicians trained in organ harvesting and the United Network for Organ Sharing (UNOS) have brought organs to recipients in an expeditious fashion. However, under the best of circumstances, transplantation had to be done within 6 hr of harvesting until a cold-storage solution was developed at the University of Wisconsin. This solution is now commercially available and permits cold-ischemia time as long as 24 hr, which means that organs can be procured anywhere and sent to a donor anywhere else in the nation. Furthermore, surgery can be scheduled at reasonable hours without disruption of hospital schedules. Cold-ischemia time can be expected to be further prolonged with even better solutions and storage devices.

PREVENTION AND CONTROL OF INFECTION

As the surgical techniques and methods of donor organ harvesting and preservation improve, infection in the immunosuppressed recipient is emerging as the major posttransplant medical problem as discussed by Klion and Fabry in Chapter 14. Many of the infectious agents plaguing victims of the acquired immunodeficiency syndrome (AIDS) also appear in the transplanted patient, and progress in preventing and controlling these will probably be accomplished in AIDS before posttransplant. In addition to opportunistic infections, the patient with a newly transplanted liver may face the problem of infection with one of the hepatitis viruses, either as a recurrence of the infection originally necessitating transplantation or as a new infection transmitted by the graft, by transfused blood, or from one of the staff caring for the patient. Infection in the biliary tree, in part due to impaired bile drainage at an anastomotic site or infection in an ischemic portion of the liver or infection of a clot in a vessel, in part due to some anastomotic mishap, cannot be considered opportunistic infections. The organisms are the same as those encountered in any postoperative infection, and treatment is with the appropriate antibiotics. Such infections will always occur, but the incidence will continue to decrease as surgical skills improve. Low doses of trimethoprim–sulfamethoxazole are routinely used to prevent bacterial infections, but how effective this really is has not been carefully evaluated.

Opportunistic infections after liver transplantation are mainly viral and fungal. The members of the herpes virus family, herpes simplex virus (HSV), varicella-zoster virus (VZV), cytomegalovirus (CMV), and the Epstein–Barr virus (EBV) are the most common and serious offenders. Acyclovir is the only drug proven to be of any value as prophylaxis, but such prevention has to be considered limited. HSV is the most sensitive, even with herpes hepatitis. The diagnosis of CMV hepatitis is best and most rapidly made on liver biopsy specimens using immunostaining with a monoclonal antibody or in situ DNA hybridization.[33] Ganciclovir has been helpful in some cases of CMV infection, including CMV hepatitis, but the drug is not well tolerated and recurrences are common. Attempts are being made to find the patients at greatest risk for CMV hepatitis. Positive donor CMV serology seems to be the most important risk factor.[34] Gammaglobulin may exert a prophylactic effect. EBV infection can cause infiltration of the graft with B lymphocytes to the point where the appearance is that of lymphoma.[35] It does not respond to any therapy, although reducing the degree of immunosuppression may bring EBV infection under control, albeit at the expense of the graft itself. The decisions are difficult indeed in the face of infections with these viruses.

Prevention of fungal infections has not been fully accomplished. Ketoconazole, which might be considered useful, inhibits cyclosporine metabolism, increasing its serum levels. Fluconazole does not have the same effect and deserves testing. Whether use of FK506 will permit such prophylaxis needs to be established. Infection with *Candida* spp. responds to amphotericin B, but if the organism is in a clot, ischemic area, or prosthetic device, the response is poor and some surgical revision with removal of the site of infection may be necessary. Amphotericin B is poorly tolerated and impairs renal function, as does cyclosporine; therefore, its administration must be carefully monitored. Safer and more rapidly acting antifungal agents are needed.

Prevention of infection and reinfection with the hepatitis viruses B and C are unsolved problems. Hepatitis B immune globulin has been used in those who are hepatitis B e antigen–positive before transplantation, but all it does is delay the infection of the graft even if it is continued indefinitely. Attempts have been made to use immune globulin and hepatitis B vaccine in various combinations, but to no avail. Attempts have also been made to rapidly vaccinate recipients who have not been exposed to the hepatitis B virus previously. No schedule of vaccination tested using less than three injections a month apart has been found efficacious. If the condition of the patient to be transplanted permits, the patient should be given three injections of vaccine a month apart before surgery with another dose at 6 or 12 months later. Thus far no prophylaxis for hepatitis C has been found. Attempts have been made at treatment with short courses of interferon alpha for as long as the patient's condition permits but this does not appear to have prevented recurrence of either hepatitis B or C infection. Trials of the use of interferon alpha after transplantation are just beginning for both hepatitis B and C, but how much such therapy will interfere with immunosuppression and whether it will be at all effective in the immunosuppressed patients remains to be determined.

DONORS

Estimates have been made that about 5000 liver transplants can be performed ultimately each year in the United States. The limiting factor is the supply of donor livers. Organ donation campaigns have been carried out across the nation and many states have instituted organ-donation statements included on drivers' licenses. More publicity and more governmental support for organ donation is needed. Some diseases like many malignancies preclude organ donation. Infection with agents for which there is no therapy, like the human immunodeficiency virus and the hepatitis viruses, also renders livers unfit for donation. Very fatty livers should not be used because these tend to function poorly at the onset. Prolonged maintenance on life-support systems makes donor organs unsuitable.

Donors of small livers are in shortest supply. To make available more organs, adult livers have been cut down to fit and have even been divided in half to make two grafts.[36] Whether a portion of the liver from a living donor is better than one from a cadaver remains to be established, but the use of living donors for children may relieve a serious problem in organ supply. Nevertheless, risk/benefit ratios will have to be carefully looked at before live donors are widely used. Donor gender does not affect the outcome of liver transplantation in children, although in adults, failure is increased when female livers are transplanted into males.[37] This may be the result of gender-specific differences in hepatocytic cell surface expressions or alterations of the hormonal milieu of the engrafted liver.

SELECTION OF RECIPIENTS

Each physician who has referred patients for transplantation or has actually performed the procedure has developed a set of personal guidelines for selection and timing, as detailed by Fabry and Klion in Chapter 6. Clearly, any patient whose life is being or soon will be threatened by liver disease is a candidate. However, some factors make noncandidates out of candidates, and some may make candidates less desirable. Absolute contraindications to transplantation are few and not universally agreed on. Active bacterial infection usually only temporarily delays the procedure until antimicrobial therapy is completed; this delay is a few days in most cases. A special problem arises with tuberculosis since therapy must be protracted and is often hepatotoxic. Furthermore, immunosuppression may limit the effectiveness of treatment and will enhance the growth and spread of the mycobacteria. Whatever is done will be a compromise at best. Active viral infections are a more common and troublesome problem, the solution of which has yet to depend on finding effective antiviral therapy.

These include infections with the human immunodeficiency virus, the hepatitis B virus, and the viruses of the herpes group. Infections with any of these adversely affects survival, sometimes to the point of declaring that serious viral infections should be absolute contraindications for transplantation. Malignant disease, when primary in the liver, is sometimes an urgent indication for transplantation and sometimes a contraindication. Results of transplantation in patients with primary malignancies of the liver are poorer as far as survival is concerned than in patients with nonmalignant disease.[38] Fibrolamellar carcinomas and epithelioid hemangioendotheliomas as well as small primary hepatocellular carcinomas should be considered indications, but patients should be informed that even with these favorable lesions, the percent survival is less than that for diffuse liver diseases. Whether the encapsulated primary cancer seen most often in the Orient should be considered an indication will have to be decided after a sufficient number have been transplanted. Large primary cancers—those that have metastasized and those that are secondary—should be contraindications. Some have been operated on, but the results are too poor to attempt surgery until tumor therapy is considerably improved. Tumors successfully treated in the patients' past with no evidence of disease over a period of several years are not contraindications. Chronic renal disease is a contraindication because of the nephrotoxicity of the immunosuppressive drugs; chronic renal failure is a more serious problem after transplantation than before.[39] The problem of pretransplant chronic renal failure can be solved by transplanting a kidney before or even at the same time as the liver. This surgical tour de force may be made more so in the diabetic in whom a pancreas may also have to be included in the already complex procedure. Cardiac impairment may be a contraindication, but before it is declared as such, the feasibility of appropriate coronary bypass, valve replacement, or even cardiac transplantation should be considered. Similar considerations can be extended to pulmonary diseases. Previous right-upper-quadrant surgery may have been so extensive to render transplantation unfeasible. Portacaval shunting has been one operation that has made the surgery most difficult and drastically has lowered the success rate. Therefore, surgeons are urged to avoid the right upper quadrant and consider early transplantation in patients with chronic liver disease. Major psychiatric problems, continuing alcohol or drug abuse, inadequate commitment to continuing medication and surveillance, and insufficient home support are frequent contraindications to transplantation. Patients with alcoholic cirrhosis who continue to drink up to the time of surgery are more likely to resume drinking after transplantation, and a minimum 6-month period of abstinence before the procedure is recommended.[40] Age limits have been changing as techniques have been improved, and several patients have received new livers after the age of 70 years. Some objections have been raised to giving an older patient a liver when the years of useful life ahead seem limited and a younger patient is denied that particular organ. Older patients can tolerate the surgery, but cardiovascular death during or after surgery is more frequent than in younger people. An important unsolved problem is the patient who has no means of paying for the procedure and the medications needed after. These societal and ethical problems need increasing discussion and decisionmaking. These are reviewed by Zinberg in Chapter 2.

Having listed some of the reasons for not providing a new liver, the reasons for doing so must also be listed. Diffuse primary liver disease that appears to be progressing and has reached a point where life will be threatened in a year or so is the best indication. Waiting until the patient's condition deteriorates is unwise because the risk of surgery increases. The likelihood of reversing any of the damage already done by medical means is too slight to warrant delay. While the search for predictors of death continues, some bedside clinical features are useful guides for selection of patients for transplants. These are increasing jaundice, increasing difficulty in performing everyday tasks, and the onset of muscle wasting. The appearance of the complications of cirrhosis, regardless of its etiology, are a reason for considering obtaining a new liver. These are bleeding esophageal varices, ascites, and encephalopathy. While a single episode of any of these can be readily treated, their occurrence together generally heralds a late and irreversible state of disease. Since earlier surgery has been associated with better survival, delaying it is inappropriate.

Liver transplantation is being performed for fulminant hepatic failure more often than previously.[41] Results are not as good as for chronic liver disease mainly because of the very unstable condition of the patient. Raised intracranial pressure because of the acute liver disease should be carefully monitored.[42]

THE FUTURE OF TRANSPLANTATION

One goal of modern hepatologic research is to make transplantation unnecessary. This is attainable but not in the near future. Therefore, the number of transplantations will increase until the limiting number is reached, at which time some sort of rationing system will have to be devised. As the number of operations rises, the skills of the teams performing them will also increase. The drugs will improve and infections will be effectively controlled. The ultimate limiting factor for society will probably turn out to be cost, which is the strongest argument for present investments in research.

REFERENCES

The number of publications related to liver transplantation are increasing at an astonishing rate so that more papers are appearing than patients transplanted. Those selected here represent a sampling of historical and current ones with no attempt at completeness and with no intention of slighting anyone.

1. Starzl TE, Brettschneider L, Putnam CW: Transplantation of the liver. In Popper H, Schaffner F: *Progress in Liver Diseases*, vol 3, pp 495–542, New York, Grune & Stratton, 1970.
2. Moore FD, Smith LL, Burnap TK, et al: One stage homotransplantation of the liver following total hepatectomy in dogs. *Transplantation* 6:103, 1959.
3. Starzl TE, Kaupp HA, Brock DR, et al: Reconstructive problems in canine liver homotransplantation with special reference to the postoperative role of hepatic venous flow. *Surg Gynec Obstet* 111:733–743, 1960.

4. Starzl TE, Marchioro TL, von Kaulla KN, et al: Homotransplantation of the liver in humans. *Surg Gynec Obstet* 117:659–676, 1963.
5. Calne RY, ed: *Liver Transplantation. The Cambridge–King's College Hospital Experiences*, p 399, New York, Grune & Stratton, 1983.
6. Otte JB, Ville de Goyet J, Alberti D, et al: The concept of the split liver in clinical transplantation. *Surgery* 107:605–612, 1990.
7. Stong RW, Lynch SV, Ong TH, et al: Successful liver transplantation from a living donor to her son. *New Engl J Med* 322:1505–1507, 1990.
8. Demetris AJ: The pathology of liver transplantation. In Popper H, Schaffner F: *Progress in Liver Diseases*, vol 9, pp 687–709, Philadelphia, Saunders, 1990.
9. Yanaga K, Lebeau G, Marsh JW, et al: Hepatic artery reconstruction for hepatic artery thrombosis after orthotopic liver transplantation. *Arch Surg* 125:628–631, 1990.
10. Kakizoe S, Yanago K, Starzl TE, Demetris AJ: Evaluation of protocol before and after reperfusion biopsies from human orthotopic liver allografts: Considerations of preservation and early immunologic injury. *Hepatology* 11:932–941, 1990.
11. Stahl RL, Duncan A, Hooks MA: A hypercoagulable state follows orthotopic liver transplantation. *Hepatology* 12:553–558, 1990.
12. Ludwig J, Gross JB Jr, Perkins JD, Moore SB: Persistent centrilobular necroses in hepatic allografts. *Hum Pathol* 21:656–661, 1990.
13. Steinhoff G: Major histocompatibility complex antigens in human liver transplants. *J Hepatol* 11:9–15, 1990.
14. Rouger P, Gugenheim J, Gane P, et al: Distribution of the MHC antigens after liver transplantation: Relationship with biochemical and histologic parameters. *Clin Exp Immunol* 80:404–408, 1990.
15. Neuberger JM, Adams DH: Is HLA matching important for liver transplantation? *J Hepatol* 11:1–4, 1990.
16. Adams D: Mechanisms of liver allograft rejection in man. *Clin Sci* 78:343–350, 1990.
17. Kabelitz D, Lobo MLS, Schuermann G, et al: Presence of γ/δ T-cell receptor-expressing T-cells in liver biopsies following liver tranplantation. *Hum Immunol* 28:167–169, 1990.
18. Hayashi S, Takagi H: Role of interleukin-2-receptor-positive cells and natural killer cells on rejected liver grafts of rats. *Hum Immunol* 28:193–197, 1990.
19. Nakhleh RF, Schwarzenberg SJ, Bloomer J, et al: The pathology of liver allografts surviving longer than one year. *Hepatology* 11:465–470, 1990.
20. Schlitt HJ, Ringe B, Wittekind C, et al: Die klinische Bedeutung der Transplatantbiopsie fuer die Behandlung lebertransplantierter Patienten. *Z Transplant-med* 1:17–26, 1990.
21. Hoeckerstedt K, Lautenschlager I, Ajonen J, et al: Diagnosis of acute rejection in liver transplantation. *J Hepatol* 6:217–221, 1988.
22. Halestrap AP, Davidson AM: Inhibition of Ca^{2+}-induced large amplitude swelling of the liver and heart mitochondria by cyclosporin is probably caused by inhibitor binding to mitochondrial-matrix peptidyl-prolyl *cis-trans* isomerase and preventing it interacting with adenine nucleotide translocase. *Biochem J* 268:153–160, 1990.
23. Kassianides C, Nussenblatt R, Palestine AG, et al: Liver injury from cyclosporine A. *Dig Dis Sci* 35:693–697, 1990.
24. Mazzaferro V, Porter KA, Scotti-Foglieni CL, et al: The hepatotropic influence of cyclosporine. *Surgery* 107:533–539, 1990.

25. Lindholm A, Henricsson S, Dahlqvist R: The effect of food and bile acid administration on the relative bioavailability of cyclosporine. *Br J Clin Pharmacol* 29:541–548, 1990.
26. Cosimi AB, Jenkins RL, Rohrer RJ, et al: A randomized clinical trial of prophylactic OKT3 monoclonal antibody in liver allograft recipients. *Arch Surg* 125:781–785, 1990.
27. Otto G, Thies J, Manner M, et al: Monoclonal antibody to interleukin-2 receptor in liver graft rejection. *Lancet* 335:1596–1597, 1990.
28. Fung JJ, Todo S, Jain A, et al: Conversion from cyclosporine to FK 506 in liver allograft recipients with cyclosporine-related complications. *Transplant Proc* 22: 6–12, 1990.
29. Shapiro R, Fung JJ, Jain AB: The side effects of FK 506 in humans. *Transplant Proc* 22:35–36, 1990.
30. McCauley J, Fung J, Jain A, et al: The effects of FK 506 on renal function after liver transplantation. *Transplant Proc* 22:17–20, 1990.
31. Groth CG, Ohlman S, Ericzon BG, et al: Deoxypergualin for liver graft rejection. *Lancet* 336:626, 1990.
32. Persson H, Friman S, Schersten T, et al: Ursodeoxycholic acid for prevention of acute rejection in liver transplant recipients. *Lancet* 336:52–53, 1990.
33. Paya CV, Holley KE, Wiesner RH, et al: Early diagnosis of cytomegalovirus hepatitis in liver transplant recipients; role of immunostaining, DNA hybridization and culture of hepatic tissue. *Hepatology* 12:110–126, 1990.
34. Gorensek MJ, Carey WD, Vogt D, Goormastic M: A multivariate analysis of risk factors for cytomegalovirus infection in liver-transplant recipients. *Gastroenterology* 98:1326–1332, 1990.
35. Randhawa PW, Markin RS, Starzl TE, Demetris AJ: Epstein-Barr virus-associated syndromes in immunosuppressed liver transplant recipients. *Am J Surg Pathol* 14:538–547, 1990.
36. Emond JC: Transplantation of two patients with one liver; analysis of a preliminary experience with "split-liver" grafting. *Ann Surg* 212:14–22, 1990.
37. Pillay P, Van Thiel DH, Gavaler JS, Starzl TE: Donor gender does not affect liver transplantation outcome in children. *Dig Dis Sci* 35:686–689, 1990.
38. Yokoyama J, Todo S, Iwatsuki S, Starzl TE: Liver transplantation in the treatment of primary liver cancer. *Hepatogastroenterology* 37:188–193, 1990.
39. McCauley J, Van Thiel DH, Starzl TE, Puschett JB: Acute and chronic renal failure in liver transplantation. *Nephron* 55:121–128, 1990.
40. Bird GLA, O'Grady JG, Harvey FAH, et al: Liver transplantation in patients with alcoholic cirrhosis; selection criteria and rates of survival and relapse. *Br Med J* 301:15–17, 1990.
41. Schafer DF, Shaw BW Jr: Fulminant hepatic failure and orthotopic liver transplantation. *Sem Liver Dis* 9:189–194, 1989.
42. LeRoux PD, Elliott JP, Perkins JD, Winn HR: Intracranial pressure monitoring in fulminant hepatic failure and liver transplantation. *Lancet* 335:1291, 1990.

— 2 —

LEGAL AND ETHICAL ISSUES

Joel M. Zinberg*

INTRODUCTION

For centuries humans have been fascinated with the prospect of transplanting body parts. As early as 700 B.C. Hindu surgeons performed skin transplants. Homer's monstrous Chimera combined the body of a goat and the head of a lion with a serpent as a tail. The mythic Chinese physician Pien Ch'iao interchanged hearts between two men, both of whom recovered after receiving a wondrous drug. In the nineteenth century, Mary Shelly in *Frankenstein* and H.G. Wells in *The Island of Doctor Moreau* combined fascination and revulsion in tales of transplantation and alteration of body parts to create new beings. More recently popular books and movies have recounted plots to murder hospital patients in order to sell their body parts for transplantation.[1]

In the past 40 years, largely because of the refinement of surgical techniques and the introduction of the highly effective immunosuppressive agent cyclosporine, organ transplantation has been transformed from science fiction to everyday surgery. The first successful kidney transplant took place in 1953.[2] A year later a transplant between monozygotic twins produced the first long-term transplant survivor.[3] By 1986 2446 nonrenal solid organ transplants (heart, liver, heart–lung, pancreas) and 8960 renal transplants were being performed annually in the United States.[4] Liver transplantation, which was first performed by Dr. Thomas Starzl in 1963,[5] has grown from an annual U.S. figure of 62 in 1982 to 2,656 in 1990.[6]

Transplantation has attracted extensive attention and elicited a plethora of legislation, regulations, comment, and controversy. Organ transplantation, and liver transplantation in particular, is a dramatic paradigm of the legal, economic, political, religious, and philosophical issues involved in providing and allocating scarce, expensive, life-saving medical technologies. A liver transplant is dra-

---

*Much of the work for this chapter was done when the author was a Silver Fellow and Lecturer in Law at the Columbia University Law School and a Rudin Fellow at the Columbia University College of Physicians and Surgeons.

matic, highly visible, and expensive, costing in excess of $235,000.[7] But in saving the life of an identified recipient society chooses to divert scarce resources from less dramatic medical and nonmedical uses (e.g., prenatal care, drug prevention and rehabilitation, mammography screening, and highway safety).

A central fact is scarcity—there are more potential recipients, i.e., persons who could benefit from a transplant (demand) than there are available organs (supply). Choosing one recipient assures that another potential recipient will die for lack of an available organ.[8] In part this scarcity is attributable to natural causes. Only persons who died in ways that did not damage the organ or create the possibility of transmitting disease to a recipient can be donors. However, a major, seldom discussed, cause of scarcity is a series of societal decisions governing the procurement (supply) of organs and the selection of recipients (or demand for organs).

Choices are made at every step. Each choice involves ethical, religious, philosophical, legal, economic, and political issues. Supply is affected by the choice of (a) the definition of death, (b) restrictions on and need for consent to donate organs, and (c) legally permissible strategies for increasing organ donation. Demand is controlled by the choice of (a) the standards for recipient eligibility, (b) the criteria for placement on transplant waiting lists, and (c) the methods of allocating available organs among persons on those lists.

These life and death decisions frequently involve "tragic choices" between deeply held values that conflict. Because these choices are so painful, society structures the decision making mechanisms to obscure the fact that choices are being made. This chapter will attempt to explicate the choices made:

> For it is in the choosing that enduring societies preserve or destroy those values that suffering and necessity expose. In this way societies are defined, for it is by the values that are foregone no less than by those that are preserved at tremendous cost that we know a society's character.[9]

I. SUPPLY

A. Donors

1. *Cadavers—The Definition of Death*

The pool of potential organ donors is limited to persons with good organ function whose organs have been donated and whose medical history excludes the possibility of transmitting disease. The earliest transplant successes involved the donation of paired organs (kidneys) by live donors. But live donors can not survive the removal of unpaired organs (liver or heart). Thus the supply of unpaired organs is limited to donation by or from dead persons. The new techniques for transplanting a lobe of liver or lung from a live donor to a related pediatric recipient have limited application.[10]

To be transplantable a functioning organ must have an adequate supply of oxygenated blood until it is harvested. The donor must be breathing and his/her heart beating. Under the traditional definition of death—permanent cessation of respiration and circulation—a potential donor who is breathing is alive. That person's organs would not be available until respiration and circulation ceased.

They would be viable only if harvested at the very instant of death. That is impractical given the need to evaluate the donor and obtain consent, the mechanics of organ removal, and the deterioration of organs during the process of dying.

The perfection of mechanical ventilation techniques and new medications enabled physicians to restore and maintain an intact cardiovascular system in patients who had irretrievably lost the capacity to breath spontaneously.[11] However, that did not alleviate the problem. It was unclear whether removing the organs of a patient who had irretrievably lost the capacity to breath spontaneously and whose respiration and heartbeat were mechanically supported would be deemed causing the patient's death.[12] Thus, if transplantation of unpaired organs was to be an available medical modality, it became necessary to expand the definition of death to include individuals whose respiration and heartbeat were mechanically maintained.[13]

The medical community urged that "irreversible cessation of all functions of the entire brain, including the brain stem" ("whole-brain death") was equivalent to the traditional cardiorespiratory definition of death, even though respiration and heartbeat was being artificially supported. The seminal 1968 Harvard study established criteria for whole-brain death.[14] The President's Commission for the Study of Ethical Problems in Medicine urged adoption of the Uniform Determination of Death Act (in 1981), which made whole brain death legally equivalent to cardiorespiratory death.[15]

Beginning in 1970, 39 states enacted laws recognizing the whole brain death standard.[16] At least four other states have adopted the standard through judicial decision.[17]

The whole brain death standard simplified the process of declaring death and harvesting transplantable organs. However, the clinical criteria are not necessarily uniform[18] nor always clearly understood.[19] The standard has been criticized because it

> principally reflects its use as an aid to decision making in intensive care and transplantation. On the conceptual level it makes less sense than either of its chief rivals: the traditional heart-lung concept [cardiorespiratory death] and the higher [neocortical] brain definition, which defines death as the loss of those brain functions that support awareness and cognition.[20]

Judicial decisions and statutes which permit withdrawal or withholding of life-sustaining medical care, including nutrition and hydration, from patients in a persistent vegetative state (neocortically dead) strongly suggest that "most involved courts, physicians, and patients' families think of the permanently unconscious [neocortically dead] patient as dead and want to stop nurturing a living corpse."[21] Thus, it is not surprising that many physicians and nurses involved with declaring death and organ donation believe that irreversible loss of all cortical function alone is sufficient to declare whole brain death.[21a]

Supplanting the whole brain death standard with a neocortical brain death standard would increase the available pool of donors. An estimated 10,000 patients in the United States are neocortically dead but are kept alive, under current standards, by artificial supports.[22] Whatever the aesthetics, a neocortical death standard is more utilitarian than the whole-brain death or cardiorespiratory death standards. It would reduce lavishing scarce resources on patients who have no possibility of recovering brain function. It would ease the trauma of the relatives' hopeless vigil. It is no less humane than watching neocortically dead patients vegetate for years until they die of other causes or obtaining a court order permitting withdrawal of nutrition and hydration and then starving them to a cardiorespiratory death.[23]

However, even with application of the whole brain death standard there could be an adequate supply if all suitable cadavaric organs were donated. (See page 18, note 41.)

2. *Anencephalics*

The acute shortage of organs for children has prompted consideration of anencephalic infants—children born with all or nearly all of the brain above the brainstem missing—as donors. "[A]nencephalic infants are currently born in sufficient numbers and with major organs of sufficient size and structural integrity to provide for a large portion of the transplantation needs in infants."[24]

Anencephalic infants have no cognition or interaction with their environment. They have a dismal prognosis, usually dying within hours, days, or rarely, weeks. There is no cure. The standard treatment is comfort care only. Transplantation might ease the parents' psychological trauma by having some good come from their tragedy. However, there are impediments to utilizing their organs.

One impediment is the whole brain death standard. Anencephalics possess a functioning brainstem. Under the whole brain death standard they are alive. Another barrier is the moral and philosophical objections. Anencephalic donation is presumably immoral because it treats human beings (the anencephalics) as means to benefit others and not as ends in themselves.[25]

In December 1987, following a successful heart transplant from an anencephalic infant and subsequent offers from 24 parents to donate their anencephalic infants' organs, Loma Linda University (in southern California) instituted a protocol that provided life support for anencephalics until whole-brain or cardiorespiratory death occurred, at which time the organs would be harvested. If death did not occur within a predetermined period, life support would be withdrawn and the infant allowed to die. The program was suspended in August 1988 because only 2 of the 12 infants admitted met the criteria for death within the specified time. No organs were procured and no transplants were performed because of difficulties in matching organs from the 2 eligible donors to recipients.[26]

The Loma Linda program attracted considerable negative publicity. It was criticized as "immoral" because it prolonged the lives of anencephalics for the sole purpose of preserving their organs for transplantation to other persons. It was criticized as "inadequate" because the organs deteriorated during the period of waiting for the anencephalics whole brain or cardiorespiratory death. The negative publicity and the practical problems have halted efforts in the United States to use anencephalics' organs.

Classifying anencephalics as dead would alleviate the shortage of transplantable pediatric organs. It would be consistent with the standards for death set by the President's Commission on Defining Death. Anencephalics "have a distinct and precisely definable condition characterized by the absence of integrative brain function, such that somatic death is uniformly imminent."[27] They are permanently and totally unconcious. They are not self-aware humans or autonomous moral agents.[28] Applying Kantian principles to prohibit transplantation from anencephalics is "a view so absorbed in principles believed to be right (or wrong) in the abstract as to fail to attend to the real and powerful concerns of the living human beings involved?"[29] Anencephalics' condition is so unique and their prognosis so uniformly dismal that they could be treated as sui generis (in a class by themselves) and transplants allowed before they meet the criteria for whole-brain death or cardiorespiratory death.

3. *Fetal Tissues*

The controversy regarding fetal tissue transplantation will only be touched on here. For the present, at least, it is not applicable to liver transplantation. Fetal tissue transplants have been suggested for patients with Parkinson's disease, Alzheimer's disease, juvenile diabetes, and immunodeficiency disorders.[30] Fetal tissue is less immunologically reactive and has greater capacity for growth and development than adult tissue.

The controversy stems from the fact that the most available source of fetal tissue is abortion. Although abortion is legal, critics and the current administration oppose anything that might encourage abortion, even though that opposition sacrifices potentially significant medical advances. It is suggested women may plan pregnancies for the sole purpose of aborting the fetus and donating the tissue or selling it. Women may be pressured to induce abortions or adopt procedures (e.g., hysterotomy) that enhance the potential usefulness of the fetal tissues but are more dangerous for the mother.

Since 1988 the federal government has banned funding fetal tissue research despite the recommendation of a 21-member National Institute of Health Human Tissue Fetal Transplant Research Panel[31] and an AMA panel[32] that potentially significant medical goals outweighed potential abuses and justified continued clinical trials. The federal ban does not bar private or state funding. However, it does remove the largest and most effective funding source.

4. *Live Donors*

Live donation was originally and is still primarily restricted to paired organs. It still accounts for approximately 25% of renal transplants.[33] The new techniques for transplanting a segment of a live adult's liver to a related pediatric recipient are potentially dangerous to the donor and do not, as yet, have a wide application.[34]

Live related donors were used in early kidney transplants to minimize immunologic mismatches. Improved immunosuppression has narrowed the gap between transplants from live and cadaver donors. The success of cadaver donation has made it unnecessary and perhaps unethical to subject living individuals to the small but real risk of live kidney donation[35] or the greater risk of live liver donation. The limited experience with live liver transplants indicates substantial donor morbidity, although there has been no donor mortality.[36] There is also the danger live donors will be coerced by relatives, physicians, or psychological and monetary incentives. Most transplant centers bar genetically unrelated live persons[37] or live persons at increased risk from donating kidneys.[38]

However, there may be psychological benefits to the live donor.[39] Surveys suggest widespread willingness to assume the risks of donating kidneys to related recipients, unrelated family members, and even to friends.[40] Live donation may improve outcomes because related donors will be a closer genetic match requiring less immunosuppression and eliminating organ ischemia associated with cadaver donors.

The scarcity of pediatric donors is another question. It translates into a 20–30% death rate for children awaiting livers. The new techniques for transplanting a segment of live adult's liver to a related pediatric recipient, although technically demanding and potentially dangerous for the donor, could ease the shortage of appropriate-size livers for children under 2 years of age who form the bulk of the pediatric liver failure population. If alternate means of increasing pediatric liver supply (e.g., anencephalics) cannot be implemented, it may be reasonable to permit fully informed adults, who have not been coerced, to assume the risks of live liver donation to related pediatric recipients.

B. Consent

The scarcity of transplantable organs is a function of the requirement for consent. Even under the current whole brain death standard there is an annual pool of 17,000–26,000 suitable cadavaric donors[41] who could probably provide enough transplantable organs to meet or exceed current demand. However, the organs cannot be transplanted without the donor's or the donor's family's consent, which, most frequently, is not given.

Alleviation of the current scarcity can best be achieved by changing the law: (a) to eliminate the need to obtain consent by presuming, in the absence of an explicit objection, that individuals consent to donate their organs at death; or (b) to permit offering commercial inducements to encourage donation. Both these suggestions are controversial. They have been denigrated as immoral without, as will be discussed below, a rational evaluation of the "moral" objections or potential benefits.

1. *The Current Procurement Mechanism*

Currently organ procurement is accomplished through a system of private, nonprofit Organ Procurement Organizations (OPOs). In May 1988 there were 71 independent or hospital based OPOs certified nationwide.[42] Each covered a designated procurement area.[43] As a condition for receiving reimbursement from Medicare or Medicaid for any medical service, each OPO[44] and hospital transplant center[45] must be a member and abide by the rules of the national Organ Procurement and Transplantation Network (OPTN) established by the National Organ Transplant Act of 1984.[46] In 1986, the Department of Health and Human Services contracted with a private, nonprofit organization [the United Network for Organ Sharing (UNOS)] to establish and run the OPTN.[47]

Hospitals are required to identify potential organ donors and notify the local OPO.[48] An OPO coordinator then appraises the potential donor's suitability and determines whether any condition (e.g., malignant tumor or HIV infection) precludes donation. If the organs are transplantable the coordinator will request consent from the donor's family and, if consent is obtained, will arrange for harvesting the donated organs and their transfer to transplant centers.

2. *The Anatomy of Consent*

Consent for organ donation is governed by the Uniform Anatomical Gift Act (hereinafter "UAGA"), which has been adopted in some form in each of the 50 states and the District of Columbia.[49] Under the UAGA, a competent adult (18 years or older) may consent to donate his organs by executing a suitable writing.[49a]

However, Americans do not believe "it is better to give (donate organs) than to receive." Few people execute organ bequests.[50] Surveys show that 93% of Americans know about and 75% approve of organ transplantation, but only 27% would donate their own organs and only 17% have completed donor cards.[51] Media campaigns have not significantly increased donation.[52]

Reluctance to donate may be due to genuine or imagined: (a) notions of bodily integrity; (b) religious objections;[53] and (c) fears of premature termination, or decreased levels, of medical care,[54] which were exemplified by a popular novel and film entitled "Coma." But perhaps most important is our inability to imagine

> Our own death . . . and whenever we make the attempt to imagine it we can perceive that we really survive as spectators. Hence . . . at bottom no one believes in his own death, or to put the same thing in another way, in the unconscious everyone of us is convinced of his own immortality.[55]

Thus, most people die intestate (i.e., without wills).[56] Even fewer execute organ donations or advance directives (e.g., living wills) to govern their medical care if they become incompetent.[57]

> [T]he typically human characteristic of procrastination and reluctance to contemplate the need for such arrangements however makes this [a living will] a tool which will all too often go unused.[58]

The UAGA recognized the problem. It provides that designated members of the family can donate the deceased's organs if an individual dies without making an organ bequest.[59] Persuading the surviving next of kin to consent to the donation is more necessary than persuading individuals to execute inter vivos organ donations because most physicians will not harvest organs without the consent of the surviving next of kin even if the decedent executed a donation that, technically, is legally binding.[60] The physician has to deal with the survivors. The decedent is gone. The survivors are now the physician's "patients" as well as potential litigants. Furthermore, transplant teams wish to avoid the negative publicity of a dispute with the survivors, which would impair procurement efforts.[60a]

3. *Requiring Routine Request*

However, there is reluctance to ask a recently bereaved family for consent to harvesting the newly departed loved one's organs. To overcome this aversion

Congress required that all hospitals, as a condition for receiving reimbursement from Medicare and Medicaid, establish "written protocols to identify potential organ donors" and to routinely make "families of potential donors . . . aware that they have an option to donate."[61] Requiring a *routine request* to donate was intended (a) to capitalize on peoples' greater willingness to donate loved one's organs rather than their own[61a] and (b) to offer purpose to the loss; and (c) to prevent foregoing organs because health professionals failed to request donation.[62] Unfortunately, and for whatever reason, these protocols have not increased the supply of transplantable organs.[63]

4. *Presumed Consent*

Creating a *new* legal presumption of consent would increase the supply—it would permit physicians or coroners to harvest organs and tissues from cadavaric donors without express consent. Organs would be (a) harvested routinely,[64] (b) harvested if the transplant team did not have notice of an objection,[65] or (c) harvested if reasonable efforts to determine whether there were objections failed.[66]

Presuming consent in the absence of actual consent or express objection has been attacked as immoral because (a) it treats the human cadaver as a source of spare parts and hospitals as chopshops,[67] (b) it impinges on the family's traditional control over disposition of the corpse, (c) it destroys the symbolism and sentiments surrounding the cadaver that help shape the lives of our people and institutions,[68] and (d) it prevents individuals from strengthening the community by altruistically donating their organs.[69]

These criticisms reflect a sentimental absorption in symbols.[70] Banning research on, or harvesting of, organs from human cadavers will "deprive living human beings of the benefits of medical knowledge and condemn unknown thousands to illness and deaths that might have been prevented. That is a poor sort of 'respect' to show a sacred symbol [the cadaver]."[71] If harvesting or research destroys the symbolism and sentiments surrounding the human cadaver, the destruction will occur with our without actual consent.

The family's traditional control over the disposition of the corpse (i.e., the next of kin's "quasi-property" right to control the disposition of a loved one's cadaver in a reasonable manner and to collect damages for interference with that right)[72] has always been regulated and limited by state law. When deemed necessary (e.g. in cases where death was not from natural causes) autopsies are required and organs and tissues are removed without consent and regardless of objection. Many states authorize coroners to harvest corneas and pituitary glands without consent in the absence of express objection[73] or if reasonable efforts to obtain consent have failed.[74] Hawaii permits removal regardless of objection. Several European countries presume consent to removal of all organs and tissues unless the decedent had previously registered an express objection.[75]

The American statutes authorizing removal of corneas without consent have survived constitutional challenges.[76] They have increased the supply of corneal tissue and have generated few objections.[77] They have not destroyed the symbolism and sentiments surrounding the cadaver.

Routinely harvesting the organs of the few decedents who qualify as donors (usually young healthy individuals who succumbed to an unexpected trauma) would be as unnoticed as compulsory autopsies. (Physical signs of harvesting would not normally be apparent to a mourner or viewer.) Requiring consent is more likely to focus attention on the harvesting and a spare-parts mentality.[78]

Generosity and altruism have not produced an adequate supply of organs. Presuming consent would increase the supply and would not prevent individuals from altruistically donating their organs. Presuming consent would make passive altruists of all potential donors and might spur voluntary altruism in other areas. But more importantly, it is oddly unaltruistic to condemn a person who desperately needs a transplant to death because voluntary altruism has not produced an organ.

There is no reliable evidence of public support for or opposition to routine salvaging organs without consent. Most people surveyed voiced no objection to their organs being taken without their consent.[79] A substantial percentage said they would donate loved one's organs. The years of experience in the twelve states that permit harvesting corneas and pituitary glands without consent suggests that presuming consent for salvaging other organs would generate few objections.[80] Persons with genuine scruples could always be given an opportunity to opt out.

However, any system of procurement requires the cooperation of medical personnel. Therefore, presumed consent would have to be explicitly enacted because unless physicians can be assured that presuming consent is legal and rid of their fear of lawsuits, they will be reluctant to salvage organs without actual consent.[81]

5. *Commercial Inducements*

The most controversial suggestion for increasing organ supply is a market for organs. A "market" means offering commercial inducements (which may have pecuniary value and may or may not include cash) to encourage people to donate organs. It does not mean a bazaar where body parts and life itself are hawked.

The National Organ Transplant Act of 1984 (the "Act") makes it a crime "for any person to knowingly acquire, receive, or otherwise transfer any human organ for valuable consideration for use in human transplantation if the transfer affects interstate commerce."[82] The prohibition and condemnation of commercial inducements was (is) justified by references to religious and philosophical principles and societal mores "which militate against regarding the body as a commodity" and the desire to "encourage altruism."[83] Commercial inducements, it is said, would be a "tawdry" affront to moral values[84] and would result in a return to the "law of the jungle."[85] Placing a price on a life saving organ encourages disrespect for and devaluation and desecration of the human body.[86]

These assertions are not supported by reasoned analysis.[86a] The Act's ban on commercial traffic in organs does not apply to blood, blood derivatives and sperm[87] because they can be replenished and donation does not compromise the health of the donor.[88] Cadavaric donation does not compromise the health of the donor, and replenishment is not an issue. Live kidney donation is not banned.

The Act only bans commercial inducements for live donation. The minimal risk of live donation "suddenly escalated into intolerable when profit became an obvious motive."[89]

It is not clear why paying for organs is more objectionable than paying for sperm, hair and skin. One might think sales of sperm, which can lead to new human lives should be more strictly regulated than commercial inducements to donate a cadaver's organs.[90]

The patronizing fear that commercial incentives will induce the poor to put themselves at risk for money may have some resonance if applied to live donation. However, it has no relevance whatsoever to cadavaric donations, which is the major source of transplantable organs. Cadavaric donations cannot compromise the health of the donor, rich or poor.

There is no reason society could not fashion adequate regulations governing live donation or foreclosing commercial incentives for live donation without banning commercial incentives for cadavaric donations. Barring the poor from selling their cadavaric organs deprives them of one of the few assets they have and impairs their autonomy.[91] If commercial incentives induce poor minorities to donate it is likely they will benefit disproportionately. Minorities, especially blacks, have less access to renal transplantation in part because fewer minority kidneys are donated making antigen matching more difficult. Increased donations by poor minorities would improve antigen matching and increase transplantation opportunities for poor minority recipients.

Richard Titmuss' 1971 study comparing the voluntary English system of blood supply and the mixed commercial and noncommercial American system prevalent around 1970[92] was influential in changing the American blood system to a largely, although not exclusively, voluntary one. It is usually cited to support the conclusion that commercial inducements will sacrifice the moral and psychological value altruistic donations have; will discourage altruistic donations;[93] will reduce the total supply of organs;[94] and will lower the quality of organs donated. Gifts, it is said, play a positive role in regulating social life and values. Gifts to strangers of significant items like body parts (organs), affirm feelings of solidarity and community in society while markets depersonalize and alienate.[95]

However, the facts did not support Titmuss's conclusions then and do not support their application to transplantation today.

The moral and psychological values of altruistic donations have not motivated broad segments of society to donate. Altruism only motivated an *aristocracy of saints*—a tiny percentage of the broad segment of English society that Titmuss studied—to donate blood.[96] Only a small percentage (3%) of the current American population donates blood. The United States purchases substantial amounts of blood products from abroad.[97] Few persons avail themselves of the moral and psychological advantages of altruistically donating their organs.

The available evidence does not establish that commercial inducements would diminish altruistic donations.[98] If, as seems likely, commercial incentives would increase the supply of transplantable organs, rejecting their use because of esoteric moral theories would be a decision to allow people to die to preserve the inviolability of the human cadaver. "One wants to remind them forcibly that while they distinguish among symbols and sentiments, there are people out there suffering and dying."[99]

The quality of donated organs need not decline under a commercial system.

Titmuss observed that commercial blood systems exhibited higher rates of hepatitis transmission. He incorrectly attributed the higher rate of post-transfusion hepatitis to the different motivations of altruistic and paid donors. A voluntary donor would refrain from giving infected blood. Paid donors would conceal their infection for pecuniary gain.

However, whether Titmuss' assumptions about human motivation are or are not correct the higher rates of post-transfusion hepatitis from commercial blood systems did not depend on whether blood was bought or donated. The rate of hepatitis transmission was a function of the blood banks' locations, the incidence of hepatitis in the donating population and the fact that at the time Titmuss wrote no hepatitis test existed. The Mayo Clinic, for example, paid sixty percent of its blood donors between 1966 and 1970 and had a very low rate of post-transfusion hepatitis.[100] Hepatitis transmission rates are high in Japan, which has a voluntary blood system, and low in Sweden, where a market system prevails.[101] The discovery and adoption of successful tests for screening hepatitis B and more recently hepatitis C and the AIDS virus (HIV) have largely eliminated these issues.

6. *Structure of a Market*

Commercial incentives to donate transplantable organs are not restricted to cash.[102] They could include, among other things, reductions in health insurance premiums;[102a] discounts or refunds of income[102b] or estate taxes;[102c] payment of the decedant's funeral expenses or medical bills;[102d] annuities for a live donor or the spouse of a deceased donor; credits for families that donate in case one later needs a transplant;[103] or any combination or permutation of these or other inducements. Commercial incentives could be used to attract live donation and cadavaric donation or only cadavaric donation.

A market for organs would be oligopsonistic, that is, it would include few buyers—basically transplant centers and private or public insurance carriers—and the actions of any one of them could affect the price. It could be readily regulated to set prices and avoid abuses.

Patients would not be buyers or bidders. Patients do not normally participate in the acquisition of the transplantable organ except in the case of a related live donor. Neither would commercial inducements appreciably increase the cost of transplantation. At most such inducements would represent a small part of the much larger physician, hospital, and drug charges a transplant entails.

II. THE NEED TO ALLOCATE

A system for allocating organs to particular recipients is necessary because the supply of organs and the resources and funding necessary to transplant them are all limited. Scarcity is a basic fact of life. All goods and services are relatively scarce; that is, the supply is not unlimited. These limited resources have to satisfy society's competing needs, such as highways, public safety, and medicine, and within medicine, competing constituencies, such as AIDS, transplantation, and cancer.

In our society most resources are allocated (rationed) by a market, based on ability to pay. However, transplants are so expensive that most recipients need financial assistance in the form of either public or charitable funding or health insurance. A market for transplants based on ability to pay might degenerate into a "ghoulish spectacle of desperately ill and, as a result, vulnerable patients bidding furiously against one another for invaluable biological materials."[104]

Allocation based on ability to pay would exacerbate the current system's potential for social and racial biases. Denying eligible individuals life-saving transplants because transplant teams were catering to wealthy recipients would not be socially acceptable.

Medical care is among those goods and services that are deemed so basic that public entitlement programs and regulations have been established to provide and fund access for those who could not otherwise afford them. However, whether such funding should provide everyone equal access to unlimited medical care or only to some, as yet undefined, level of "adequate" medical care (which may or may not include transplants) are important questions that are beyond the scope of this chapter. This chapter examines the allocation of available organs among potential recipients within the current system's constraints.

The Current System

A patient suffering from end-stage organ disease must first be identified as a potential recipient, referred to a transplant program, and must be willing to undergo transplantation. The patient must then apply to and qualify for placement on one or more transplant centers' waiting list(s). The transplant center will also place the patient on a central registry maintained by UNOS.[105] Finally, the patient must be selected from the transplant center's list when an organ becomes available.

1. *The First Stage*

If the patient is among the millions of Americans who have limited or no access to a physician because they are uninsured (30–35 million)[106] or underinsured (27 million),[107] or because there is a shortage of knowledgeable medical personnel in their community, they will never get past the first stage.[108] There are also groups, particularly some minorities, who will not participate in transplantation as donors or recipients.[109] They distrust the medical care system in general and perceive racial, economic, or other biases in the transplantation referral process.

2. *Admission to a Waiting List*

Each transplant center maintains a waiting list and formulates its own criteria for admission to that list.[110] A patient admitted at one center may be rejected at another.[111] There is little accountability, and arbitrary decisionmaking can occur.[112]

Admission Criteria. Most transplant center criteria are presumably based on medical factors. But there is no consensus as to which medical factors are the appropriate criteria or their relative importance. Also, how strictly a center adheres to its criteria depends on (a) the availability of organs and financing, (b) the experiences and predelictions of the transplant team, and (c) the applicant's condition.[113]

Chronological age, for example, is usually a criterion. Ostensibly it correlates with the success of the medical outcome. However, age criteria vary from center to center and from organ to organ. The patient's physiological condition is a more reliable predictor of the medical outcome than age. Many centers are raising age limits and transplanting healthy older patients. Age criteria may mask a center's covert judgment that older persons deserve a lower priority because they have less time left to live and have already enjoyed a longer life.[114]

Some ethicists urge that scarcity and intergenerational fairness justify setting explicit age limits as has been done in England.[115] However, in the United States that would probably elicit a storm of public outrage and be defeated by the senior citizens' powerful political lobby.

Medical Contraindications. Centers also differ as to medical contraindications. For example, there is no reliable evidence that success differs significantly between alcoholics and nonalcoholics. Nevertheless, some centers reject alcoholics. Most centers will transplant recovering alcoholics, but require proof of current abstinence. The required period, the evidence of abstinence, and the rigor with which it is checked vary from center to center. Some centers transplant unreformed alcoholics on the theory transplantation is the ultimate sobering experience.

Rejecting alcoholics usually represents a judgment that alcoholics have low social worth and are responsible for their disease.[115a] The aversion to the alcoholics' self-destructive behavior is understandable. However, diagnosing social worth and assigning fault is not the particular competence of the medical profession and can mask racial and social bias and other prejudices. Alcoholism and lack of social worth are not synonymous. It would be a shame to give the sober village idiot a higher priority than a brilliant alcoholic. Categorical rejection also ignores the variable susceptibility of different groups (e.g., American Indians) to alcoholism.

Identical arguments for restricting access to life-saving medical resources (e.g., ICU beds, expensive chemotherapeutic drugs and antibiotics) were made and rejected with respect to AIDS-infected homosexuals and drug addicts and also with respect to cardiac patients who, despite multiple warnings, continued to be overweight smokers. Arguably, livers are scarcer than the resources necessary to treat AIDS.[115b] However, unlike AIDS, a transplant can potentially cure alcoholic liver disease, and the scarcity of organs can be alleviated by altering the process of organ procurement.

However, UNOS regulations to the contrary notwithstanding, neither ethical principles nor common sense require ignoring social worth. There should, for example, be no objection to giving the President priority over an alcoholic drifter or most, if not all, other potential recipients.

Psychosocial Assessments. Most transplant centers use a psychosocial assessment to predict the patients' ability to (a) tolerate the emotional stress of transplantation and (b) comply with the postoperative immunosuppressive drug regimen all transplant patients will be on for the rest of their lives. The assessment usually evaluates the patient's age, education, occupation, financial situation, family and emotional support system, and general level of functioning.[116]

There is no reliable evidence these assessments accurately predict compliance.[117] They can mask racial and social bias and other prejudices[118] and should be used with caution. For example, the level of the potential recipient's education may have less to do with the ability to tolerate the emotional stress and postoperative regimen than with physicians' preference for saving educated persons most like themselves.[118a]

Ability to Pay. A critical problem is cost. Transplants are expensive and most centers do not accept candidates who cannot demonstrate ability to pay.[119] For most recipients funding depends on a patchwork of public[120] and private insurance programs.[121] But many insurance programs do not cover transplants or provide inadequate coverage. For example, to date, Medicare coverage has been so restrictive that Medicare has not funded a single liver transplant and covers immunosuppressive drugs for only one year.[122] Medicaid programs in 48 states cover liver transplantation, but 11 limit it to children only and 10 others provide inadequate funding.[123]

To obtain funding desperate patients often publicize their plight. Some centers encourage financially indigent patients to do just that.[124] The strategy often succeeds because society has great difficulty ignoring the publicized life-threatening need of an identified person in immediate peril (e.g., the little girl trapped in a well shaft).[125] Almost invariably public empathy translates into resources diverted to save the individual, disregarding the fact that this deprives unpublicized candidates of their turn and depletes funding for less emergent procedures that will benefit a large number of unpublicized persons (e.g., prenatal care). The tragic choice to forego other uses of scarce medical resources is hidden because the deprivation affects future and unidentified persons.

When states have tried to channel their limited resources away from transplants to less costly procedures that will benefit a greater number of lives, they have ignited intense controversy. In 1987 Oregon halted Medicaid funding of liver, heart, and bone marrow transplants in favor of expanding services for low-income children and prenatal care. An emotionally charged debate ensued.[126] The initial cutoff of funds was partially reversed after publicity about patients dying for lack of transplant funding. Oregon is now attempting to devise a plan prioritizing medical procedures and funding those above a certain level of cost-effectiveness. They hope it will expand coverage and control the expenditures level. However, it will require permission from the Health Care Financing Agency or Congress to deviate from the federally mandated Medicaid package. The fate of this plan and of transplant funding in Oregon remains to be seen.[127]

3. *Selection from a Waiting List*

Local Primacy. When an organ becomes available, it is first offered to the local transplant center or to a shared list of recipients within a defined procurement area.[128] If the organ is not used locally, it is offered to the regional list and then the national list.[129] There is an exception in connection with kidney transplants. If all six measured HLA antigens of the donor kidney's match a potential recipient on the national UNOS list, the kidney must be offered to that recipient.[130]

Originally organs were offered locally for logistical reasons. Hearts and livers would decay if the time between procurement and transplant exceeded a few hours. That is no longer the case. The length of time organs can be preserved has been extended. However, organs are still offered locally, even though local preference may divert organs from patients who would have a better outcome, because it is assumed local priority increases organ procurement; i.e., transplant teams try harder to obtain organs for their own patients.[131] Whether local preference does adversely affect outcomes or does increase the supply are unanswered empirical questions.

Selection Criteria. UNOS has a point system to rank patients' selection for each kind of organ. For nonrenal organs the controlling factor is medical urgency. For kidneys the quality of the antigen (HLA) match is almost always controlling. However the point system notwithstanding, the final decision is the prerogative of the transplant surgeon and physicians responsible for the care of the patients and they have vast discretion.[132]

Potential liver recipients are awarded points based on (a) medical urgency, (b) time waiting, and (c) blood type identity. Medical urgency almost invariably garners more points than blood type identity. Time waiting is a makeweight. The most seriously ill patients are placed in status 4 and always taken first, regardless of other factors.[133]

Urgency. In heart, lung, and liver transplantation urgency is important because there is no alternative treatment and transplant personnel want to save each patient in their care. However, giving priority to the sickest candidates may not maximize the medical outcome. Patient survival, graft survival (the length of time the transplanted organ functions before being rejected by the patient's immune system), and the post-transplant quality of life are much worse for sicker patients.[134] Sicker patients incur higher costs and require longer postoperative hospitalization and more extensive treatment.[135]

Healthier patients usually have a longer survival, incur less costs, and enjoy a better quality of life. Prioritizing sicker patients means that healthier patients have to wait. As they wait the once healthier patients get sicker, their chances of a successful transplant deteriorate or disappear, and sometimes they die. Once again society makes a tragic choice:

> Not to use an available organ in the patient with an urgent need condemns that patient to death, yet using an organ in such a patient results in an outcome far poorer than would be achieved if that organ were given to a recipient in better condition.[136]

Transplant surgeons, understandably, feel a special commitment to their sickest patients and to patients they have operated on. Thus, when a liver transplant fails the recipient is placed in the "most urgent" category despite the fact that retransplants are only about one-half as successful as primary transplants and invariably involve extended and expensive care.[137] Surgeons have transplanted second and third livers into one patient while an equally eligible patient waits and sometimes dies while on the list.[138]

Retransplanting livers probably denies other candidates equitable access to the available supply of scarce organs. It may be warranted in certain circumstances such as primary nonfunction of the liver. But there is no present limit on the number of retransplants a patient can receive. Currently, 23.9% of liver transplants are retransplants and 18.5% of kidney transplants are retransplants.[139]

CONCLUSION

Liver transplantation can be considered as two parallel tracks: organ procurement and organ allocation. Choices are made at each step that affect the supply and allocation of organs. However, the most pressing problem is the inadequate supply of transplantable livers. Three strategies would probably greatly increase that supply.

The first strategy would replace the requirement of express consent to the harvesting of a decedent's organs with a presumption of consent. Requiring express consent wastes more than two-thirds of eligible cadavaric organs. Most eligible cadavaric donors are young healthy individuals who died suddenly and unexpectedly as a result of trauma. Most people, and young healthy people in particular, are unlikely to have contemplated their own death or considered organ donation during life. Recently bereaved families are burdened with grief, shock, anger, and real or imagined religious and moral conceptions about the symbolism of the decedent's cadaver which may confound consideration of organ donation. Required request protocols have not increased donation. Presuming consent would make donation routine and eliminate the anxieties provoked by having to make decisions at an inopportune time. The opportunity for individuals or their families to opt out would avoid offending anyone who had genuine objections to cadavaric organ donation.

A second strategy would use commercial incentives to encourage cadavaric organ donation. Objections to commercial incentives relate to risks associated with live donation and allocation based on ability to pay. Incentives limited to promoting cadavaric organ donation probably would increase the supply of organs without posing any risk to the donor's health. Commercial incentives would not be used to allocate organs. Potential recipients would not be bidders or buyers. The market would be oligopsonistic. There would be few buyers. The price (incentives) could be readily regulated and controlled by the government, UNOS or the transplant centers.

A third strategy would add neocortical death to the traditional cardiorespiratory (heart–lung) definition and the whole brain death concept. This would be consistent with most persons' view of death, simplify the problems of dealing with permanently vegetative, noncognitive patients and increase the supply of organs.

Persons in a permanent vegetative state have lost all cognition. They cannot interact with their surrounding environment. Their prognosis is dismal to nonexistent. Even though they continue to breathe and their hearts continue to beat, most people regard them as dead (or living corpses). This is evidenced by numerous litigations by families, and now physicians, requesting courts to order the removal of all life support and discontinuance of nutrition and hydration in order to starve the living corpse to a cardiorespiratory death. Adopting a neocortical death standard would add the 10,000 or more individuals in a permanent vegetative state to the pool of eligible donors and also facilitate the use of anencephalics' organs for pediatric transplants and fetal tissues for research and transplantation. However, a neocortical standard would require careful delineation and regulation.

Finally, attention could be directed to tuning up the allocation system by ascertaining (a) whether local primacy actually encourages more aggressive local efforts to secure organ donations and increases the supply, (b) whether the current UNOS point system, which is strongly weighted toward medical urgency, reduces efficiency by allocating organs to the sickest candidates least likely to benefit from them while other potential recipients die, (c) what criteria are appropriate for selecting transplant recipients and how they should be applied, and (d) what criteria are appropriate for limiting retransplantation and how they should be applied. But most important perhaps is increasing the supply of organs. If we can increase the supply these allocation questions will probably be more easily solvable.

REFERENCES AND NOTES

1. Cook R: "Coma" (as both a book and a movie).
2. Evans R, et al: The National Heart Transplantation Study: Final Report, vol 1, pp 2–7 (Seattle, Batelle Human Affairs Research Centers, 1984); Hamilton, Kidney transplantation: a history. In Morris P: *Kidney Transplantation: Principles and Practice* 2d ed, 1984.
3. Murray: Remembrances of the early days of renal transplantation, 13 (Suppl. 1) *Transplant Proc* 9: 1981.
4. *Scientific and Clinical Status of Organ Transplantation: Report for 1987*, US Department of Health and Human Services, October 1988, Table I-1, p 13 (hereinafter DHHS).
5. Starzl TE, et al: Evolution of liver transplantation, *Hepatology* 2:614, 1982.
6. DHHS, *supra* note 4, Table I-1 and Cade F, Laudicina S, Transplantation White Paper, Fig 1, p 2 (Annenberg Washington Program in Communications Policy Studies of Northwestern University, 1991) (hereinafter "White Paper").
7. White Paper, *supra* note 6, Fig 10, p. 16.
8. White Paper, *supra* note 6, at 3; Organ Transplantation: Issues and Recommendations, Report of the Task Force on Organ Transplantation, US Department of Health and Human Services, April 1986, at 27 (hereinafter "TASK FORCE").
9. Calabresi G, Bobbitt P: *Tragic Choices*, Norton, New York, 1978, p 17.
10. Broelsch CE, Edmond JC, et al: Application of reduced-size liver transplants as split grafts, auxiliary orthotopic grafts, and living related segmental transplants. *Ann Surg* 212:368–377, 1990; Medical news and perspectives: mother to child: first living donor lung transplant, *JAMA* 264:2724, 1990. *See infra* pp. 17–18.
11. President's Commission for Study of Ethical Problems in Medicine and Biomedical and Behavioral Research. *Defining Death: Medical, Legal, and Ethical Issues in the Determination of Death*, 3:21–24 (1981) (hereinafter "President's Comm'n").
12. *Strachan v John F Kennedy Memorial Hosp*, 109 N.J. 523, 532, 538 A.2d 346, 350 (1988).
13. TASK FORCE, *supra* note 8, p. 29; *People v Eulo* 63 N.Y.2d 341, 352, 482 N.Y.S.2d

436 (1984) ("The immediate motive for adopting this position was to ease and make more efficient the transfer of donated organs").

14. Report of Ad Hoc Committee of Harvard Medical School to Examine the Definition of Brain Death, A definition of irreversible coma. *JAMA* 205:337, 1968.
15. President's Comm'n; *supra* note 11, pp. 55–84; 12 ULA 270 (1986).
16. New York State Task Force on Life and the Law, *The Determination of Death,* 4 (1986) (hereinafter "NYS Task Force").
17. TASK FORCE, *supra* note 8, p 29.
18. Plum F, Posner J: *The Diagnosis of Stupor and Coma,* 3d ed, Tables 20, 21, pp 314–323, 1982.
19. Younger S, Landefeld C, Coulton CJ, Juknialis BW, Leary M: Brain death and organ retrieval: a cross-sectional survey of knowledge and concepts among health professionals. *JAMA* 261:2205, 2208, 1989.
20. Wikler D, Weisbrod A: Editorial: appropriate confusion over "brain death." *JAMA* 261:2246, 1989.
21. Zinberg J: *Decisions for the Dying: An Empirical Study of Physicians' Responses to Advance Directives, Vermont L Rev* 13:445, 454 n 28, 1989; Smith DR: Legal recognition of neocortical death. *Cornell L Rev* 71:850, 1986.

21a. Younger, *supra* note 19.

22. *Am Med News,* March 28, 1986, p 1, col 1.
23. See *In re* Quinlan, 70 N.J. 10, 355 A.2d 647, *cert. denied,* 428 U.S. 922, 1976 (Ms Quinlan lived more than 10 years in a vegetative state without respirator); *Brophy v New England Sinai Hospital,* 398 Mass. 417, 497 N.E.2d 626, 1986. (allowing removal of nutrition and hydration for a vegetative patient to starve to death).
24. Botkin JR: Anencephalic infants as organ donors. *Pediatrics* 82:250, 251–252, 1988; see also Truog RD, Fletcher JC: Anencephalic newborns: Can organs be transplanted before brain death? *New Engl J Med* 321:388, 1989; but cf. Medearis DN, & Holmes LB: On the use of anencephalic infants as organ donors. *New Engl J Med* 321:391, 1991.
25. This argument relies on Immanuel Kant's categorical imperative: "Act so that you treat humanity, whether in your own person or in that of another, always as an end and never as a means only." *Kant, Foundations of the Metaphysics of Morals,* p 47 (LW Beck, trans, Liberal Arts Press, 1959).
26. Truog & Fletcher, *supra* note 24; Peabody JL, Emery JR, Aswhwal S: Experience with anencephalic infants as prospective organ donors. *New Engl J Med* 321:344, 1989.
27. Truog & Fletcher, *supra* note 24, p 389.
28. Walters JW, Ashwal S: Organ prolongation in anencephalic infants: ethical and medical issues. *Hastings Ctr Rpt* 19, 21, Oct/Nov 1988.
29. Ethics and Social Impact Committee, Transplant Policy Center: Anencephalic Infants as Sources of Transplantable Organs. *Hastings Ctr Rpt* 28, 29, Oct/Nov 1988.
30. Lindvall O, Rehncrona S, Gustavii B, et al: Fetal dopamine-rich mesencephalic grafts in Parkinson's disease. *Lancet* 1483, 1988; Pearce J: Adrenal and nigral transplants for Parkinson's disease. *Br Med J* 296:1211, 1988.
31. Consultants of the Advisory Committee to the Director of the National Institutes of Health, *Report of the Human Fetal Tissue Transplantation Research Panel,* Washington, DC; National Institutes of Health, 1988.
32. Council on Scientific Affairs and Council on Ethical & Judicial Affairs. Medical

applications of fetal tissue transplantation. *JAMA* 263:565, 1990; see also British Medical Association, BMA guidelines on the use of fetal tissue. *Lancet* 1119, 1988.

33. TASK FORCE, *supra* note 8, pp 35–36.
34. Voelker R: Surgeons urge caution on repeating live-donor liver tissue transplant. *Am Med News* Dec 15, 1989, 2, col 2.
35. Ibid, 34; Starzl TE; Living Donors: con. *Transplantation Proc* 19:174, 1987.
36. Broelsch CE, Emand JC, Whittington PF, Thistlethwaite JR, Baker AL, Lichtor JL: Application of reduced-size liver transplants as split grafts, auxiliary orthotopic grafts, and living related segmental transplants, *Ann Surg* 212:368, 1990.
37. Spital A: Unconventional living kidney donors: attitudes and use among transplant centers. Transplantation 48:243, 1989; Stiller CR: Living related donation. *Transplantation Proc* 17:85, 1985.
38. Spital A, Spital M: Donor's choice or Hobson's choice? *Arch Int Med* 145:1297, 1985.
39. Fellner CH, Marshall JR: Kidney donors—the myth of informed consent. *Am J Psychiat* 126:1245, 1970 (donor's report increased self-esteem).
40. Spital A, Spital M: Kidney donation: attitude findings. *Transplant Proc* 20:383 (Suppl 1), 1988.
41. TASK FORCE, *supra* note 8, p 35.
42. The number of OPAs decreased in 1988 for the first time because of federal pressure to consolidate OPAs; see Prottas: The organization of organ procurement. 14 *J Health Politics, Policy & Law* 14:41, 49, 1989.
43. The Omnibus Budget Reconciliation Act of 1986 allowed certification of only one OPA per "service area," a term that was undefined in the statute; 42 USC s1320b-8(b)(2).
44. Omnibus Budget Reconciliation Act of 1986, Publ L No 99-509, s9318, 100 Stat 2009 (1986); Social Security Act s1138(b)(1)(D).
45. Ibid; Social Security Act §1138(a)(1)(B); 53 *Fed Reg* (*Federal Register*) 6526, 6530, 1988.
46. Pub Law No 98-507, 98 Stat 2344 (1984), 42 USC §273–274d.
47. UNOS was a central computer registry of potential kidney recipients that had evolved from the Southeast Organ Procurement Foundation (SEOPF), an organ-sharing group established in the southeast in 1976
48. Social Security Act at §1138(a)(1)(A).
49. Uniform Anatomical Gift Act (hereinafter "UAGA") 8A U.L.A. 15, 15–16 (listing the statutes for the jurisdictions that adopted the UAGA); Lee W, Kissner: Organ donation and the Uniform Anatomical Gift Act. *Surgery* 100:867, Tables I–VI (describing and comparing the provisions of the state versions of the UAGA). An amended version of the UAGA was approved in 1987 but thus far has not been widely adopted by the states; Uniform Anatomical Gift Act (1987), 8A U.L.A. 2 (Suppl 1989).

49a. UAGA §2(a), 8A U.L.A. 15, 34 (1983). The donation may include all or part of the body and may specify the donee including particular hospitals, medical schools, physicians, or recipients and the purpose of the gift, including research, education, or transplantation. UAGA §3, 8A U.L.A. 15, 41.

50. In most states fewer than 10% of persons have signed donor cards and 3% were carrying cards at the time of their death.
51. TASK FORCE, *supra* note 8, p 38.

52. Caplan A: Requests, gifts, and obligations: the ethics of organ procurement, *Hastings Cent Rep* 18(Suppl 2):49, 50, 1986.

53. TASK FORCE, *supra* note 8, p 38. See also May: Religious justifications for donating body parts. *Hastings Cent Rep* 15:38, 1985; Frenkel D: Transplants. In N. Rakover N: *Jewish Law and Current Legal Problems*, p 195, 1983.

54. This is the most frequently cited reason for not giving permission to donate organs. See TASK FORCE, note 8 (above), p. 38. This concern is particularly strong among minorities and may partially explain their lower donation rates. See also Developments in the law—Medical technology and the law v. organ transplantation. *Harv Law Rev* 103:1519, 1614, 1618–1619, 1990 (hereinafter HARVARD).

55. Freud S: Thoughts for the Times on War and Death. In *Great Books of the Western World* 54:761, 1952.

56. Dukeminier: Supplying organs for transplantation. *Mich L Rev* 68:811, 829, 1970 (80% of people die intestate).

57. Zinberg J: Decisions for the dying: an empirical study of physicians' responses to advance directives. *Vermont L Rev* 13:445, 450–451, 1989.

58. *Barber v Superior Court*, 147 Cal. App. 3d 1006, 1015, 195 Cal. Rptr. 484, 489, 1983.

59. UAGA §2(b), 8A ULA 15, 34–35 (1983).

60. White Paper, *supra* note 6, p 7; TASK FORCE, note 8, p 29; UAGA §2. Donor cards are legally binding in 48 states. Florida and New York allow specified family members to veto the deceased's decision to donate. See Fla Stat Ann §732.912(3) (West Suppl 1989); NY Pub Health Law §4301(3) (McKinney 1985 & Suppl 1991); Overcast, Evans, et al: Problems in the identification of potential organ donors: misconceptions and fallacies associated with donor cards. *JAMA* 251:1561, 1984; 1561 (survey indicates surgeons in 46 states and the District of Columbia require family approval even if donor documentation is available).

60a. Childress J: Ethical criteria for procuring and distributing organs for transplantation. *J Health Politics Policy & Law* 14:87, 92, 1989; Overcast, *supra* note 60, pp 1561–1562.

61. *Fed Reg* 53:6526, 6527 (March 1, 1988); "Required request" or "routine inquiry" was first proposed in 1984 by Arthur Caplan; see Caplan A: Organ procurement: it's not in the cards. *Hastings Cent Rep* 14:6, 1984.

61a. Veatch R: *Death, Dying, and the Biological Revolution.* p 216 (rev ed 1989) (characterizing routine request as a scheme to obtain organs from individuals "who are statistically known to be unwilling to donate"); 73% of people are willing to donate the organs of a loved one but only 27% would donate their own; see TASK FORCE, *supra* note 8, p 38. Over 60% of families asked consented to donate. Caplan A: Requests, gifts, and obligations: the ethics of organ procurement. *Transplant Proc* 18:49, 53 (Suppl 2 June), 1986.

62. TASK FORCE, *supra* note 8, p 32.

63. HARVARD, *supra* note 54, pp 1620–1621; Diethelm: Ethical Decisions in the history of organ transplantation. *Ann Surg* 211:505, 514, 1990; NYS Task Force, note 16, p 24; The Distribution of Organs for Transplantation: Expectations and Practices, Report of the Inspector General of HHS (Aug 1990) on C-4 at p 4, and n 21. Required request statutes in 28 states have had only limited results. Gerson: Refining the law of organ donation: lessons from the French law of presumed consent. 19 *NYU J Int Law & Pol* 19:1013, 1987.

64. See Jonsen A: Transplantation of fetal tissue: an ethicist's viewpoint. *Clin Res* 36:215, 1988; Dukeminier, Sanders: Supplying organs for transplantation. *Mich L*

Rev 68:811, 1970; Note: compulsory removal of cadaver organs. *Columbia L Rev* 69:693, 1969 (proposing legislation requiring compulsory removal of organs regardless of objection).

65. Muyskens JL: An alternative policy for obtaining cadaver organs for transplantation. *Phil & Pub Aff* 8: 88, 99, 1978 (individuals during or their next of kin have the burden of making objection to donation known; this scheme allows objection by next of kin to trump decedent's consent); Sanders Dukeminier: Organ transplantation: a proposal for routine salvaging of cadaver organs. *New Engl J Med* 279:413, 1968 (individual or next of kin have burden to object except next of kin do not have veto power.); cf Note: Consent and organ donation. *Rutgers Computer & Tech L J* 11:559, 571, 1985 (only decedents while alive should be allowed to object to donation).
66. The Uniform Anatomical Gift Act proposed in 1987 includes a section requiring coroners to make reasonable efforts to obtain consent for donation and only presume consent for those bodies under their jurisdiction when these efforts have failed. See 8 ULA 2 (Suppl 1989) §4(a)(2).
67. May W., Attitudes toward the newly dead. *Hastings Ctr Studies* 1:3, 6, 1972.
68. Ibid, p 5; May W: Religious justifications for donating body parts. *Hastings Ctr Rpt* 31:38, 1985.
69. Ibid, pp 38, 41 ("organized giving . . . encourages a pattern of giving that will have positive moral consequences for the society at large"); Ramsey P: *The Patient as a Person* 210 (1970). ("The routine taking of organs would deprive individuals of the exercise of the virtue of generosity").
70. Feinberg, The mistreatment of dead bodies. *Hastings Ctr Rpt* 31:32, 1985.
71. Ibid, p 34.
72. *Strachan v John F Kennedy Memorial Hosp* 538 A 2d 346, 350 (N.J. 1988); *Whitehair v Highland Memorial Gardens,* 327 SE 2d 438, 440–401 (W.Va. 1985); *Leno v St. Joseph Hosp* 302 NE 2d 58, 59 (IL 1973).
73. Note: "She's got Bette Davis eyes": Assessing the nonconsensual removal of cadaver organs under the takings and due process clauses. *Columbia L Rev* 90:528, 535 n 35, 1990 (listing state presumed consent statutes that limit acquisition only where coroner has positive knowledge of dissent; coroners need not inquire).
74. Ibid, p 536 n 39 (listing state presumed consent statutes that require coroner to make reasonable effort to obtain consent).
75. Swerdlow J: *Matching Needs, Saving Lives: Building a Comprehensive Network for Transplantation & biomedical research* 19 (1989) ("more than a dozen countries . . . have adopted 'presumed-consent' laws, under which everyone is designated a donor unless they register their refusal").
76. *Arnaud v Odom* 870 F.2d 304, 311 (5th Cir 1989); *State v Powell,* 497 So2d 1188, 1192, 1193 (Fla. 1986); *Georgia Lions Eye Bank v Lavant* 335 SE 2d 127, 128, 225 Ga 60 (1985), cert den 475 US 1085.
77. Childress, *supra* note 60a, pp 97–98; TASK FORCE, *supra* note 8, p 30. Presumed consent for solid organs in European countries has also been effective. Childress note 60a, p 96.
78. Muyskens JL: An alternative policy for obtaining organs for transplantation. *Phil & Pub Aff* 8:88, 98, 1978.
79. In a 1985 Gallup poll 86% opposed removing organs from persons who did not sign donor cards without consulting the next of kin. See Childress, note 60a, p 97. But 63% would not object if their own organs were donated even if they had not given permission. Ibid, p 94. Combining these results with the professed willingness

of 73% to donate loved ones organs (TASK FORCE, p 38), it is hard to see who would object.

80. Editorial: Implied consent for cadaveric organ donation. *JAMA* 251:1592, 1984. (It would be a mistake to assume "that implied consent statutes would create controversy and a public outcry.")
81. Several European countries allow routine retrieval of organs if there are no known objections by the decedent or the family, e.g., France, Israel, Finland, Italy, Spain. Nevertheless, physicians continue to seek family approval before retrieval. See Cantaluppi, Scalamogna, Ponticelli: Legal aspects of organ procurement in different countries. *Transplant Proc* 16:102, 1984.
82. 42 USC §274e (Suppl V, 1987). Violations carry a maximum penalty of a $50,000 fine and a 5-year prison sentence. Ibid, s 274e(b). Several states also limit the sale of organs. HARVARD, p 1623, n 54.
83. TASK FORCE, *supra* note 8, p 96.
84. May, *supra* note 68, p 41.
85. Sir Roy Calne, quoted in Organs for sale: from marketplace to jungle. *Hastings Ctr Rpt* 1986.
86. Murray T: On the human body as property: the meaning of embodiment, markets, and the meaning of strangers. *JL Reform* 20:1055, 1079, 1987. Determining a price for a life saving good calls attention to the fact that the good and the life it will save are not priceless. See *Tragic Choices,* note 9 (above), pp 32, 39.

86a. Neither the United States Senate, House, nor the Task Force offered any analysis beyond the assertion that commercialization was bad. See Senate Rpt No 382, 98th Congress, 2d Sess 16, reprinted in 1984 *US Code Cong & Admin News* 3975, 3982; House Conf Rpt No 1127, 98th Cong, 2d Sess 16, reprinted in 1984 *US Code Cong Admin News* 3989, 3992; Task Force, note 8 (above), p 96. Hansmann has pointed out a different sort of risk. Introducing markets into the previously nonmarket transaction of living-related donor kidney transplants might create severe strains on the moral fabric of the families involved. It may become difficult to charge a relative for a kidney and yet expect free moral and other support from that person. In addition, the existence of a market would mean that there is an opportunity cost to providing free organs to your relatives. See Hansmann R: The economics and ethics of markets for human organs. *J Health Politics, Policy & Law* 14:57, 77–78, 1989.

87. 42 USC §274e.
88. Senate Report, 1984 *US Code Cong & Admin News* 3982.
89. Caplan AL: Blood, sweat, tears, and profits: the ethics of the sale and use of patient derived materials in biomedicine. *Clin Res* 33:448, 450, 1985.
90. Scott: *The Human Body as Property* 179–197; Hansmann, *supra* note 86a, p 77.
91. Engelhardt argues that autonomy, the free choice of rational persons, includes the right to sell oneself. See Engelhardt H: *The Foundations of Bioethics* 127–135, 366, 1986.
92. Titmuss R: *The Gift Relationship: From Human Blood to Social Policy*. New York, Pantheon, 1971.
93. Ibid, p 239.
94. Ogden DA, MD, (President of the National Kidney Foundation), testifying before the House Committee on Energy and Commerce, Report on HR (House of Representatives) 5580, HRPT 98-769 (May 15, 1984).
95. Murray T: Gifts of the body and the needs of strangers. *Hastings Ctr Rpt* 30:35–37, 1987.

96. [I]n the United Kingdom the percentage of the eligible population that gives blood is actually very small, only 6 percent. . . . The picture of a broadly altruistic society seems somewhat blurred when we realize what a small fraction of the population is in fact functioning altruistically. . . . Indeed, the small number of blood donors in the United Kingdom suggests, if I were to generalize as freely as Titmuss does, the idea of an aristocracy of saints. See Arrow K: Gifts and exchanges. *Phil. & Pub Aff* 1: 1972.

97. The New York Blood Center Fact Sheet, p 1. Blood is purchased from Europe. See *The New York Blood Center Annual Report,* 1988/89, p 22. Most blood plasma is obtained from prisoners and paid donors. Ibid, p 140.

98. See Oswalt: A review of blood donor motivation and recruitment. *Transfusion* 17:124, 1977 (reviewing the empirical literature); Upton: Altruism, attribution and intinsic motivation in the recruitment of blood donors. In *Selected Reading in Donor Motivation and Recruitment,* Vol II, ed American Red Cross, 1973.

99. Feinberg, note 70 (above), p 34; Note: Compulsory removal of cadaver organs. *Columbia L Rev* 69:693, 705, 1969.

100. Eckert: Blood, money, and monopoly. In *Securing a Safer Blood Supply,* Vol I, pp 6–27 (esp 21–22), 1985.

101. Caplan, note 89 (above), p 450.

102. Schwindt, Vining: Proposal for a future delivery market for transplant organs. *J Health Politics, Pol & Law* 11:483, 1986. See also Brams: Transplantable human organs: should their sale be authorized by state statutes? *Am J Law & Med* 3:183, 1977.

102a. Hansmann, note 86a (above).

102b. A proposal in Connecticut called for a refund of $10 of the driver's license renewal fee for individuals who agree to donate their organs. Ibid, p 63.

102c. Former Representative Crane proposed a $25,000 tax deduction per organ donated. See May, note 86, (above), p 41. This proposal would have more value for a rich decedent than a poor one.

102d. HARVARD, *supra* note 54, p 1628; Hansmann, *supra* note 86a, p 62.

103. May, note 68 (above), p 41; Dukeminier, Sanders: Supplying organs for transplantation. *Mich L Rev* 68:811, 848–849, 1970.

104. Caplan, *supra* note 89, p 449.

105. United Network for Organ Sharing, *UNOS Policies* 3.1.

106. Moyer: A revised look at the number of uninsured Americans. *Health Aff* 8:102, 1989; Davis: National initiatives for care of the medically needy. *JAMA* 259:3171, 1988.

107. Farley: Who are the underinsured? *Milbank Mem Fund Q* 63:476, 499, 1985. (Tens of millions are underinsured with inadequate protection against large medical bills.)

108. Braverman et al: Adverse outcomes and lack of health insurance among newborns in an eight-county area of California, 1982–1986. *New Engl J Med* 321:508, 1989. The poor are half as likely to have visited a physician prior to a medical emergency as are persons with high incomes. Bayer R: Introduction. In Bayer R, Caplan A, Daniels N: *In Search of Equity,* pp. ix, xviii, 1983. Lack of information among patients and physicians may limit access to transplantation. TASK FORCE, *supra* note 8, p 87.

109. Only 10% of black dialysis patients opt for kidney transplantation as compared to 20% of whites. See Callender: Organ donation in the black population: Where do we go from here? *Transplant Proc* 19(Suppl 2): 36, 37, 1987. Blacks are less

inclined to donate organs than are other groups. See *The Distribution of Organs for Transplantation: Expectations and Practices* (HHS, Office of Inspector General, August 1990); Callander, p 36. Cf, Hagle, Rosenberg, Lysz, et al: Racial perspectives on kidney transplant donors and recipients. *Transplantation* 48:421, 423, 1989. (Blacks donate kidneys at rates comparable to whites.)

110. The only restrictions on these criteria are general federal antidiscrimination statutes. HARVARD, *supra* note 54, pp 1630–1631.

111. NYS Task Force, *supra* note 16, p 108.

112. HARVARD, *supra* note 54, pp 1635–1636.

113. NYS Task Force, *supra* note 16, pp 108–109.

114. Koenig : As liver transplants grow more common, ethical issues multiply: by operating on the elderly, Thomas Starzl steps up patient-selection debate. *Wall St J*, Oct 14, 1986, p 1, col 1; TASK FORCE, note 8 (above), p 90.

115. Callahan D: Rationing medical progress: the way to affordable health care *New Engl J Med* 322:1810, 1990. Aaron HA, Schwartz WB: *The Painful Prescription: Rationing Hospital Care* (Washington, DC, Brookings Institution, 1984); Aaron HA, Schwartz WB: Rationing health care: the choice before us. *Science* 247:418, 1990. Former Governor Lamm of Colorado suggested that old people had a duty to die and get out of the way. See *NY Times*, March 29, 1984, p A16, col 5.

115a. Moss A, Siegler M: Should alcoholics compete equally for liver transplantation? *JAMA* 265:1295, 1991.

115b. Ibid, p 1296.

116. NYS Task Force, *supra* note 16, pp 109–111; House, Thompson: Psychiatric aspects of organ transplantation. *JAMA* 260:535–536, 1988; Christopherson: Cardiac transplantation: a psychological perspective. *Circulation* 75:57–58, 1987.

117. Evans, Yagi: Social and medical considerations affecting selection of transplant recipients: the case of heart transplantation. In Cowan D, Kantorowitz J, Moskowitz J, Rheinstein P: *Human Organ Transplantation: Societal, Medical-Legal, Regulatory, and Reimbursement*, pp 27, 37, 1987.

118. *See* Brock: Ethical issues in recipient selection for organ transplantation. In Mathieu D: *Organ Substitution Technology: Ethical, Legal and Public Policy Issues*, pp 86, 89–90, 1988; Merriken, Overcast: Patient selection for heart transplantation: When is a discriminating choice discrimination? *J Health Politics Policy & L* 10:7, 11, 1985.

118a. Fox R, Swazey J: *The Courage to Fail*, 2d ed, pp 231–233, 1978.

119. Some have termed this the "green screen." See Caplan A: Obtaining and allocating organs for transplantation. In *Human Organ Transplantation*, note 117 (above), pp 5, 6.

120. Schuck: Government funding for organ transplants. *J Health Politics, Policy & Law* 14:169, 170–173, 1989; Rettig P: The politics of organ transplantation: a parable of our time. *J Health Politics, Policy & Law* 14:191, 218, 1989; NYS Task Force, note 16 (above), p 113.

121. Transplants are so expensive that private individual funding is extremely rare.

122. An expansion of Medicare coverage was proposed. See Medicare program; criteria for medicare coverage of adult liver transplants, proposed notice. *Fed Reg* 55:8545 (March 8, 1990). A final ruling was published in the *Federal Register* on April 12, 1991 but coverage has been delayed by Medicare review and approval of the transplant programs.

123. White Paper, note 6 (above), 10–11.

124. NYS Task Force, *supra* note 16, p 112.

125. See Fried C: The value of life. *Harv L Rev* 82:1415, 1969.

126. *Medicaid Coverage and Payment Policies for Organ Transplants: Findings of a National Survey*, pp 18–23 (Intergovernmental Health Policy Project, George Washington University, Washington, DC, Nov 1988); Welch H, Larson E: Dealing with limited resources: the Oregon decision to curtail funding for organ transplantation. *New Engl J Med* 319:171, 1988.

127. Lund D: No decision yet on "complex" Oregon Medicaid plan. *Am Med News*, Sept 16, 1991, p 6, col 1.

128. United Network for Organ Sharing, *UNOS Policies* (June 20, 1989) 3.5, 3.5.1 (kidneys); 3.6, 3.6.1 (livers). Patients are allowed to list themselves on multiple local waiting lists. See *UNOS Policy* 3.2. This policy has been criticized for giving the wealthy and well informed who are more likely to have the resources to list themselves at several centers. See NYS Task Force, note 16 (above), p 93.

129. *UNOS Policies* 3.5.6; the country is divided into 11 regions.

130. *UNOS Policies* 3.3.

131. NYS Task Force, note 16 (above), p 118.

132. *UNOS Policies* 3.5 (kidneys), 3.6 (extrarenal organs except hearts and lungs), 3.7 (hearts, lungs, and heart–lung combinations).

133. *UNOS Policies* 3.6.4.1, 3.6.5.1 in *UNOS Update*, Nov 1990, pp 18, 19.

134. In liver transplantation, the most critically ill recipients had a survival rate less than half that of patients well enough to be at home awaiting a transplant. See TASK FORCE, *supra* note 8, p 88. In heart transplantation urgent priority patients had twice the mortality of healthier patients. See Stevenson et al: Urgent priority transplantation: When should it be done? *J Heart Transplant* 6:271, 1987.

135. Slater, Klein, & Gray: Review: Clinical orthotopic cardiac transplantation. *Am J Surg* 153:582, 1987.

136. TASK FORCE, *supra* note 8, p 88.

137. Gutkind L: *Many Sleepless Nights*, pp 240–242, Norton, New York, 1988; Starzl T, Demettis A: Liver transplantation: a 31-year perspective (part III). *Current Prob Surg* 27:183, 218, 1990. ("No liver transplant surgeon of whom we are aware would countenance the concept of patient abandonment implicit in a policy that precludes or even discourages retransplantation in a patient who is potentially salvageable.")

138. Gutkind, *supra* note 137.

139. Retransplant rates for each organ: United States Data, October 1, 1987 through September 30, 1988. *UNOS Update* 5:6 (Oct/Nov, special edition), 1989.

—3—

WHO GETS A DONOR LIVER? ALLOCATING SCARCE RESOURCES

Lynn Rogut and Maureen Rueger

INTRODUCTION

Liver transplantation is one of the most complex surgical procedures performed today. A similar degree of complexity also applies to the process by which a potential transplant candidate receives a donor liver due to the scarcity of these life-saving resources. This chapter provides a description of that process and discusses a unique organization in place in New York that plays a major role in liver transplant patient selection and review and the equitable allocation of donor livers.

NATIONAL ORGAN PROCUREMENT AND TRANSPLANTATION NETWORK

In order to understand how a particular patient actually gets a donor liver, some background information on the structure of organ procurement and transplantation is required. These services are highly regulated by the federal government making them somewhat unique within the spectrum of our health care system in the United States. Federal regulation was first initiated in 1972 with the passage of amendments to the Social Security Act, which established the End-Stage Renal Disease Program and provided Medicare reimbursement for kidney transplant procedures and procurement.[1] During the early 1980s, Congress became more deeply involved when several transplant candidates and their families, desperate to obtain donor organs before it was too late, appealed to their elected representatives and the media for help. One such example was a family who appealed directly to President Ronald Reagan. On one of his weekly radio broadcasts in 1983, the President pleaded for a donor liver for this family's infant who ultimately died before one became available.[2] Out of concerns over the allocation of donor organs that are an extremely scarce resource, the role of the media in their allocation, the shortcomings of the existing system, and the need to undertake efforts to increase organ procurement, Congress passed the National Organ Transplant Act [PL (Public Law) 98-507] in 1984. Prior to this piece of legislation, there was virtually no regulation or government oversight of transplantation or organ procurement except in a few states.

The 1984 Act directed the Secretary of Health and Human Services (HHS) to establish a national organ procurement and transplantation network (OPTN). The reason for creating the network was to develop a nationwide system for matching donor organs with transplant candidates, thereby increasing access and reducing organ wastage. Additional objectives were the adoption of quality standards for organ acquisition and their transportation; collection, analysis, and publication of data; and provision of information on organ donation.

> The legislation also prohibited the purchase of donor organs, created a scientific registry of organ transplant recipients and established a task force to advise Congress on the medical, legal, ethical, economic and social issues arising from organ procurement and transplantation activities.[3]

After receiving the task force's advice in early 1986, Congress passed the Omnibus Budget Reconciliation Act (PL 99-509), which had several provisions related to transplantation and organ procurement. One required all hospitals participating in the Medicare and Medicaid programs to implement policies to identify potential organ donors and to request donation from their next of kin.[4] This provision, known as "required request," was specifically enacted for the purpose of increasing the pool of available donor organs. A second provision required organ procurement organizations (the nonprofit organizations that procure organs for transplantation in the United States) to meet specific standards in order to become eligible to receive Medicare reimbursement. A third required all hospitals performing organ transplants to be members of the OPTN and to abide by its rules.[5] The United Network for Organ Sharing was selected by HHS to establish and operate the national network in 1986.

United Network for Organ Sharing (UNOS)

UNOS is a nonprofit organization located in Richmond, Virginia whose members as of May 1991 included 261 qualified transplant centers, 51 independent organ procurement organizations, and 46 histocompatibility laboratories in the United States.[6] It is governed by a 36-member board of directors including transplant physicians and surgeons, organ procurement representatives, transplant coordinators, laboratory directors, transplant patients and family members, and public members from the fields of ethics, religion, behavioral science, and law.

"The organization's overall mission is to improve the effectiveness of human organ donation, procurement, distribution and transplantation."[7] In carrying this out, UNOS establishes policies for distributing organs equitably; develops and implements quality standards for procurement, laboratory testing, and distribution and transportation of organs; establishes qualification requirements for its members' professional staff; collects, analyzes, and publishes data; considers ethical issues; and serves as an informational resource for its members, other health care professionals, and the public.

UNOS operates the OPTN and the US Scientific Registry for Organ Transplantation through contractual arrangements with HHS. The contracts are cost-sharing in nature and are financed by payments from HHS and fees collected by UNOS for registering transplant candidates on its nationwide waiting lists for donor organs.

Waiting Lists and Organ Allocation

Policies for the allocation of cadaver organs to transplant candidates in the United States are established by UNOS. According to a provision of the Omnibus Budget Reconciliation Act of 1986, all hospitals performing organ transplants are required to abide by the rules of the OPTN or face potential loss of Medicare reimbursement. Although, at the time of this writing, OPTN policies have not yet been published in the *Federal Register* and therefore do not legally qualify as federal rules and regulations, the U.S. transplant community adheres to them on a voluntary basis. To rectify the current voluntary nature of OPTN policies, the process for their publication in the *Federal Register* has been initiated but may not be completed until 1993. However, the fact remains that there are rules and the rules are followed.

As part of its efforts to carry out its mission, UNOS maintains computerized nationwide waiting lists of all transplant candidates for each organ (heart, heart–lung, kidney, liver, lung, and pancreas) and operates a system for matching organs to individuals on the lists. All transplant candidates and all cadaver and living-related donors in the United States must be registered with UNOS.[8] The UNOS Organ Center in Richmond houses a mainframe computer that performs the matching of donor organs with transplant candidates. The computer system is accessible 24 hr per day and serves as the nationwide linkage between organ procurement organizations and transplant centers. UNOS' Organ Center has specialists that also assist with the placement, distribution, and transportation of organs available for use outside the local geographic area where they are being procured.

Over 22,800 organ transplant candidates were listed with UNOS as of April 1991, 80% of whom were waiting for donor kidneys (see Exhibit Table 3-1). More than 1,300 of these patients were waiting for donor livers to become available. Preliminary data reveal a total of only 4,357 cadaver donors nationally in 1990, which resulted in the performance of 2,647 liver transplants for the year.[9] The number of cadaver donors whose livers can be used for transplantation is limited by acceptance criteria such as age, history of alcohol and drug abuse, adequate liver function, exposure to hepatitis, and other medical characteristics. Another nine liver transplants were performed in 1990 using liver segments from living-related donors. As of December 31, 1989, the median waiting time for a donor liver was approximately three months, with 35% of the patients waiting longer than 6 months.[10] Over 300 new liver transplant candidates are now being registered with UNOS monthly.

TABLE 3-1. United Network for Organ Sharing National Waiting Lists, April, 1991

Organ	*Patients*	*Additions*[a]
Kidney	18,270	1,153
Heart	1,997	308
Heart–lung	175	13
Liver	1,388	328
Lung	431	63
Pancreas	581	62
Total	22,842	1,927

[a]New candidates added during the month.
Source: United Network for Organ Sharing, *UNOS Update*, 7 (May 1991), 19.

The process by which a patient with end-stage liver disease becomes a liver transplant recipient begins with referral to a liver transplant center for evaluation. On completion of the evaluation by a multidisciplinary team of medical professionals, the patient is presented at the center's regularly scheduled recipient conference and reviewed for potential candidacy. If accepted, the patient is registered with UNOS and placed on the waiting list as a liver transplant candidate. The patient's position in the queue for a given donor liver is dependent on the geographic area in which the organ is procured and the candidate's blood type, size (height and weight), medical urgency status, and length of time waiting.

Although the United States has a national OPTN and a nationwide system for allocating donor organs, the system is not nationalized in the true sense of the word. Cadaveric livers procured in the United States are distributed to candidates awaiting transplantation according to a local–regional–national geographic scheme. Following the identification of an organ donor by hospital personnel, the liver is first offered to patients of transplant centers served by the same organ procurement organization as the donor hospital. The number of patients a local liver will be offered to depends on the length of the waiting list and the definition of the term local in that specific geographic area. Variations in its meaning are the result of a broad definition of "local" in UNOS Policies.[11] If there is no patient in the local area (however defined) who is a suitable recipient, the liver is then offered to patients of transplant centers in the region in which the organ procurement organization is located. Fortunately, the regions are very clearly defined: there are 11 in the United States (see Fig. 3-1). If there is no patient in the region who is a suitable recipient, the liver is offered to patients in need nationwide.

Within this geographic scheme, a point system is used to rank patients locally, regionally, and nationally. At the start of the allocation process for a specific donor liver, points are assigned to each transplant candidate of the appropriate height and weight for blood type compatibility, time waiting, and medical urgency status. This last variable has the greatest weight in the allocation algorithm. Sicker patients receive more points for medical urgency, leading to a relatively higher ranking on the list. The weighting given to medical urgency in donor liver allocation is somewhat controversial and is currently being ana-

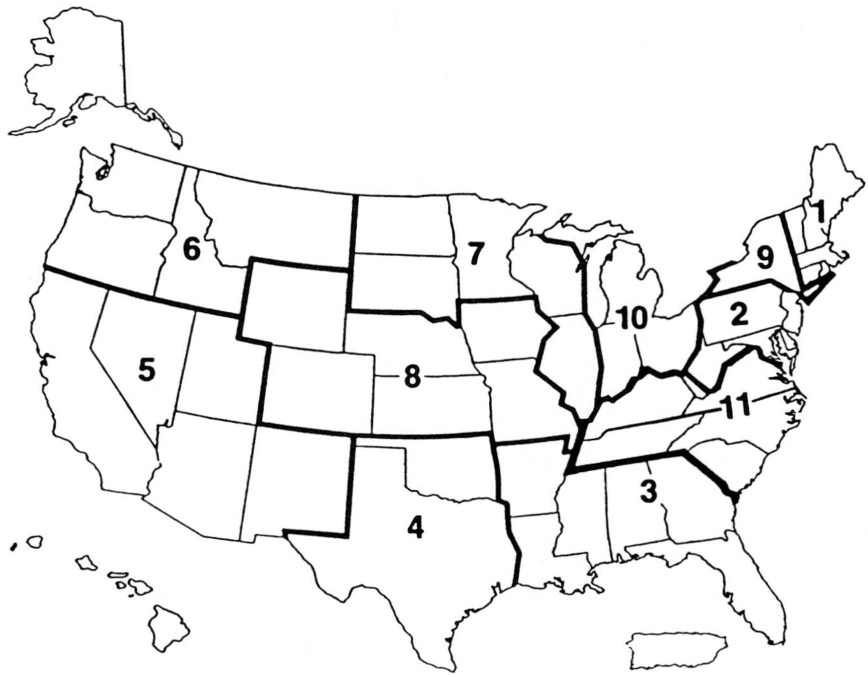

Source: UNOS Update, 5 (Oct./Nov. 1989): 4.

Figure 3-1. UNOS regional map.

lyzed and considered at the national level from both equity and efficacy perspectives.

There are four categories used to define medical urgency ranging progressively in their severity as follows:

Status	*Definition*
1	Patient's level of functioning and overall health status are not yet affected by underlying liver disease
2	Patient requires ongoing and frequent medical care; brief hospitalizations may be necessary
3	Patient is hospitalized and cannot be discharged
4	Patient is in the intensive-care unit (ICU) from either acute or chronic liver failure and has a life expectancy of <7 days[12]

Combining both the geographic scheme and the algorithm for candidate characteristics, a donor liver is allocated locally first to patients in the ICU with a life expectancy of <7 days (status 4). If there are no candidates of this type, the liver is offered to other local candidates in descending sequence of their rank on the list. If the donor is not accepted locally, it is offered to regional status 4 patients, then to all other regional patients, then to national status 4 patients and finally to all other patients nationwide.[13] Whether to accept a given donor liver for particular patients is the prerogative of the patient's transplant surgeon and/or physician.[14] Once accepted, the transplant surgeon determines who will perform the procurement surgery.

National Allocation System

As mentioned previously, UNOS is charged with overseeing the equitable distribution of donor organs for transplantation. The organization was required by its 1991 OPTN contract with HHS to assess the effectiveness and practicality of the present organ allocation system and the feasibility of a fully nationalized system.[15] An ad hoc Studies Oversight Committee was formed and determined that allocating organs on the basis of a single national waiting list is not feasible at the present time due to organ preservation issues including excessive ischemic time, cost considerations and the impracticality of a national cross-matching (antibody) system for kidneys. Ethical and patient advocacy issues are being studied by other UNOS committees.

LIVER TRANSPLANT CONSORTIUM

The process of donor liver allocation in New York differs from that in most other areas of the nation. This is due to the existence of the New York Center for Liver Transplantation, Inc., (NYCLT), a consortium of five academic medical centers that have or are developing state-approved liver transplant programs. NYCLT is relatively unique: there are only three other transplant consortia in existence nationwide (in Ohio, Boston and Washington, DC).

Clinical Policy and Organ Allocation in New York

The New York consortium plays a major role in liver transplant patient selection and review and the allocation of donor livers. When NYCLT was established in December 1988, its five members (The Mount Sinai Hospital, New York University Medical Center, The Presbyterian Hospital in the City of New York, State University of New York Health Science Center at Brooklyn, and Westchester County Medical Center) agreed to implement common clinical policies and procedures and a single waiting list for their liver transplant candidates. Due to the scarcity of donor livers, a set of diagnostic indications for transplantation was agreed upon and transplantation for more controversial indications was limited to consortium-wide protocols. As a result of these decisions, NYCLT began to guide and oversee the candidate selection activities of its member transplant centers.

Appropriate indications for liver transplantation are determined and modified by NYCLT's Clinical Policy Committee which also develops protocols for those which are more controversial. The Committee's 25 members include transplant surgeons, hepatologists, nurse coordinators and organ procurement representatives. All transplant candidates are reviewed at the committee's monthly meetings where cases are discussed and treatment advice is exchanged. This multi-institutional interaction provides a very unique benefit to patients and serves as a forum for achieving consensus on controversial issues. In addition to these activities, a uniform database has been implemented through the Committee, providing significant potential for future clinical research applications.

A single statewide waiting list for liver transplant candidates in New York was officially created in August 1990 as a result of the consortium's efforts. This mechanism provides an exemption from the local–regional–national allocation scheme discussed earlier in this chapter and required the approval of UNOS. Since New York State comprises its own UNOS region (Region 9), donor livers are now allocated first regionally or statewide and then nationally. Local allocation within the state has been eliminated. The point system used to rank patients regionally is identical to the one discussed earlier in this chapter. When a donor liver becomes available through an organ procurement organization in New York State, it is first offered statewide to patients in the ICU with a life expectancy of <7 days (status 4) and then to all other New York patients in descending order of their rank on the list.

The benefit of the single list is that it provides access for liver transplant candidates in the state to all donor livers procured by organ procurement organizations located in the state. It therefore can be described as "patient-driven" rather than "transplant center-driven." From a statewide perspective, a single list is considered a more equitable distribution scheme since all patients are treated equally by virtue of being in a single queue. If more than one patient on the list is eligible to receive a specific donor liver, the recipient is chosen following discussion among the liver transplant program directors involved. As a result of these procedures, interinstitutional conflicts over the use of donor livers have been completely avoided. If a donor liver cannot be used by any transplant candidate in the state, it is then offered through UNOS to out-of-state patients on the national waiting list. Allocation of donor livers in New York is monitored by UNOS.

Quality Assurance (QA)

In addition to its member hospitals' own activities for assuring the delivery of high-quality care to surgical patients, NYCLT has developed and implemented a multiinstitutional quality assurance plan for liver transplantation. Through its QA Committee, the consortium reviews all patient mortalities, retransplants, surgical procedures requiring >50 units of blood, and returns to the operating room for biliary complications. Corrective actions are recommended for any problems identified. After a specified period of time, the implementation and effectiveness of the recommendations are evaluated by the Committee.

SUMMARY

The allocation of donor livers to patients in need of transplantation is a complex process that occurs in accordance with policies determined by the national OPTN operated by UNOS. Cadaveric livers procured in the United States are distributed to transplant candidates on the waiting list according to a local–regional–national geographic scheme. Ranking on the list for a given donor liver is dependent on a candidate's blood type, size (height and weight), medical urgency, and length of time waiting. Continued monitoring activities and refinement of the allocation process to ensure equitable distribution are carried out by UNOS.

The donor liver allocation process in New York is somewhat different than in most other regions of the United States. This is due to the existence of NYCLT, a liver transplant consortium, and its efforts to create a single waiting list and organ-sharing arrangement for liver transplantation statewide. New York's donor liver allocation scheme provides equitable access for all liver transplant candidates in the state by virtue of their being in a single queue.

NYCLT plays both coordinating and oversight roles in the delivery of liver transplant services in the state. Because of its involvement in both candidate selection and donor allocation decisions, the consortium serves as a forum for achieving consensus on the painful decisions and judgments required by a field in which lifesaving resources are extremely scarce.

REFERENCES

1. Task Force on Organ Transplantation, *Organ Transplantation, Issues and Recommendations, Report of the Task Force on Organ Transplantation.* Washington, US Government Printing Office, 1986, p 16.
2. The Partnership for Organ Donation, Inc., *Solving the Organ Donor Shortage,* Boston, 1991, p 3.
3. UNOS, Health Resources and Services Administration and the Division of Organ Transplantation, *Annual Report on the US Scientific Registry for Organ Transplantation and the Organ Procurement and Transplantation Network, 1988 and 1989,* August 1990, p 1.
4. US General Accounting Office, *Heart Transplants: Concerns about Cost, Access, and Availability of Donor Organs.* Washington, DC, US Government Printing Office, 1989, p 11.
5. Ibid.
6. UNOS, *Facts about Transplantation in the US,* Richmond, May 1991.
7. UNOS, *Annual Report for the Years 1988 and 1989,* Richmond, 1990, inside cover.
8. UNOS, *UNOS Policies,* Richmond, June 1989, pp 4, 13.
9. UNOS, *Facts about Transplantation in the US,* Richmond, May 1991.
10. UNOS, Health Resources and Services Administration and the Division of Organ Transplantation, *Annual Report on the US Scientific Registry for Organ Transplantation and the Organ Procurement and Transplantation Network, 1988 and 1989,* August 1990, p 137.
11. "A local area shall be either the individual transplant center recipient list or a shared list of the recipients within a defined procurement area and shall be no larger than the OPO and service area designated by HCFA." UNOS, *UNOS Policies,* Richmond, June 1989, p 9.
12. UNOS, *UNOS Update,* Nov 6, 1990, p 18.
13. Ibid, p 9.
14. Ibid, p 6.
15. UNOS, *UNOS Update,* April 7, 1991; p. 2.

— 4 —

THE ROLE OF THE PHYSICIAN IN THE DONOR PROCESS

Abraham Zifroni

The number of solid organ donors in the United States has not increased in the last 3 years, and has stabilized around 4000 a year, while at the same time, the recipient waiting list has grown by almost 30% per year, numbering 20,457 as of April 1990, at which time 909 people on the list were awaiting liver transplantation. The most tragic consequence of organ shortage is that 24.3% of patients listed for liver transplantation die within 12 months without the benefit of receiving a new organ.[1] Therefore, it is of utmost importance to be familiar with the donation process, to identify potential suitable donors in the critically ill, and to manage them properly so that the supply of proper organs for transplantation can be increased.[1a]

This chapter describes the donation process; evaluation, and management of organ donors, and assessment and preservation of the donor liver.

THE DONATION PROCESS

Any seriously injured head-trauma patient should be considered a potential donor, and the possibility of donation should always be regarded as a logical step in the algorithm of care. Potential donors may be identified among those who have suffered spontaneous intracranial hemorrhage, acute neurologic or neurosurgical traumas, gunshot wounds to the head, primary brain tumors, metabolic disorders, cerebral anoxia from diverse causes, or drug overdose.[2] Primary care physicians can discuss organ donations during routine office visits with their patients. The patients can express their wish either in a living will or on their driver's license. Neither of these are legally binding, but can provide directions for their next of kin or for the custodian named in their Health Care Proxy.

In a hospital setting recognition of the potential donor by health-care professionals treating critically ill patients is the beginning of the process of organ procurement.

BRAIN DEATH

The first step following identification of the potential organ donor is assessment of the clinical signs of brain death. Brain death has been defined by the President's Commission for the Study of Ethical Problems in Medicine and Biomedical and Behavioral Research as the condition in which there is an irreversible loss of all functions of the entire brain, including the brain stem, for 6–24 hr.[3]

To be declared brain-dead, a patient must meet accepted clinical criteria for brain death. The exact criteria may vary from state to state, but they usually include lack of spontaneous movements or movements elicited by painful stimuli to the face or trunk; the absence of nonspinal-cord reflex activity and the absence of brain stem reflexes (Table 4-1).[4] Diagnosis of apnea is established when there is no respiratory effort after disconnection from the respirator for 10 min, despite arterial $p_{CO_2} > 60$ mmHg.

A period of observation might be needed to confirm the irreversibility of neurologic functions. If the diagnosis is uncertain or there exist confusing secondary conditions (i.e., hypoxia after head injury), it is recommended to wait 12–24 hr after the patient first meets the clinical criteria of brain death to make the final declaration.[4]

Alcohol, barbiturates, other neurodepressant drugs, neuromuscular blocking agents, and metabolic abnormalities, such as those seen in hepatic or renal failure, can reversibly impair brain function and mimic the clinical picture of brain death. In case of doubt, more studies might be needed to confirm the diagnosis of brain death. Confirmatory tests include cerebral blood flow studies, such as radionuclide arteriography, demonstrating irreversibility of brain dam-

TABLE 4-1. Clinical Criteria for Brain Death

No spontaneous movement
No response to painful stimuli
No reflex activity unless of spinal cord origin
No brainstem reflexes
No pupillary response to light
No oculocephalic reflex ("doll's eyes")
No oculovestibular reflex (no movement of the eyes after irrigation of each ear drum with 50 mL of ice water)
No corneal reflex
No gag reflex
No cough reflex after passing a cannula into the tracheobronchial tree with or without irrigation
Positive apnea test (no respiratory effort when p_{CO_2} >60 mmHg; O_2 given via tracheal canula to prevent hypoxia)

age by showing absent cerebral blood flow. Conventional contrast four-vessel angiography, which is complex, costly and potentially damaging, has been used mostly in Europe. Electrocerebral silence, demonstrated by EEG, suggests the diagnosis of brain death, but does not establish it because reversible inactivity (e.g., from intoxication, hypothermia) cannot be differentiated.

DONOR ASSESSMENT

A thorough history and physical examination are essential to the initial assessment of donor suitability. A number of underlying conditions exclude a potential donor from further consideration: septicemia, chronic liver disease, AIDS, viral hepatitis, viral encephalitis, Guillain-Barré syndrome, current intravenous drug abuse, active tuberculosis, malignancy outside the central nervous system, and severe hepatic trauma (Table 4-2). The presence of infection is not an absolute contraindication to transplantation, unless it is uncontrolled by treatment or intraabdominal.

In previous years, age has been considered a major criterion for donor acceptance with application of arbitrary age limits. However, recent data indicate that satisfactory graft function and survival can be achieved using donor livers older than 50 years, provided that other generally accepted donor criteria are satisfied.[1,5] Because of the risk of pulmonary infections developing in the ICU, it is preferred that the donor has been intubated for <5 days.

Parameters included in donor assessment are height, weight, and chest circumference to match liver size of recipient. Compatibility of ABO blood type, but not HLA, is an important consideration in matching.

While liver function studies are routinely included in the donor evaluation (Table 4-2), they have not been shown to predict allograft function accurately. Marked elevations in serum aminotransferase levels can occur in donors subjected to transient periods of shock or asystole. However, if enzyme elevations decrease with time, the liver usually can be used. Newer methods for testing pretransplant liver function are being investigated. One of them, based on the formation of the lignocaine metabolite monoethylglycinexylidide (MEGX), has

TABLE 4-2. Complete Evaluation of the Potential Liver Donor

Serology for HBsAg, HCV, VDRL, HIV, CMV
ABO typing
Documented cause of brain death
No obvious malignancy outside central nervous system
Normal or near normal AST, ALT, bilirubin, or elevations decreasing with time
Absence of prolonged hypoxia
Absence of severe hepatic trauma
Absence of systemic sepsis

Source: Policy and Procedure Manual, New York Center for Liver Transplantation, Inc. (NYCLT), 1990.

been suggested to predict early hepatic graft survival.[6] Another test that appears to have prognostic value is the lecithin: cholesterol acyltransferase (LCAT) activity, shown to correlate with posttransplant allograft function.[7]

MEDICAL MANAGEMENT OF DONOR

Once brain death has been diagnosed, immediate attention must be given to the maintenance of organ function. The principal goals of medical management include early recognition and treatment of hemodynamic instability, maintenance of a systemic perfusion pressure to maximize posttransplantation allograft function, and prevention and treatment of complications.[8] Maintenance of skin integrity, regulation of body temperature, lubrication and protective closure of the eyes, manual lung inflation, and frequent airway suctioning to prevent atelectasis and pneumonia are all important aspects of general intensive care.

Because of the exquisite sensitivity of the liver to ischemia, systolic blood pressure should be maintained above 80 mmHg. Hypotension is treated primarily by repleting existing volume deficits with blood, colloids, and crystalloids. If vasopressor therapy is required, dopamine is preferred because of its potential for maintaining renal and mesenteric blood flow, and can be administered at doses up to 10μg/kg per minute. However, since dopamine in higher doses interferes with portal vein flow, and can cause hepatic arterial vasoconstriction,[9] an effort to decrease its requirement should be made. To prevent hepatic edema, central venous pressure should be monitored so as not to exceed 8–10 mmHg.

The development of diabetes insipidus is common in brain-dead organ donors, because the destruction of the hypothalamic–pituitary axis causes a decrease in circulating antidiuretic hormone. This condition is treated with vasopressin to avoid excessive volume losses and electrolyte disturbances and to maintain hemodynamic stability. A synthetic analogue of arginine vasopressin, desmopressin, might be preferred to other vasopressin preparations because of its low pressor/antidiuretic ratio is less likely to reduce total hepatic blood flow.[9]

Mechanical ventilation is required in all brain-dead donors to support systemic oxygenation and maintain acid–base (pH) balance. Supplemental oxygen is administered to maintain an arterial oxygen saturation of at least 95% and $p_{O_2} > 70$ mmHg. Higher concentrations of inspired oxygen are preferred to the use of high levels of positive end-expiratory pressure in the maintenance of arterial saturation so that the deleterious effect of positive end-expiratory pressure on hepatic perfusion is minimized.[10]

ASSESSMENT OF THE DONOR LIVER

Evaluation of the donor liver prior to implantation into the recipient consists of clinical and laboratory assessment of the donor as well as visual (gross) histologic inspection of the organ. Undetected preexisting chronic disease has been distinctly uncommon in livers that have passed through the donor screening process.[11] However, the pathologist is often requested to evaluate a donor liver by frozen section before implantation because of suspicious physical appearance or agonal events in the donor. The surgeon performing the donor operation may notice rounded borders, a yellow discoloration on finger pressure, or hepatomegaly suggesting a steatotic graft. An apparently firm liver may show severe hydropic degeneration on a frozen section. The presence of severe macrovesicular fatty infiltration or hydropic degeneration predict poor graft function, and donor livers with these histologic patterns should not be transplanted. On the other hand, livers with mild (<30% of hepatocytes with fatty infiltration) or moderate steatosis (30–60% of hepatocytes involved) function adequately and can be used.[12,13] Organs with nonspecific reactive hepatitis, small noncaseating granulomas, and other mild nonspecific changes are routinely used and have not caused problems. Usually, small focal nodular hyperplasia lesions are removed before implantation.[14]

There are rare reports of an unrecognized malignancy,[15] congenital factor XI deficiency,[16] and Gilbert's syndrome[17] transferred with the donor liver.

PRESERVATION OF THE DONOR LIVER

An effective transportation and distribution system of donor organs requires a simple method to preserve the organ outside the body for an extended period. A prolonged preservation period allows the surgeon to perform liver transplantation on a nonemergency basis.

The interval between cessation of donor circulation and cooling of the liver with preservation fluid is called *warm-ischemia time.* The storage time after instillation of preservation fluid plus the time to sew in the liver and restore its portal flow after removing it from an ice chest is termed *cold-ischemia time.* Under conditions of heartbeating brain-death procurement, and with modern techniques of multiple-organ procurement, there is virtually no warm ischemia. Thus, most clinical reports refer to the time from devascularization in the donor to reperfusion in the recipient as cold-ischemia time.

In the first heterotopic liver transplants, performed in dogs, Goodrich found 33 min to be the limit of warm ischemia tolerated if transplantation was to be successful.[18] Later, in developing a technique for orthotopic transplantation, tolerance of the liver to hypoxia was extended by using peritoneal cooling with iced saline in the donor. Starzl used cooling of the donor in an ice bath and an in situ flush of chilled Ringer's lactate via the portal vein,[19] subsequently, core cooling remained the first step in the preservation of all whole-organ grafts.

Extension of the safe period of liver preservation beyond that provided by initial cooling has depended on one of two approaches. The first approach was to perfuse the organ continuously ex vivo with a cold perfusate primed with blood and oxygenated within a hyperbaric chamber.[20] As this approach proved to be complex, an alternative of simple cold storage with specific solutions has evolved. Schalm in 1969 introduced a plasma-based solution, which has been the preferred method of preservation in the United Kingdom. Collins solution, or the modified Euro-Collins solutions, has been used as the standard for liver

TABLE 4-3. Composition of Preservation Solutions[a]

Constituent	*RL*	*EC*	*UW*
Electrolytes			
Calcium (m*M*/L)	1.5	—	—
Chloride (m*M*/L)	109	15	—
Magnesium (m*M*/L)	—	—	5
Sodium (m*M*/L)	130	10	30
Potassium (m*M*/L)	4	115	120
Anions			
Bicarbonate (mM/L)	—	10	—
Lactate (mM/L)	28	—	—
Lactobionate (mM/L)	—	—	100
Phosphate (mM/L)	—	57.5	25
Colloids and impermeants			
Hydroxyethyl starch (g/L)	—	—	50
Raffinose (g/L)	—	—	17.8
Others			
Glucose (g/L)	—	194	—
Adenosine (mM/L)	—	—	5
Allopurinol (mM/L)	—	—	1
Glutathione (mM/L)	—	—	3
Insulin (U/L)	—	—	100
Antibiotic and steroids			
Sulfamethoxazole (mg/L)	—	—	40
Trimethoprim (mg/L)	—	—	8
Dexamethasone (mg/L)	—	—	8
Osmolality (mOsm/L)	273	375	325
pH	6.3	7.4	7.4

[a]RL = Ringer's lactate, EC = Euro-Collins, UW = University of Wisconsin.

preservation in the United States, allowing for a safe cold storage up to 8 hr.[21] Euro-Collins solution attempts to oppose ionic shifts across the cell membrane by mimicking intracellular ionic concentrations: high concentration of potassium and low concentration of sodium and chloride (Table 4-3). In addition, it contains high concentration of glucose to suppress cell swelling.

The introduction of UW (University of Wisconsin) solution in 1987 by Belzer and associates has been a major advance in liver preservation in the last decade. Clinical studies have shown extended cold-storage preservation[22,23] and improved graft function despite increased cold-ischemia time.[24] UW solution contains lactobionate and raffinose as impermeants to suppress hypothermia-induced cell swelling, the colloid hydroxyethylstarch to provide oncotic pressure and allopurinol and glutathione as antioxidants (Table 4-3). The most remarkable impact of UW solution on liver transplantation is the extended preservation time, which effectively increases the capability for long-distance liver procurement and sharing and has the potential to increase the efficiency of using the scarce resource of donor organs.

REFERENCES

1. Alexander JW, Vaughn WK: The use of "marginal" donors for organ transplantation. The influence of donor age on outcome. *Transplantation* 51:135–141, 1991.

1a. Evans RW, Orians CE, Ascher NL: The potential supply of organ donors, *JAMA* 267:239–246, 1992.

2. Warren J, Gill B (eds): *Guidelines for Hospital Administration for Implementing Required Request*, pp 1–36, Alexandria, VA, American Council on Transplantation, 1987.

3. Report of the medical consultants on the diagnosis of death to the President's Commission for the Study of Ethical Problems in Medicine and Biomedical and Behavioral Research: guidelines for the determination of death. *JAMA* 246:2184–2186, 1981.

4. Kaufman HH, Lynne J: Brain death. *Neurosurgery* 19:850–856, 1986.

5. Wall WJ, Mimeault R, Grant DR, et al: The use of older donor livers for hepatic transplantation. *Transplantation* 49:377–381, 1990.

6. Oellerich M, Burdelski M, Ringe B, et al: Lignocaine metabolite formation as a measure of pre-transplant liver function. *Lancet* 1:640–642, 1989.

7. Higashi H, Yanaga K, Shimada M, et al: Plasma lecithin/cholesterol acyltransferase (LCAT) activity in multiple-organ donors: a predictor of allograft viability in clinical liver transplantation. *Transplant Proc* 22:433, 1990.

8. Darby JM, Stein K, Grevnik A, et al: Approach to management of the heartbeating "brain dead" organ donor. *JAMA* 261:2222–2228, 1989.

9. Richardson PDI, Witherington PG: Liver blood flow: Effects of drugs on hormones in liver blood flow. *Gastroenterology* 81:356–375, 1981.

10. Matuschak GM, Pinsky MR, Rogers RM: Effects of positive end-expiratory pressure on hepatic blood flow and performance. *J Appl Physiol* 62:1377–1383, 1987.

11. Eggink HF, Hofstee N, Gips CH, et al: Histopathology of serial graft biopsies from liver transplant recipients. *Am J Pathol* 114:18–31, 1984.

12. D'Alessandro AM, Kalayoglu M, Sollinger HW, et al: The predictive value of donor liver biopsies for the development of primary nonfunction after orthotopic liver transplantation. *Transplantation* 51:157–163, 1991.

13. Adam R, Reynes M, Johann M, et al: The outcome of steatotic grafts in liver transplantation. *Transplant Proc* 23:1538–1540, 1991.

14. Starzl TE, Demetris AJ (eds): Early graft function pp 43–45. In: *Liver Transplantation. A 31-Year Perspective*. Chicago, Year Book Medical Publishers, Inc. 1990.

15. Marsh JW, JR, Esquivel CO, Makowka L, et al: Accidental transplantation of malignant tumor from a donor to multiple recipients. *Transplantation* 44:449–450, 1987.

16. Dzik WH, Arkin CF, Jenkins RL: Transfer of congenital factor XI deficiency from a donor to a recipient by liver transplantation (letter). *New Engl J Med* 316:1217–1218, 1987.

17. Henne-Bruns D, Kremer B: Manifestation of Gilbert syndrome (Meulengracht disease) following orthotopic liver transplantation: a rare cause of postoperative hyperbilirubinemia. *Klin Wochenschr* 66:596–598, 1988.

18. Goodrich EO Jr, Welch HF, Nelson JA, et al: Homotransplantation of the canine liver. *Surgery* 39:244, 1956.

19. Starzl TE, Kaupp HA Jr, Brock DR, et al: Reconstructive problems in canine liver homotransplantation with special reference to the postoperative role of hepatic venous flow. *Surg Gynecol Obstet* 111:733–743, 1960.

20. Brettschneider L, Daloze PM, Huguet C, et al: The use of combined preservation techniques for extended storage of orthotopic liver homografts. *Surg Gynecol Obstet* 126:263–274, 1968.
21. Benichou J, Halgrimson CG, Weil R III, et al: Canine and human liver preservation for 6-18 hours by cold infusion. *Transplantation* 24:407–411, 1977.
22. Kalayoglu M, Sollinger WH, Stratta RJ, et al: Extended preservation of the liver for clinical transplantation. *Lancet* 1:617–619, 1988.
23. Todo S, Nery J, Yanaga K, et al: Extended preservation of human liver grafts with UW solution. *JAMA* 261:711–714, 1989.
24. Cofer BC, Klintmalm GB, Howard TK, et al: A comparison of UW solution with Euro-Collins preservation solution in liver transplantation. *Transplantation* 49:1088–1093, 1990.

— 5 —

TRANSPLANT BIOLOGY

Kirk Sperber and Lloyd Mayer

Liver transplantation provides treatment for fatal end-stage liver disease. Once in place, transplanted livers provide a challenge to clinical immunologists. Because transplanted livers are subjected to different types of injuries (intraoperative ischemia, drug toxicity, mechanical cholestasis from suboptimal biliary anastomoses, transfusion-associated viral hepatitis, and immunologic rejection), a clear understanding of the nature of the rejection process has been slow to emerge.[1] Recent studies at both the light and electron-microscopic levels have now clearly established that the intrahepatic bile duct epithelium is the initial target of the immune response in liver allograft rejection.[2,3] The dominant histologic picture is a progressive, nonsuppurative destructive cholangitis with preservation of the hepatic parenchyma.[1-10] The picture is strikingly similar to immunologically mediated events seen in primary biliary cirrhosis[11] and in the hepatic component of the graft versus host reaction,[12] a common consequence of bone marrow transplantation. In addition, some patients develop segmental disease of the larger intra- and extrahepatic bile ducts that resembles sclerosing cholangitis.[1-10]

In order to understand the immunologic consequences of liver transplantation, it will be useful to review some fundamental principles of transplantation.

LAWS OF TRANSPLANTATION

The laws of transplantation are guidelines used to predict successful transplantation. These observations were initially formulated by C.C. Little in 1914 and codified into five laws of transplantation.[16,17] Although these observations were based on animal model systems, they are still useful for understanding human transplant immunology. These laws are summarized as follows:[18]

1. *Transplants within inbred strains will succeed.* Transplants between genetically identical members of the same species will be accepted. The only excep-

tion to this is transplants from males to females who may be rejected through Y chromosome incompatibility.

2. *Transplants between outbred strains will fail.* Members of genetically unrelated strains will always reject the transplanted organ.
3. *Transplants from a member of an inbred parental strain to an F1 (first-generation offspring from genetically distinct strains) will succeed, but those in the reverse direction (from an F1 offspring to one of the original parental strains) will fail.* Offspring of two genetically distinct inbred strains of mice will inherit the entire genetic material of both parental strains. Thus, transplants from any one of the parental strains to the F1 generation will succeed. In contrast, transplants in the reverse direction from the F1 animal (which has genetic material from the one unrelated parental strain) to the other parental strain will fail.
4. *Transplants from F2 and all subsequent generations to F1 animals will succeed.* Grafts of subsequent offspring of F1 mice will succeed when transplanted back to the F1 generation. The F1 parental line contains all of the original genetic material.
5. *Transplants from inbred parental strains to F2 generations will usually, but not always, fail.* Because of chromosomal segregation in subsequent generations, occasional homozygotes will be obtained which contain all of the genetic of one parent and will not be rejected by the original parent line but the majority of the progeny will express incompatible histocompatibility antigens that will be rejected.

By themselves these laws provide little insight into the genetic basis for rejection. However, C.C. Little's contribution to our understanding of transplantation was his hypothesis that there are multiple genetic loci (histocompatibility antigens) with codominant expression (i.e., products of both genes are equally expressed) that are responsible for organ transplantation rejection.[19] Incompatibility of any product of a histocompatibility locus in the donor, but not the recipient, can lead to organ rejection.[20-22] These ideas have become the basis of our current thinking in organ transplantation. Little's hypothesis leads directly into further analysis of the surface glycoproteins, which form the basis of the major histocompatibility complex (MHC), which in turn is directly responsible for rejection. The MHC complex is a series of cell surface molecules present on nucleated cells.[23]

Analysis of the "major" histocompatibility locus quickly led to the recognition that this was not a single locus but rather a complex of several loci which are important in clinical transplantation.[24,25] There are 3 loci within the MHC complex: class I molecules, the classical transplantation molecules expressed on all nucleated cells (HLA ABC in humans); class II molecules, which are present on cells responsible for presentation of antigen to T-cells (HLAD in man); and class III molecules, which do not appear to play any role in antigen recognition.[20-25]

Although recognized because of their importance in the rejection of transplanted organs, the MHC did not evolve for this purpose. Rather, MHC molecules are essential for the recognition of foreign antigens by both cytotoxic and helper T-cells. The name major histocompatibility merely reflects the historic nature of

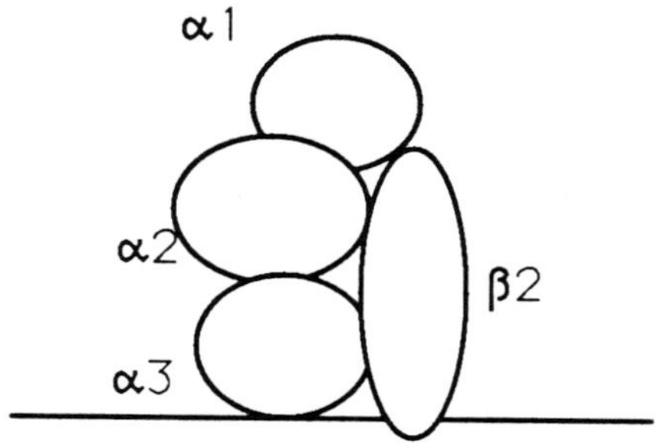

MHC class I

Figure 5-1. Schematic representation of a class I molecule. It is composed of two chains, alpha (α) and beta (β). The alpha chain has three domains, α-1, α-2, and α-3, which bear the antigenic determinants. The beta chain is nonpolymorphic and is called B2 microglobulin.

their discovery. The MHC exhibits extraordinary polymorphism which provides a survival advantage in being able to respond to a broad variety of foreign antigens. The large number of alleles that are encoded by each locus combined with the presence of at least six individual loci provide an enormous variety of MHC types and make the likelihood of achieving an exact match for a transplanted liver virtually impossible.[20-25] It will be instructive at this point to review the structure of some elements of the MHC antigens, the class I and class II antigens.

Class I Antigens

Class I molecules consist of three separate alleles—HLA A, HLA B, HLA C (HLA = human leuckocyte antigen)—each of which consist of a two-chain structure.[26] The heavy or alpha chain of each HLA molecule is a polymorphic glycoprotein [molecular weight (MW) = 44,000] of 338 amino acids which is encoded by genes on chromosome 6. It is subdivided into three regions:[27] an extracellular region, a transmembrane region, and an intracellular region (Fig. 5-1). The extracellular region can be further divided into three regions: α-1, α-2 and α-3.[28] The second chain is non-convalently linked, nonpolymorphic (MW 12,000) protein, which is called *B2 microglobulin*. The entire molecule is anchored in the cell membrane by the alpha chain. The α-1 and α-2 regions of the class I antigens are polymorphic.[26-28]

Class I molecules bind to intracellular antigen, forming a complex that is then expressed on the cell surface and can be recognized by the T-cell receptor. Without class I molecules, no recognition would take place. In viral infection, viral proteins are produced in the cell, bind to class I antigens, and are presented to cytotoxic CD8 T-cells[31,32] after being coexpressed on the cell surface. Antigen recognition and subsequent cell killing will occur only if the viral antigens are

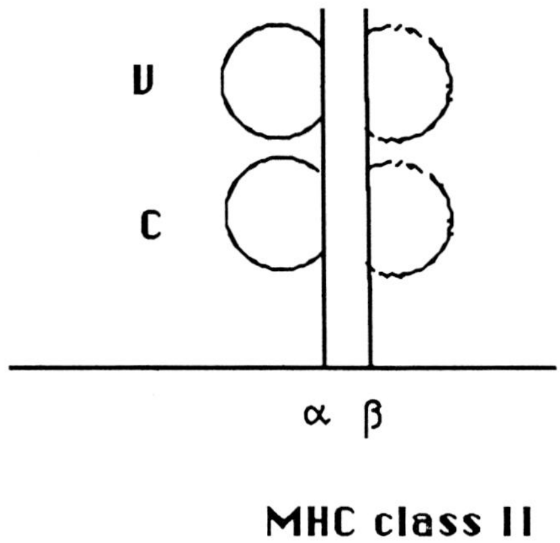

Figure 5-2. Schematic representation of a class II molecule consisting of an alpha and a beta chain in noncovalent association that has a proximal constant domain (C) and a variable distal domain (V). The structure of class II molecules is similar to immunoglobulins, which may relate to the ability of both to bind to peptides.

complexed to class I antigens. This phenomenon is termed MHC restriction and occurs not only in the course of a normal immune response to a variety of viral infections, but in organ transplantation also. In transplantation, donor class I molecules are recognized as foreign antigens against which host responses are generated during graft rejection.[33–35]

Class II Antigens

The basic structure of class II molecules is similar to class I in that it is a two-chain structure with an alpha (α) (or heavy) and a beta (β) (or light) chain[36] (Fig. 5-2). The chains are noncovalently linked; however, unlike class I antigens, the exact three-dimensional arrangement of these molecules is still unknown. Each chain consists of external domains, a transmembrane domain, and a cytoplasmic tail. The distal external domains show marked diversity in amino acid composition, which accounts for variability in peptide binding, while the proximal external domains as well as the transmembrane and intracytoplasmic portions are well conserved.[36]

The human HLA class II antigens are composed of three alleles, DR, DQ, and DP, which are located on the short arm of chromosome 6. The DR, DQ, and DP class II antigens are members of the immunoglobulin supergene family and demonstrate significant homology with different domains of class I molecules and the immunoglobulin heavy and light chains.[38] The class II molecules are also structurally related to immunoglobulins, which may relate to their ability to bind to peptide antigens. Their organization into the polymorphic (first) and conserved (second) domains is similar to the variable and constant regions of immunoglobulin molecules.[38] Class II molecules are more potent antigens in stimulating rejection than class I molecules. This is demonstrated in the mixed-lymphocyte reactions where antibodies against class II antigens and not class I antigens block proliferation of responder T-cells[39–40] that are stimulated by donor monocytes expressing both foreign (or mismatched) class I and Class II antigens.[42]

The tissue distribution of class I and class II molecules is different. Class I antigens are present on nearly all nucleated cells of the body[43] but may be sparse on antigen presenting cells which have considerable quantities of class II antigens.[44] Class II antigens have more limited expression on macrophages, B lymphocytes, and dendritic cells. Class II antigen expression on some tissues, such as epithelium, is not constant but is dependent on gamma (γ) interferon stimulus.[45-47] In the liver, class I antigens are strongly expressed on bile duct epithelium and while present in small quantities, are not easily detected on normal hepatocytes.[48,49] The absence of class I antigens on normal hepatocytes is believed to be extremely important: the liver in this "privileged" state does not elicit a strong allogeneic T-cell response leading to rejection. The presence of class I antigens on biliary epithelium may serve to direct the attack of sensitized cytotoxic T-cells to this site. Class II antigens are expressed predominantly on the various populations of sinusoidal cells including both Kupffer and endothelial cells.[48,50] A variety of hepatobiliary diseases have an abnormal distribution of class I and class II antigens. This confuses the role HLA determinants may play in the initial phases of hepatic allograft rejection. Unlike renal and cardiac transplantation, where class I and class II histocompatibility is associated with better graft acceptance, class I and class II histocompatibility between donor and recipient does not predict a successful liver allograft. In fact, routine HLA tissue typing between donor and recipient is not performed preoperatively.

Minor Histocompatibility Antigens

It became apparent that not all renal transplant rejection could be explained by disconcordances of the major (class I and class II) histocompatibility antigens.[51-53] These observations led to the discovery of minor histocompatibility antigens, which are defined as antigens capable of causing cell-mediated graft rejection different from MHC products. The exact biochemical nature of these antigens is not well understood. It appears that there is a chromosomal association between major and minor histocompatibility antigens.[54-56]

BLOOD GROUP ANTIGENS

Blood group antigens (ABO) do not evoke cell-mediated response and hence do not play a major role in cellular rejection of organ transplantation. Humoral responses are important in the acute rejection of highly vascular grafts like the kidney because vascular endothelium express ABO antigens on their surface.[57,58] However, hyperacute rejection in liver transplantation is uncommon and occurs only when the recipient has preformed antibodies to donor antigens. Even then the liver is relatively resistant to hyperacute rejection. This may be due to either insensitivity of the transplanted organ to preformed antibodies or that the size of the liver graft may dilute the concentration of antibody levels. ABO compatibility, and not class I or class II typing, is the major criterion used for tissue typing in liver transplantation.

MECHANISMS OF GRAFT REJECTION

Transplanted livers will be rejected if donor class I and class II antigens are expressed on the cell surface in a form accessible to the host's immune system.[60] Foreign Class II antigens are potent stimulators of cellular responses. The T-cell response to transplanted donor class I and class II antigens can be divided into phases: (1) a sensitization phase where recipient cell populations are expanded in response to exposure to donor alloantigens and (2) an effector phase characterized by cellular rejection of the graft.

The initial cells activated in transplant rejection require the presence of donor antigen presenting cells (APCs) such as monocytes, which express class II antigens.[60] Pretreatment of donor livers of animal models with anti-class II and antimonocyte antibodies results in prolonged graft survival.[61] These APCs also produce "second signals," including interleukin-1, which serve as cofactors for proliferation of B- and T-cells.[62] The activation of the CD-4 T helper inducer cells is critical to rejection. These cells release interleukin-2 (IL-2),[63] which regulates subsequent T-cell and B-cell growth. As a consequence of this interaction between donor class II and class I antigens and recipient T-cells, clonal proliferation of donor-specific T- and B- cells occurs.[64-68] These activated T-cells then migrate to the liver and cause tissue damage in the transplanted liver.

As described above, effector T-cells (CD-4 and CD-8) recognize distinct MHC molecules.[64-68] Cytotoxic CD-8 cells recognize class I antigen-bearing cells,[69,70] whereas helper CD-4 cells recognize class II antigen-bearing cells[71,72] (Fig. 5-3). Although both cell types can destroy the transplanted liver by direct cytotoxicity,[73-78] more importantly they release gamma interferon. Gamma interferon has two key consequences in liver transplant rejection: it induces class I antigen expression on hepatocytes, rendering them more susceptible to infiltrating T-cells, and it activates monocytes that can nonspecifically destroy the graft. T-cells can destroy the transplanted liver directly or stimulate monocytes to nonspecifically destroy tissue.[73-78] Other lymphokines produced by activated T-cells include IL-4 and IL-5, which are important in directing immunoglobulin production and development of antibody-dependent cell-mediated cytotoxicity.[79,80] These experimental findings are confirmed by immunohistochemical staining of rejected livers. T-lymphocytes account for 50–90% of the infiltrating cell population.[2,3]

Early liver rejection in man is characterized by infiltration of the bile ducts and portal triads with mononuclear cells. Late rejection is characterized by the loss of bile ducts,[2,3] suggesting that the bile duct epithelium is important in the rejection process. As described earlier, bile duct epithelial cells express class I antigens.[33] Like epithelial cells from other organs, bile duct epithelial cells can express immunoregulatory molecules, class II antigens, especially after gamma interferon stimulation. In some cases, expression of class II antigens is thought to result in the presentation of "self" antigens to T-cells, eventuating in an autoimmune disorder like Grave's disease,[80] Kawasaki's disease,[81] and diabetes.[82] Another scenario involves the role of the epithelial cell as a true antigen-presenting cell, processing and presenting foreign antigen to immunocompetent T-cells.[39] In the case of rejection, foreign class II represents self (nonpolymorphic portions of the molecule) and nonself (polymorphic portions of the molecule), although presentation of "self" antigens or antigens to which we are normally

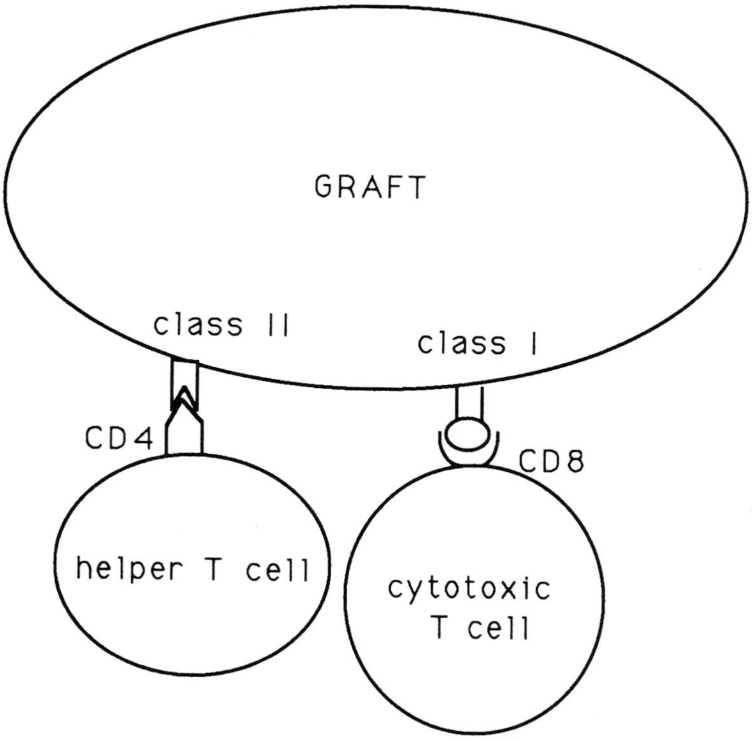

Figure 5-3. Schematic representation of class I and class II recognition by host T-cells that mediate the rejection process. Cytotoxic T-cells recognize class I antigens, which are present on all nucleated cells but have limited expression on hepatocytes. Helper T-cells recognize class II antigens, which are present on donor macrophages, T-cells, and B-cells that have been transplanted with the liver.

tolerant could occur. In the liver, then, regionalized expression (bile ducts) of class I and class II molecules would seem to explain the pattern of cellular infiltrates that mediate the rejection process and the lack of class I antigen on hepatocytes correlates with initial lack of hepatocyte destruction and cellular infiltrates.[33]

Liver transplantation may be associated with some degree of graft-versus-host (graft–host) disease because the transplanted liver contains large numbers of lymphoid cells. Although transplantation of the liver can take place[83] in the face of blood group incompatibilities. there is evidence that long term survival is diminished.[84] In fact, an antibody-dependent hemolysis of recipient red blood cells mediated by transplanted donor B cells and graft–host disease has been described in ABO-incompatible liver transplants.[85,86]

Animal Models

While histologic studies of rejected human donor livers are important in understanding the rejection process, animal model systems have been developed to better understand early events in rejection. Liver allografts do not always obey the laws of transplantation. In many species, including monkeys,[87] pigs,[88,89] and certain strains of rat,[90-92] transplanted livers survive without immunosuppression. In other species, such as the baboon[93] and the dog,[94] liver grafts are typically rejected in the absence of immunosuppression. The basis of this permissive state is uncertain. Much of the initial work has been done with rat model systems which are easier to work with because of the availability of many strains. These rodent model systems involving livers transplanted between different strains of rats provide important insights into mechanisms of rejection. In these studies livers that are transplanted between selected rat strains have a 95% survival rate whereas skin, heart, and kidney grafts transplanted within the rat strains are promptly rejected.[95,96] In addition, between certain rat strains liver allografts are not only accepted indefinitely, but convey onto the recipient animals the ability to accept other grafts (skin and kidney) that are rejected in non-liver-transplanted animals.[97,98] These animals studies suggest that the liver deletes alloreactive T-cells that mediate rejection not only of the liver but of other organs as well.[99] Several groups have reported that this loss of allograft reactivity can be transferred by serum to other amimals.[100] While these model systems are interesting and could potentially provide insight into human liver transplant rejection, a permissive state is not observed with human liver transplantation.[101]

PRINCIPLES OF IMMUNOSUPPRESSIVE THERAPY

Different stages of an immune response differ in susceptibility to immunosuppressants. In general a primary immune response is more readily inhibited than a secondary response.[121] The primary rejection of a liver allograft is easily impaired by a combination of azathioprine and corticosteroids, while a presensitized recipient (second rejection) requires more intensive immunosuppression.[122]

Cellular events associated with the rejection process can be divided into two phases: the inductive and effector phases.[123] The first process involves the presentation of the liver allograft antigens to the host immune system. This phase is characterized by rapid proliferative expansion of antigen reactive sensitized T- and B-cells.[124] Thereafter, the reaction is considered to have entered an established phase.[124] Most cytotoxic agents are highly effective in the induction phase but are less active once the response has entered the established phase.[126] The effectiveness of an immunosuppressive agent is dependent on the timing between the administration of the immunosuppression and the antigen exposure.[127] On the basis of the above findings, immunosuppressive agents can be divided into two groups: (1) agents that exert maximum immunosuppressive activity when administered just before antigen challenge—these agents which are much less effective when administered after introduction of the antigen, include steroids and cytoxan;[105,128,129] and (2) drugs that exert immunosuppressive properties only if administered after antigen challenge and includes methotrexate and azathioprine.[130]

Immunosuppressive drugs can exert differential toxicity for T- and B-cells. For example, cyclophosphamide preferentially reduces the number of B-cells rather than T-cells, and because of this, more profoundly inhibits antibody production.[131] Clinically, cyclophosphamide would be more effective in inhibiting antibody mediated rejection[128] than, for example, azathioprine, which preferentially inhibits T cell mediated responses.[132]

IMMUNOSUPPRESSIVE THERAPY

Unlike liver transplants in some animal model systems which do not evoke an allogeneic rejection response, cell-mediated rejection regularly occurs in transplanted human livers and requires immunosuppressive therapy to prevent loss of the allograft.[1,101] Over the past 20 years compounds that block distinct aspects of the immune response have been developed. The success of these drugs have been directly responsible for the marked increase in liver transplantation over the past 10 years.[1] Unfortunately, immunosuppression is not specific for the transplanted organ but is global, which results in complications.[102,103] Immunosuppressive agents can be divided into several groups: corticosteroids, cytotoxic agents, immunomodulators, and antilymphocyte antibodies. Since each of these agents affect different aspects of the rejection process, they can be used in combination to improve graft survival and reduce toxicity.[104]

Corticosteroids

Corticosteroids have many effects on the immune system, which can be broadly divided into three general categories: (1) the effect on circulating leukocytes, (2) the ability to alter specific cellular function, and (3) other activities.[105]

Circulating Leukocytes

Within 24 hr after bolus of steroids, there is a prompt increase in the number of circulating neutrophils followed by a concomitant decrease in the total number of lymphocytes, monocytes and eosinophils.[106,107] This effect appears to be due to an increase in the release of neutrophils from marrow reserves and a decrease in neutrophil migration to sites of inflammation.[108]

In contrast, corticosteroids cause a marked reduction in the number of circulating lymphocytes.[109] In humans, unlike in animal species (mice, rats, and rabbits), corticosteroids are not lympholytic but cause a sequestration of lymphocytes into lymphoid tissue, including the bone marrow and lymph nodes.[105] Circulating levels of CD-4 T-cells are reduced to a greater extent than are CD-8 cytotoxic T-cells, while B-cells are only modestly reduced after steroid therapy.[107] Another important steroid effect is profound monocytopenia.[107] Eosinophils and basophils are also markedly reduced because of redistribution.[107]

Cellular Functions

Neutrophil activity, including the release of microsomal proteolytic enzymes such as collagenase, are decreased by steroids, while chemotaxis is generally not affected accounting in part for the steroid antiinflammatory activity.[108]

T-lymphocyte function is significantly altered by steroids. Proliferation is markedly inhibited by steroids probably due to an impairment in synthesis and secretion of IL-2. Mitogen-induced T-cell proliferation is blocked by corticosteroids by inhibiting entry of cells into the G1 phase and an arrest in the progression of activated lymphocytes from the G1 phase to the S (DNA synthesis) phase.[107] Proliferation is also decreased by diminished production of IL-1 by monocytes, a critical growth factor for T-cells.[108] Corticosteroids do not affect gamma-interferon production or *macrophage inhibition factor* (MIF)[105] synthesis. Corticosteroids have less of an effect on B-cells, but high-dose therapy can reduce serum concentration of IgG as well as the IgG subclasses.[110,111]

NK Cells and Monocytes

Monocytes and tissue macrophages are markedly affected by corticosteroids. Bactericidal activity, antigen presentation, and migration in response to a chemotactic stimulus are suppressed.[108] Fc-receptor expression and complement receptor expression important in immune complex clearing are also inhibited by corticosteroid therapy.[108] In contrast, corticosteroids do not alter natural-killer (NK) cell activity or antibody-dependent cellular cytotoxicity (ADCC).[105]

Cytotoxic Agents

Cytotoxic drugs also prevent liver allograft rejection. Although initially introduced as chemotherapic agents for malignancy, these drugs possess the pharmacologic property of killing cells capable of self-replication (such as lymphocytes).[112-114] There are three cytotoxic drugs in use for immunosuppression: cyclophosphamide, azathioprine, and methotrexate. These drugs affect all cells of the immune system and increase susceptibility to both opportunistic infections and certain malignancies.[115]

Rapidly proliferating cells like intestinal mucosal cells, hematopoietic stem cells, and germ cells are killed[116]: bone marrow suppression, gasrointestinal toxicity, and infertility are predictable side effects.[117] Drug toxicity is related to the effect of the drugs on specific phases of the mitotic cycle.[118] Azathioprine and methotrexate are phase-specific and are toxic to cells in the S (DNA synthesis) phase, while cyclosphosphamide is cycle-specific since it is toxic for cells in all phases of mitosis.[119] Cyclophosphamide is more toxic for proliferating cells than for resting cells.[120]

Azathioprine

Azathioprine is a phase-specific drug.[133] It is a purine antagonist, which is similar in structure to 6-mercaptopurine.[134] Its major activity is to block DNA synthesis by competitive inhibition of the synthesis of inosinic acid, the precursor to adenylic and guanylic acids.[135] This, in turn, inhibits cell replication and explains the phase specificity of this agent.[136] Azathioprine preferentially inhibits T-cells. B-cell proliferation is also affected so that both humoral and cellular responses can be inhibited.[137] NK and ADCC activities are also inhibited by this drug.[138]

Combination of azathioprine and corticosteroids has been a standard therapy for inhibition of acute liver transplant rejection. Short courses of azathioprine do not reduce circulating numbers of T- or B-cells but rather inhibit clonal proliferation and therefore total immunoglobulin levels and antigen-specific antibodies are not decreased.[140]

Cyclophosphamide

This immunosuppressive, cycle-specific agent has a greater effect on B-cells than on T-cells.[131] Because of its greater anti-B-cell activity, it has more suppressive activity for humoral responses rather than for cellular responses.[141] Cyclophosphamide can be administered either orally or intravenously and is inactive until it is metabolized by the liver.[142] The predominant effect of this drug is to crosslink DNA, causing either immediate cell death or death during a subsequent mitosis.[143] If DNA repair mechanisms are efficient and the crosslinking is repaired, the affected cell will survive.[144] B-cells are more readily affected than T-cells because B-cells are less able to recover from DNA crosslinking.[145] Cyclophosphamide causes a dose-dependent lymphopenia. Significant side effects associated with this therapy are suppression of hematopoiesis, gastrointestinal symptoms, including diarrhea and stomatitis, infertility,[146] hemorrhagic cystitis, and alopecia.[146] There is also an increased incidence of non-Hodgkins lymphoma and acute myelogenous leukemia with long-term therapy.[147]

Methotrexate

Methotrexate, like azathioprine, is a potent inhibitor of DNA synthesis and is an S-phase-specific agent.[149] It is a specific inhibitor of dihydrofolate reductase, the enzyme necessary to convert folic acid to tetrahydrofolate, which is necessary for thymidine synthesis.[148] It is used in the treatment of primary biliary cirrhosis, rheumatoid arthritis, psoriasis, bronchial asthma, and other autoimmune diseases. Methotrexate has also been used to prevent graft–host disease in bone marrow transplantation.[150] Significant toxicities associated with its use include hepatic fibrosis and hypersensitivity.[151]

Immunomodulators

Cyclosporine A

Cyclosporine A (CsA) is a novel drug that has a unique activity distinct from all immunosuppressive agents.[152] This drug selectively inhibits helper T-cell activity and granulocyte and monocyte[153] function. Cyclosporine acts by impairing helper T-cell activity without killing target lymphocytes[154-157] and has become the standard immunosuppressive agent in preventing liver allograft rejection. CsA is a undecapeptide that is obtained as a metabolite of the soil fungus *Tolypocladium inflatum* Gams.[152] It inhibits the activities of helper T-cells and not suppressor T-cells, allowing cyclosporine to inhibit helper T-cell-dependent allograft rejection.[158-160] Additionally, it acts at an early stage of the developing rejection response.[161-164] Cyclosporine inhibits IL-2 synthesis and secretion[160,165] and impairs the ability of T-cells to respond to IL-2 by decreasing IL-2 receptor expression.[166] Through its effect on helper T-cells, cyclosporine restricts the generation of antigen-specific cytotoxic T-cell activities, which is dependent on IL-2.[154-156,161] NK activity is preserved, while T-cell-dependent antibody responses are inhibited.[167-169] Synergistic effects of cyclosporine with other immunosuppressive agents have been observed. Cyclosporine has been used in conjunction with corticosteroids because of their different effects on the growth and proliferation of T-cells.[170] Corticosteroids inhibit IL-1 synthesis from monocytes, a necessary cofactor for a T-cell response, while cyclosporine blocks IL-2 synthesis.[170] The development of cyclosporine along with improved surgical techniques have been largely responsible for the increased success of liver transplantation.[1] Cyclosporine is not toxic to bone marrow.[171–174] Renal insufficiency is the major complication of therapy,[175-179] which is reversible if the medication is stopped promptly.[180-182] Reversible liver toxicity is also common with cyclosporine therapy.[183-187] As with cyclophosphamide treatment, the development of B-cell lymphomas is a major side effect of long-term therapy because of diminished T-cell surveillance.[188-191] Other complications include gingival hyperplasia, seizures, and hirsutism.[192-193]

FK506

FK506 is a novel macrolide product of *Streptomyces tukubaesinsis* that was first discovered in 1987.[194-196] This drug is 100 times more potent than cyclosporine in inhibiting the secretion of IL-2 and gamma interferon from helper T-cells.[197-201] FK506 also inhibits mixed lymphocyte reactions,[199] T-dependent humoral responses,[200] cytolytic T-cell responses,[196] and allograft rejection.[202] The main action of this drug appears to be the inhibition of maturation of precursor cytotoxic T-cells by blocking either IL-2 secretion or IL-2R (IL-2 receptor) expression.[200-203] It does not affect the lytic action of the cytotoxic lymphocytes.[198] FK506 does not inhibit IL-2- or IL-6-driven proliferation of cloned B-cells.[201] Thus it appears that FK506 inhibits T-cell proliferation during the recognition and induction phase of the allograft reaction but not the proliferation that is seen after the production and binding of cytokines.[204,205] The activities of this drug are not limited to T-cells. It has been demonstrated that FK506 can inhibit IL-1 release from monocytes.[206] FK506 can also suppress allograft rejection in transplant model systems of liver, heart, and kidney in the rat,[207-209] dog, and monkey.[210–212] The principal side effects of FK506 are a low-grade nephrotoxicity and neurotoxicity, including paresthesias, insomnia, headaches, expressive dysphasia, mood changes, and anorexia.[213-215] Initial clinical trials have reported encouraging results using FK506 for both kidney and liver transplantation, although the therapeutic index is narrow and toxicity is a potential problem.[213,216]

In addition to its use as a sole agent to suppress rejection of allografts, there is in vitro evidence that synergism exists between FK506 and cyclosporine. This synergistic effect has been demonstrated in vivo using canine renal and rat liver allografts where lower doses of FK506 and cyclosporine suppressed rejection.[217,218] This approach is exciting and may lead the way for improved combination therapy at less toxic doses of both drugs.

Antilymphocyte Antibodies

Another mechanism of preventing rejection is to specifically remove the cells responsible for its induction.[219] Polyclonal antibodies directed against T-cell-specific antigens are effective immunosuppressants in animal model systems. Their primary effect is to impair cell-mediated responses.[220] Clinically they induce lymphopenia and can be quite effective[221] in immunosuppression. However, there are several problems associated with the use of polyclonal anti-T-cell sera. A specific clinical effect cannot be predicted because of nonstandardization of preparations. The antibodies are not selective for T-cells, and there is cross-reactivity with many other cells and platelets, which can lead to thrombocytopenia. Heterologous serum can lead to a host humoral response resulting in a serum sickness.[222] More recently specific monoclonal antibodies (viz., OK T3) have been used to prevent graft rejection.[223] These monoclonal antibodies have the advantage of greater specificity and more accurate quantitation but are also limited in their usefulness. One constant problem is that monoclonal antibodies of murine origin are recognized by the host as foreign. Anti-murine antibodies are generated after one course of therapy.[223] The presence of antimurine antibodies precludes its usefulness for recurrent administration since immune complexes are cleared rapidly before the immnosuppressive effect is seen. The rational for monoclonal therapy is quite compelling. Antibodies to the IL-2R, to CD-4, or to helper T-cells are highly effective in preventing graft rejection (blocking activated inductive and effector cells.[224] Recent attempts to "humanize" these monoclonal antibodies by genetic engineering (to prevent their recognition and removal) have met with some success.[225]

CONCLUSION

Liver transplantation provides a definitive treatment for otherwise fatal end-stage liver disease. Liver allografts, partially due to the lack of expression of histocompatibility antigens, are generally less immunogenic than other organs such as the kidney and skin. Despite this "privileged state," liver allografts are still rejected. As our understanding of the inductive and effector mechanisms of rejection has increased, we have been able to develop specific therapies to regulate immune responses against the allograft. A clearer picture of the rejection process will allow us to tailor suitable immunomodulator therapy to promote graft survival.

REFERENCES

1. Starzl TE, Iwatsuki S, Van Thiel DH, Gartner JC, Zitelli BJ, Malatack J, Schade RP, Shaw BW, Hakala TR, Rosenthal JT, Porter KA: Evolution of liver transplantation. *Hepatology* 2:614–636, 1982.
2. Vierling JM, Fennell RH: Histopathology of early and late human hepatic allograft rejection: Evidence of progressive destruction of interlobular bile ducts. *Hepatology* 5:1076–1082, 1985.

3. Fennell RH, Vierling JM: Electron microscopy of rejected human liver allografts. *Hepatology* 5:1083–1087, 1985.
4. Wight DGD: Pathology of rejection. In Calne RY: *Liver Transplantation,* pp 247–277, New York, Grune & Stratton, 1983.
5. Calne R: Hepatic transplantation. *Springer Semin Immunopathol* 3:385–393, 1980.
6. Roddy, H, Putnam CW, Fennell RH: Pathology of liver transplantation. *Transplantation* 22:625–630, 1976.
7. Fennell RH, Shikes RH, Vierling JM: Relationship of pre-transplant hepatobiliary disease to bile duct damage occurring in the liver allograft. *Hepatology* 3:84–89, 1983.
8. Eggink HF, Hofster N, Gips CH, et al: Histopathology of serial graft biopsies from liver transplant recipients. *Am J Pathol* 114:18–31, 1984.
9. Snover DC, Sibley RF, Freese DK, et al: Orthotopic liver transplantation: a pathological study of 63 serial liver biopsies from 17 patients with special reference to the diagnostic features and natural history of rejection. *Hepatology* 4:1212–1222, 1984.
10. Demetris AJ, Lasky S, Van Thiel DT, et al: Pathology of hepatic transplantation. A review of 62 adult allograft recipients immunosuppressed with a cyclosporine/steroid regimen. *Am J Pathol* 118:151–161, 1985.
11. Baggenstass AH, Faulk WT, Butt HR, Bahn RC: The pathology of primary biliary cirrhosis with emphasis on histogenesis. *Am J Clin Pathol,* 42:259, 1964.
12. Shulman HM, Sharma P, Amos D, et al: A coded histologic study of hepatic graft-versus host disease after human bone marrow transplantation. *Hepatology* 8:463–470, 1980.
13. Gibson T, Medawar PB: The fate of skin homografts in man. *J Anat* 77:299, 1943.
14. Medawar PB: The behavior and fate of skin autografts and skin homografts in rabbits. *J Anat* 78:176–199, 1944.
15. Medawar PB: Second study of behavior and fate of skin homo-grafts in rabbits. *J Anat* 79:157, 1944.
16. Little CC, Typpe EE: Further studies on inheritance of susceptibility to a transplantation tumor of Japanese waltzing mice. *J Med Res* 33:393, 1916.
17. Little CC: The genetics of tumor transplantation. In Snell GD: *Biology of the Laboratory Mouse,* 1 ed, pp 279–309, New York, Dover, 1941.
18. Winn HJ: Laws of transplantation. In *Human Immunogenetics.* New York: Marcel Dekker, 1988.
19. Little CC: A possible Mendelian explanation for a type of inheritance apparently non-Mendelian in nature. *Science* 40:904–906, 1914.
20. Amos DB, Ward FE: Immunogenetics of the HLA system. *Phys Rev* 55:206–246, 1979.
21. Shejgaard A, Haugl M, Jersild C, Platz P, Ryder LP, Nielsen LS, Thomsen M: The HLA System. An introductory survey. *Monographs in Human Genetics,* Vol. 7, Basel, S Kargel, 1979.
22. Medawar PB: The immunology of transplantation. In *The Harvey Lectures* 1956–57, New York, Academic Press, 1957.
23. Shrefflen DC, David CS: The H-2 major histocompatibility complex and the immune response region: Genetic varations functions, and organization. *Adv Immunol* 20:125, 1975.
24. Dorf ME (ed): *The Role of the Major Histocompatibility complex in Immunobiology,* New York, Gorbound JTPM Press, 1981.

25. Gotze D, (ed): *The Major Histocompatibility System in Man and Animals,* Berlin, Springer-Verlag, 1977.
26. Moller G: Molecular genetics of Class I and Class II MHC antigens. *Immunol Rev* 84:1, 1985.
27. Bjorkman PJ, Saper MA, Samraoui B et al: Structure of the human Class I histocompatibility antigen HLA-A2. *Nature* 329:506, 512, 1987.
28. Moller G: Molecular genetics of Class I and Class II MHC antigens. *Immunol Rev* 85:1, 1985.
29. Townsend ARM, Gotch FM, Davey J: Cytotoxic T cells recognize fragments of the influenza nucleoprotein. *Cell* 42:457–467, 1985.
30. Maryanski JC, Pala P, Corradir G, Jordan BR, Cerottini JC: H-2 restricted cytolytic T cells specific for HLA can recognize a synthetic HLA peptide. *Nature* 324:578–579, 1986.
31. Gooding LR, O'Connell KA: Recognition by cytotoxic T Lymphocytes of cells expressing fragments of the SV40 tumor antigen. *J Immunol* 131:2580–2586, 1983.
32. Braciale TJ, Braciale VL, Winkler M, Stroynowski I, Hood L, Sambrvak J, Gethering MJ: On the role of the transmembrane anchor sequence of influenza hemaglutinin in target cell recognition by Class I MHC-restricted hemagglutinin-specific cytolytic T lymphocytes. *J Exp Med* 166:678–692, 1987.
33. DeVas R, DeWolf-Peeters C, Van der Oord JJ, Desmet V: Ultrastructure immunocytochemical demonstration of HLA Class I antigens in human pathological liver tissue. *Hepatology* 6:1071–1075, 1985.
34. Mason DW, Dallman MJ, Arthur RP, Manus PJ: Mechanisms of allograft rejection: The role of cytotoxic T cells and delayed type hypersensitivity. *Immunol Rev* 77:177, 1984.
35. Steinmuller D: Which T cells mediate allograft rejection. *Transplantation* 40:229–233, 1985.
36. Moller G, Structure and function of HLA-DR. *Immunol Rev* 66:1, 1982.
37. Hanser TH, Sacks DH: The major histocompatibility complex. In Paul WE, *Fundamental Immunology* New York, Raven Press, 1989.
38. Robinson MA, Kermit TJ: Major histocompatibility complex antigens and genes. In Paul WE: *Fundamental Immunology,* New York, Raven Press, 1989.
39. Mayer L, Shlien R: Evidence for function of Ia molecules on gut epithelial cells in man. *J Exp Med* 166:1471–1483, 1987.
40. Bach FH, Hirschhorn K: Lymphocyte interaction: a potential histocompatibility test in vitro. *Science* 143:462–466, 1964.
41. Bair B, Vaz MR, Lowenstein L: The development of large immature mononuclear cells in mixed lymphocyte cultures. *Blood* 23:108–116, 1964.
42. Hayrz P, Defendi V: Mixed lymphocyte cultures produce effector cells: model in vitro for allograft rejection. *Science* 168:133–135, 1970.
43. Harris HW, Gill TJ: Expression of class I transplantation antigens. *Transplantation* 42:109, 1986.
44. Daor AS, Fuggle SV, Falene JW, Tieng A, Morris PJ: The detailed distribution of MHC class II antigens in normal human organs. *Transplantation* 38:293, 1984.
45. Wimar K, Curran U, Forsum L, Klareskug V, Malmnas-Tjernlund L, Rask L, Tragarsh L, Peterson PA: Occurrence of Ia antigens on tissues in normal human nonlymphoid origin. *Nature* 276:711, 1978.
46. Selley WJ, Paulten LW, Hobbs S, Jewell DP: Expression of HLA-DR antigens by

colonic epithelial cells in inflammatory bowel disease. *Clin Exp Immunol* 44:453, 1981.

47. Geppert TD, Lipsky PE: Antigen presentation by interferon gamma treated endothelial cells and fibroblasts: differential ability to function as antigen presenting cells despite comparable Ia expression. *J Immunol* 135:3750, 1985.
48. Van der Oord JJ, Denset VJ: Destruction patterns of major histocompatibility antigens in normal and diseased liver. *Lehe, Mager, Dam* 14:244–254, 1985.
49. DeVas R, DeWolf-Peetyers C, Van der Oord JJ, Desmet VJ: Ultrastructured immunohistochemical demonstration of HLA class I antigens in human pathological liver tissue. *Hepatology* 5:1071–1075, 1985.
50. Thomas HC, Shiptor V, Montano C: The HLA system: its relevance to the pathogenesis of live disease. In Popper H, Schaffner, F: *Progress in Liver Disease,* 7th ed, pp 517–527, Orlando, FL, Grune & Stratton, 1982.
51. Loveland B, Simpson E: The non-MHC transplantation antigens: neither weak nor minor. *Immunol Today* 7:223–229.
52. Graff RJ, Baily AW: The non-H-2 histocompatibility loci and three antigens. *Transplant Rev* 15:26, 1973.
53. Rooperian DC, Orosz C, Bach FH: Responses against single minor histocompatibility antigens. I. Functional immunogenetic analysis of cloned cytolytic T cells. *J Immunol* 131:2135–2140, 1983.
54. Rooperian DC, Widne MN, Orosz C, Bach F: Responses against single minor histocompatibility antigens II. Analysis of cloned helper T cell. *J Immunol* 132:1080–1084, 1984.
55. Tekolf WA, Shaw S: Primary in vitro generation of cytotoxic cells specific for human minor histocompatibility antigens between HLA-identified siblings. *J Immunol* 132:1756–1760, 1984.
56. Czitron AA, Gascoigne NR, Edwards S, Waterfield AJ: Introduction of minor alloantigen-specific T cell subsets in vivo: recognition of processed antigen by helper not by cytotoxic T cell precursors. *J Immunol* 133:33–39, 1984.
57. Oriol R: Tissular expression of ABH and Lewis antigens in humans and animals. Expected value of different anemic models in the study of ABO incompatible organ transplants. *Transplant Proc* 19:4416, 1987.
58. Szulman AE: The histologic distribution of the blood group substances in man as disclosed by immunofluorescence. II. The H antigen and its relation to A and B antigens. *J Exp Med* 115:977–996, 1962.
59. Paul LC, Baldwin WM, Von Es LA: Vascularendothelial alloantigens in renal transplantation. *Transplantation* 40:117, 1985.
60. Chen HD, Raab S, Silvers WK: Influence of major-histocompatibility-complex-compatible and incompatible Langerhan's cells on the survival of H-Y incompatible skin grafts in rats. *Transplantation* 40:194, 1985.
61. Auchincloss H, Sacks AH: Transplantation and graft rejection In Paul WE: *Fundamental Immunology,* p 809, New York, Raven Press, 1989.
62. Lowry RP, Gurley KE, Forbes RDC: Immune mechanisms in organ allograft rejection: T cell delayed-type hypersensitivity and lymphotoxicity in heart graft rejection. *Transplantation* 36:391–401, 1983.
63. Mizuochi T, Omo S, Malek TR, Singh A: Characterization of two distinct primary T cell populations that secrete interleukin 2 upon recognition of class I or class II major histocompatibility antigens. *J Exp Med* 163:603–619, 1986.
64. Mizuochi T, Golding H, Rosenberg AS, Glimicher L, Malek TR, Singh A: Both

L3T4$^+$ and Lyt-2$^+$ helper T cells initiate cytotoxic T lymphocyte responses against allogenic major histocompatibility antigens but not against trinitrophenyl-modified self. *J Exp Med* 162:427–443.

65. Spent J, Schaefer M: Properties of purified T cell subsets. I. In vitro responses to class I and class II H-2 alloantigens. *J Exp Med* 162:2060–2080, 1985.

66. Mizouchi T, Minitz TI, McCarthy S, Andryplak PM, Kung J, Gress RA, Singh A: Differential helper and effector responses of Lyt-2 T cells to H-2 Kb mutant (Kbm) determinants and the appearance of thymic influence on antiKbm CTL responsiveness. *J Immunol* 137:2740–2747, 1986.

67. Golding H, Mizouchi T, McCarthy JA, Cleveland CA, Singh A: Relationship among function, phenotype and specificity in primary allospecific T cell populations. Identification of phenotypically identical but functionally distinct primary T cell subsets that differ in the recognition of MHC class I and MHC class II allodetermination. *J Immunol* 138:10–17, 1987.

68. Singh A, Munitz TI, Golding H, Rosenberg AS, Mizouchi T: Recognition requirements for the activation, differentiation and function of T helper cells specific for class I MHC alloantigens. *Immunol Rev* 98:143–170, 1987.

69. Zinkermagel RM, Daughterty PC: Restriction of in vitro T cell-mediated cytotoxicity in lymphocytic choriomeningitis within a synergeneic or semiallogeneic system. *Nature* 248:701–702, 1974.

70. Shearer GM, Rhen T, Garborium CA: Cell mediated lympholysis of trinitrophenyl-modified autologous lymphocytes. Effector cell specificity to modified cell surface components controlled by the H-2K and H-2D serological regions of the murine major histocompatibility complex. *J Exp Med* 141:1348–1364, 1975.

71. Swierkosz JE, Rock K, Manack P. Kapplen JW: The role of H-2 linked genes in helper T cell function. II. Isolation of antigen pulsed macrophages of two separate populations of F_1 helper T cells each specific for antigen and one set of parental H-2 products. *J Exp Med* 147:554, 1978.

72. Singh AS, Hathcock KS, Hodes RJ: Cellular and genetic control of antibody response V. helper T cell recognition of H-2 determinant or accessory cells but not B cells. *J Exp Med* 149:1208, 1979.

73. Cerrattini JC, Brunner KT: Cell mediated cytotoxicity allo-graft rejection and tumor immunity. *Adv Immunol* 18:67, 1974.

74. Loveland BE, Hogarth PM, Ceredig R, McKenzie IFC: Cells mediating graft rejection in the mouse. I. Lyt-1 cells mediate skin graft rejection. *J Exp Med* 153:1044–1057, 1981.

75. Tyler JD, Galli SJ, Snider ME, Dworski AM, Steinmiller D: Cloned Lyt-2 cytolytic T lymphocytes destroy allogeneic tissue in vivo. *J Exp Med* 149:57–67, 1984.

76. LeFrancais L, Berson MJ: A rexamination of the role of Lyt-2 positive T cells in murine skin graft rejection. *J Exp Med* 159:57–67, 1984.

77. Mason DW, Morris PJ: Effective mechanisms of allograft rejection. *Ann Rev Immunol* 4:119–145, 1986.

78. Thomas FT, Thomas JM, Ganghoff O, Gross V: Mechanisms of cell-mediated rejection in kidney, GM Williams, JF Burdick, K Solley: *Transplant Rejection*, pp 29–54, New York: Marcel Dekker, 1985.

79. Mizel SB: The interleukins. *FASEB J* 3:2379, 1989.

80. Burman KD, Baker JR: Immune mechanisms in Grave's disease. *Endocr Rev* 6:183, 1985.

81. Leung DYM, Siegel RL, Grady S, Krensky A, Meade R, Reinerz EL, Geha R: Immu-

noloregulatory abnormalities in Kawasaki disease. *Clin Immunol Immunopathol* 23:100–112, 1982.

82. Burman DK, Baker JR: Immune mechanisms in Grave's disease. *Endocrinol Rev* 6:183–355, 1984.
83. Gordon RD, Fung JJ, Markas B, Fax I, Iwatsuki S, Esquirel CO, Tzakis A, Todo S, Starzl T: The antibody crossmatched in liver transplanation. *Surgery* 100:707–715, 1986.
84. Gordon RD, Iwatsuki S, Esquivel CO, Tzakis A, Todo S, Starzl TE: Liver transplantation across ABO blood groups. *Surgery* 100:342–348, 1986.
85. Ramsey G, Nusbacher J, Starzl TE, Linsay GD: Isohemagglutinin of graft origin after ABO-unmatched liver transplantation. *New Engl J Med* 311:1167–1170, 1984.
86. Burdich JF, Vogelsang GB, Smith WJ: Severe graft-versus-host disease in a liver transplantation recipient. *New Engl J Med* 318:689–691, 1988.
87. Calne RY, Davis RD, Pena JR, et al: Hepatic allograft and xenografts in primates. *Br J Med* 1:103, 1967.
88. Cordier C, Garnier H, Clat JP, et al. La Greffe de foie orthopique chez le parc; premier resultats. *Mem Acad Chim* 92:27, 1966.
89. Calne RY, White HJO, Yaffa DE et al: Prolonged survival of liver transplants in the pig. *Br Med J* 4:645, 1967.
90. Zimmerman FA, Butcher GW, Davies HS, Brons G, Kamada N, Turel O: Techniques of orthotopic liver transplantation in the rat and some studies of the immunologic responses to fully allogeneic liver grafts. *Transplant Proc* 11:571, 1979.
91. Kamada N, Brons G, Davis HffS: Fully allogeneic liver grafting in rats induces a state of systemic nonreactivity to donor transplantation antigens. *Transplantation* 29:429, 1980.
92. Haussin D, Gigou M, Franco D, Bismuth H: Specific transplantation tolerance induced by spontaneously tolerated liver grafts in inbred strains of rats. *Transplantation* 29:418, 1980.
93. Myburgh JA, Smith CA, Mieny CJ, Mason A: Hepatic-allotransplantation in the baboon: III. The effects of immunosuppression and administration of donor specific antigens after transplantation. *Transplantation* 12:202, 1971.
94. Moore FD, Smith LL, Burnoys TK, et al: One stage homotransplantation of the liver following total hepatectomy in dogs. *Transplantation* 6:103, 1959.
95. Zimmerman FA, Butcher GW, Davies HffS, et al: Techniques for orthotopic liver transplantation and some studies of the immunologic responses to fully allogeneic grafts. *Transplant Proc* 11:571, 1979.
96. Kamada N, Davies HffS, Rosner BJ: Fully allogeneic liver grafting and the induction of donor specific unreactivity. *Transplant Proc* 13:837, 1981.
97. Kamada N, Brons, Davies HffS: Fully allogeneic liver grafting in rats induces a state of systemic nonreactivity to donor transplantation antigens. *Transplantation* 29:429, 1980.
98. Kamada N, Davis HffS, Rosner BJ: Reversal of transplantation immunity by liver grafting. *Nature* 292:840, 1981.
99. Davis HffS, Kamada N, Rosner BJ: Mechanisms of donor-specific unresponsiveness induced by liver grafting. *Transplant Proc* 15:831–835, 1981.
100. Kamada N, Brons G, Davies HffS: Fully allogeneic liver grafting in rats induces a state of systemic nonreactivity to donor transplantation antigens. *Transplantation* 29:429–431, 1979.
101. Russel PS: Some immunological considerations in liver transplantation. *Hepatology* 4:76S–78S, 1984.

102. Penn I: The occurrence of malignant tumors in immunosuppressed states. *Prog Allergy* 37:259, 1986.

103. Schein PS, Winokur Sh: Immunosuppressive and cytotoxic chemotherapy: long term complications. *Ann Int Med* 82:84, 1975.

104. Fahey JL, Sarna G, Gale RP et al: Immune interventions in disease, *Ann Int Med* 106:257, 1987.

105. Claman NH: Glucocorticosteroids I. Anti-inflammatory mechanisms II. The clinical response. *Hosp Prac* 18:123–143, 1983.

106. Cupps TR, Fauci AS: Corticosteroid-mediated immunoregulation in man. *Immunol Rev* 65:133, 1982.

107. Meuleman J, Katz P: The immunologic effects, kinetics and use of glucosteroids. *Med Clin N Am* 69:805, 1985.

108. Parrillo JE, Fauci AS: Mechanisms of glucocorticoid action on immune processes. *Ann Rev Pharmacol Toxicol* 19:179, 1979.

109. Zweiman B, Atkins PC, Bedard PM: Corticosteroid effects on circulating lymphocyte levels in normal humans. *J Clin Immunol* 4:141, 1984.

110. Posey WC, Nelson HS, Pearlman DS: The effects of acute corticosteroid therapy for asthma on serum immunoglobulin levels. *J Allergy Clin Immunol* 62:340–348, 1978.

111. Settipane GA, Pudupaakkan RK, McGavan JH: Corticosteroid effect on immunoglobulins. *J Allergy Clin Immunol* 62:162–166, 1978.

112. Sartorelli AC, Johns DC, (eds): *Antineoplastic and Immunosuppressive Agents*, Berlin, Springer-Verlag, 1975.

113. Chabner BA, Collins JM (eds): *Cancer Chemotherapy*, Philadelphia, Lippincott, 1990.

114. Handschumacher RE: In Gilman A, Rull T, Nies AS, Taylor P: *Goodman and Gilman's Pharmacologic Basis of Therapeutics*, New York, Pergamon Press, 1990.

115. Penn I: Cancer is a complication of severe immunosuppression. *Surg Gynecol Obstet* 162:603–616, 1986.

116. Calabresi PA, Chabner BA: In Gilman A, Rull T, Nies AS, Taylor P: *Goodman and Gilman's Pharmacological Basis of Therpeutics*. New York, Pergamon Press, 1990.

117. Calabresi PA, Schein PS, Rosenberg SA: *Medical Oncology*. New York, Macmillan, 1985.

118. Chabner BA (ed): *Pharmacological Principles of Cancer Chemotherapy*, Philadelphia, Saunders, 1982.

119. Chabner BA, Allegra CJ, Curt GA, Clenderium NJ, Baran J, Kaizumi S, Drake JC, Jolinet J: Polyglutamation of methotrexate. Is methotrexate a prodrug? *J Clin Invest* 76:907–912, 1985.

120. Wheeler GP: Some biochemical effects of alkylating agents. *Fed Proc* 26:885–892, 1967.

121. Mitchell MS, Fahey JL (eds): *Immune Suppression and Modulation*, Vol 4 of *Clinics in Immunology and Allergy*, Philadelphia, Saunders, 1984.

122. Calne RW: The initial study of the immunosuppressive effects of 6-mercaptopurine and azathioprine in organ transplantation and a few words on cyclosporine. *J Surg* 4:637–640, 1982.

123. Spreafico F, Tagliabue A, Vecchi A: In Sirais CP, Rola-Plesczynski R: *Chemical Immunodepressants in Immunopharmocology* Amsterdam, Elsevier, 1982.

124. Braun DP, Harris JE: Modulation of the immune response by chemotherapy. *Pharmacol Therap* 14:89–122, 1981.

125. Winkelstein A: Immunosuppressive Therapy in Terr A, Stites D: *Immunology*, Norwalk, CT, Appleton-Lange, 1990.

126. Winkelstein A: Differential effect of immunosuppressives on lymphocyte function. *J Clin Investigation* 53:2293–2299, 1983.

127. Berenbaum MC: Time-dependent and selectivity of immunosuppressive agents. *Immunology* 36:355–365, 1979.

128. Ahmed AR, Hombal SM: Cyclophosphamide (cytoxan). *J Am Acad Dermatol* 11:1115, 1984.

129. Turk JL, Parker D: Effect of cyclophosphamide on immunological control mechanisms. *Immunol Rev* 65:99, 1982.

130. Scherbaum I, Ambrosius H: Comparative investigations of quantitative determinations of cell mediated immunity by skin test, macrophage migration inhibition assay and lymphocyte transformation test in guenea pigs. *Allergy Immunol* 24:278–286, 1979.

131. Cupps TR, Edgar LC, Fauci AS: Suppression of human B lymphocytes by cyclophosphamide. *J Immunol* 128:2453, 1982.

132. Oger JJ-F, Antel JP, Kuo HH, Aranson HGK: Influence of azathioprine on in vitro immune function in multiple sclerosis. *Ann Neurol* 111:177–181, 1977.

133. Elion GB, Hitchings GH: Metabolic basis for the actions of analogs of purines and pyrimidines. *Adv Chemother* 2:91–177, 1965.

134. Elion GB: Biochemistry and pharmacology of purine analogs. *Fed Proc* 26:898–904, 1967.

135. Carrico CK, Sartorelli AC: Effects of 6-thioguanine on mqacromolecular events in the regenerating rat liver. *Cancer Res* 37:1868–1875, 1977.

136. McCormick JJ, Sartorelli AC: Purine antimetabolites. In Chabner BA: Pharmacologic Principles of Cancer Treatment, Philadelphia, Saunders, pp 213–228, 1982.

137. Elion GB, Hitchings GH: Azathioprine. In Sartorelli AC, Johns DC: *Antineoplastic and Immunosuppressive Agents, Handbook der Experimentellem Pharmakalolgie*, Vol 38, pp 403–525, Berlin, Springer-Verlag, 1975.

138. Moreau JF, Ythier A, Soulillau JP: Natural killer activity in kidney allograft recipients *Transplant Proc* 13:1610–1613, 1981.

139. Najarian JS, Sutherland DER, Simmons RL, et aL: Ten year experience with renal transplantation in juvenile onset diabetes *Ann Surg* 190:487–500, 1979.

140. Wolberg G: Antipurines and purine metabolism In Bray MA, Morley J: *The Pharmacology of Lymhocytes, Handbook of Experimental Pharmacology*, Vol 85, pp 517–533, Berlin, Springer-Verlag, 1980.

141. Hengst JCD, Kempf T: Immunomodulation by cyclophosphamide. In *Immune Suppression and Modulation Clinics in Immunology and Allergy*, Philadelphia, Saunders, 1983.

142. Colvin M: The alkylating agents. In Chabner BA: *Pharmacological Principles of Cancer Treatment*, Philadelphia, Saunders, 1982.

143. Ludlum DB, Tony WP: DNA modification by the nitrosoureas: chemical nature and cellular repair In Muggia EM, Nishoff M: *Cancer Chemotherapy*, Vol II, pp 141–154, Boston, Martinus Nijhoff, 1985.

144. Wheeler G, Alexander TA: The effects of nitrogen mustard and cyclophosphamide upon the synthesis of DNA in vivo and in cell free preparations. *Cancer Res* 29:98–109, 1969.

145. Turk JL, Paulter A: Selective depletion of lymphoid tissue by cyclophosphamide. *Clin Exp Immunol* 10:285–295, 1972.

146. Trompeter BS, Evans Pr, Barratt TM: Gonodal function in boys with steroid resistant nephrotic syndrome treated with cyclophosphamide. *Lancet* 1:1177–1179, 1981.
147. Kahn MF, Arlet J, Bloch-Michel H: Leucemies aigues apres traitment par agents cytotoxiques en rheumatologie 19 observations chez 2006 patients. *Nouv Presse Med* 8:1393–1937, 1979.
148. Weinstein GD: Methotrexate. *Ann Int Med* 86:199–204, 1977.
149. Skipper HT, Schnobel FM: Quantitative and cytokinetic studies in experimental tumor models. In Holland JF, Frei E: *Cancer Medicine,* 2d ed, pp 663–684, Philadelphia, Lea & Febiger, 1982.
150. Tugwell P, Bennett K, Gent M: Methotrexate in rheumatoid arthritis. *Ann Int Med* 107:358–366, 1987.
151. Roenigh HH, Auerbach R, Maibach HI, Weinstein GD: Methotrexate in psoriasis: revised guidelines. *J Am Acad Dermatol* 19:145–156, 1988.
152. Borel JF, Feurer C, Gubler HU, Stahelin G: Biological effects of cyclosporin A: a new antilymphocyte agent. *Agents Actions* 6:468–475, 1976.
153. Tosato G, Pike SE, Koski IR, Blease RM: Selective inhibition of immunoregulatory cell functions by cyclosporin *A. J Immunol* 128:1986–1991, 1982.
154. Wang, BS, Heacock EH, Collins KH, Hutchinson IF, Tilney NL, Mannich SA: Suppressive effects of cyclosporin A on the induction of alloreactivity in vitro and in vivo. *J Immunol* 127:89–93, 1981.
155. Hess AD, Tutschka PJ: Effect of cyclosporin on human lymphocyte response in vitro: I. CsA allows for the expression of alloantigens-activated suppressor cells while preferentially inhibiting the induction of cytotoxic effector lymphocytes in MLR. *J Immunol* 124:2601–2626.
156. Hess AD, Tutschka PJ Santos GW: Effect of cyclosporin A on human lymphocyte responses in vitro: III. CsA inhibits the production of T lymphocytes growth factors in secondary mixed lymphocyte reactions but does not inhibit the response of primed lymphocytes to TCGF. *J Immunol* 128:355–359, 1982.
157. Hess AD, Tutschka PJ, Pu Z, Santos GW: Effect of cyclosporin A on human lymphocyte responses in vitro IV. Production of T cell stimulatory growth factors and development of responsiveness to the growth factor in CsA-treated primary MLR cultures. *J Immunol* 128:360–367, 1982.
158. Orosz CG, Fidelius RF, Rooperian DC, Widmer MB, Ferguson RM, Bach FH: Analysis of cloned T cell function I: Dissection of cloned T cell proliferation responses using cyclosporin A. *J Immunol* 129:1865–1868.
159. Orosz CG, Rooperian DC, Widmer MB, Ferguson RM, Bod FH: Analysis of cloned T cell function by cyclosporine. *Transplantation* 36:706–711, 1983.
160. Wang BS, Heacock EH, Zheng CX, Tilney NL, Mannick JA: Restoration of allogeneic responsiveness to lymphocytes from cyclosporin A treated animals with interleukin-2. *Transplantation* 33:454–456, 1982.
161. Wang BS, Zheng CX, Heacock EH, Tilney NL, Strom TB, Mannick JA: Inhibition of the production of a soluble helper mediator by cyclosporine A results in the failure to generate alloreactive cells in mixed lymphocyte culture. *Clin Immunol Immunopathol* 27:160–169, 1983.
162. Abb J, Abb H, Dunhardt F: Effect of cyclosporine on the production of interferon by human peripheral blood lymphocytes in vitro. *Antiviral Res* 2:361–367, 1982.
163. Reim GH, Coch LA, Vilech J: Gamma interferon synthesis by human thymocytes and T lymphocytes inhibited by cyclosporine A. *Science* 221:63–65, 1983.
164. Hess AD, Tutschka PJ, Santos GW: Effect of cyclosporine A on human lymphocyte responses in vitro II. Induction of specific alloantigens unresponsiveness mediated by nylon wool adherent suppressor cells. *J Immunol* 126:961–968, 1981.

165. Bunges D, Hardt C, Rollinghof M, Wagner H: Cyclosporine mediates immunosuppression of primary cytotoxic T cell responses by impairing the release of IL-1 and IL-2. *Eur J Immunol* 11:657–661, 1981.

166. Miyawaki T, Yachie A, Ohzeki S, Nagaki T, Taniguchi N: Cyclosporine A does not prevent expression of Tac antigen, a probable TCGK receptor molecule, on mitogen stimulated human T cells. *J Immunol* 130:2737–2742, 1983.

167. Kunkl A, Klaus GG: Selective effects of cyclosporine A on functional B cell subsets. *J Immunol* 125:2526–2532, 1980.

168. Paavonen T, Hayry A. Effect of cyclosporine A on T-dependent and T-independent immunoglobulin synthesis in vitro. *Nature* 287:542–544, 1982.

169. Muraguchi A, Bulter L, Kehrl JHG, Falhoff RJ, Fauci AS: Selective suppression of an early step in human B cell activation by cyclosporine A. *J Exp Med* 158:690–702, 1983.

170. Larsson EL. Cyclosporine A and dexamethasone suppress T cell responses by selectively acting at distinct sites in the triggering process. *J Immunol* 124:2828–2833, 1980.

171. Thomson AW, Whiting PH, Cameron ID, Lessels SE, Simpson JG: A toxicological study in rats receiving immunotherapeutic doses of cyclosporine A. *Transplantation* 31:121–124, 1981.

172. Gordon MH, Singh JW: Selective effects of cyclosporine on colony forming lymphoid and myeloid cells in man. *Nature* 279:433–434, 1979.

173. Berger R, Majdic O, Meingassne JG, Knapp W: In vitro effects of cyclosporine A (CsA) on human hematopoetic cell lines. *Immunopharmacology* 5:123–127, 1982.

174. Kellman A, Goldman JM: Effects of cyclosporine A on human granulopoiesis in vitro. *Transplantation* 30:386–387, 1980.

175. Felchner SM, Van Buren ME, Kerman RH, Kahan BD: The nephrotoxicity of cyclosporine in renal transplant recipients. *Transplant Proc* 15:2689–2694, 1983.

176. Devineni R, McKenzie J, Duplan J, Keown P, Stillen C, Wallace AC: Renal effects of cyclosporine: clinical and experimental observations. *Translant Proc* 15:2695–2698, 1983.

176. Powell-Jackson PR, Young B, Calne RY, Williams R: Nephrotoxicity of parenterally administered cyclosporine after orthotopic liver transplantation. *Transplantation* 36:505–508, 1983.

178. Klintmalin GB, Iwatsuki K, Starzl TE: Nephrotoxicity of cyclosporine A in liver and kidney transplantation patients. *Lancet* 1:470–471, 1981.

179. Simonton SC, Rynasiewicz J, Sibley RK: Light and electron microscopic features of experimental cyclosporine A nephrotoxicity. *Lab Invest* 43:78A–79A, 1983.

180. Flechner SM, Van Buren CT, Kerman R, Kahan BP: The effect of conversion from cyclosporine to azathioprine immunosuppression for intractable nephrotoxicity. *Transplant Proc* 15:2869–2873, 1983.

181. Canafax DM, Sutherland DE, Ascher NL, et al: Cyclosporine nephrotoxicity in renal allograft recipients: conversion to azathioprine to improve renal function. *Transplant Proc* 15:2874–2877, 1983.

182. Klintmalm G, Ringden O, Groth CG: Clinical and laboratory signs in nephrotoxicity and rejection in cyclosporine-treated renal allograft recipients. *Transplant Proc* 15:2815–2820, 1983.

183. Klintmalm GB, Iwatsuki S, Starzl TE: Cyclosporine A hepatotoxicity in 66 renal allograft recipients. *Transplantation* 32:488–489, 1981.

184. Rodgers RS, Turney JH, Haines I, Michael J, Adu D, McMaster P: Cyclosporine and liver function in renal allograft recipients. *Transplant Proc* 15:2754–2756, 1983.

185. Schade RR, Gugliemi A, Thgiel DH, et al. Cholestasus in heart transplant recipients treated with cyclosporine. *Transplant Proc* 15:2757–2760, 1983.

186. Atkinson K, Biggs J, Dodds A, Concannon A: Cyclosporine associated hepatotoxicity after allogeneic bone marrow transplantation in man: differentiation from other causes of post-transplant liver disease. *Transplant Proc* 15:2761–2767, 1983.

187. Loertschler R, Thiel G, Harder F, Brunner FP: Persistent elevation of alkaline phosphatase in cyclosporine A treated renal transplantation recipients. *Transplantation* 36:115–116, 1983.

188. Thiu S, Calne RY, Naginton J: Lymphoma in renal allograft patients treated with cyclosporine A as one of the immunosuppressive agents. *Transplant Proc* 13:359–364, 1981.

189. Rosenthal JT, Iwatsuki S, Starzl TE, Taylor RJ, Hakala TR: Histiocytic lymphoma in renal transplant patients receiving cyclosporine. *Transplant Proc* 15:2805–2807, 1983.

190. Beveridge T, Krupps P, McKibbin C: Lymphoma and lymphoproliferative lesions developing under cyclosporine therapy [Letter]. *Lancet* 7:788, 1984.

191. Penn I: Malignancies following use of cyclosporine A in man. *Cancer Surv* 1:621–624, 1982.

192. Joss DV, Barrett AJ, Kendra JR, Lucas CF, Desai S: Hypertension and convulsions in children receiving cyclosporine A. *Lancet* 2:829–830, 1982.

193. Durrant S, Chipping PM, Palmer S, Gordon-Smith EC: Cyclosporine A, methylprednisolone and convulsions [Letter]. *Lancet* 2:829–830, 1982.

194. Kino T, Katanaka H, Migata S, et al: FK506, a novel immunosuppressant isolated from Streptomyces. *J Antibiot (Tokyo)* 40:1256, 1987.

195. Sawada S, Suzuki G, Kawase Y, et al: Novel immunosuppressive agents FK506: in vitro effects on cloned T cell lines. *J Immunol* 139:1797, 1987.

196. Zeevi A, Duquesnoy R, Eiras G, et al: Immunosuppressive effect of FK506, *Transplant Proc* 19:40, 1987.

197. Ochiai T, Nakajima K, Kino T, et al: Studies of the induction and maintainance of long term acceptance by treatment with FK506 in heterotropic cardiac allotransplantation in rats. *Transplantation* 44:734, 1987.

198. Morris RE, Hoyt EG, Murphy MP, Shorthouse R: Immunopharmacology of FK506. *Transplant Proc* 21:1042–1044, 1989.

199. Thomson AW, Woo SJ, Nason NU, Whiting PH: Immunosuppressive activity T cell subsets, analysis and acute toxicity of FK506 in rats. *Transplant Proc* 21:1048–1049, 1989.

200. Tocci MJ, Matkovitch DA, Collins KA: FK506 selectively inhibits expression of early T cell activation genes. *J Immunol* 143:718, 1989.

201. Yoshimura N, Matsui S, Hamashima T: Effect of a new immunosuppressive agent FK506 on human lymphocyte responses in vitro. Inhibition of IL-2 and gamma interferon but not B cell stimulating factor 2. *Transplantation* 47:34, 1989.

202. Sawada S, Suzuki G, Kawase Y, Takaku F: A novel immunosuppressive agent FK506. *J Immunol* 139:1797, 1987.

203. Zeevi A, Duquesnoy R, Eiras E et al: *Surg Res Commun* 1:315, 1987.

204. Takagishi K, Yamamoto M, Nishimira A, Yamasaki G, Kanazawa N, Hotokebuchi T, Kaibara N: Effects of FK506 on collagen arthritis in mice. *Transplant Proc* 21:1053–1055, 1989.

205. Yashimura N, Matsui S, Hamashima T, Lee CJ, Oka T: A new immunosuppressive agent FK506 inhibits the expression of alloantigen activated suppressor cells as well as the induction of alloreactivity. *Transplantation* 21:1047–1047.

206. Keicho N, Sawada S, Kitamura K, Yotsumato H, Takaku F: Effects of an immunosuppressant, FK506, on interleukin 1a production by human macrophages and a macrophage like line U-937. *Cellular Immunol* 1332:285–294, 1991.

207. Murase N, Kim DG, Todo S, Cramer DV, Fung J, Starzl TE: FK506 suppression of heart and liver allograft rejection. *Transplantation* 50:739–744, 1990.

208. Inagaki K, Fukuda Y, Sumimoto K, Matsuno K, Ito H, Takahashi M, Dahi K. Effect of FK506 and 15-deoxyspergualin in rat orthotopic liver transplantation. *Transplant Proc* 21:1069–1071.

209. Tsuchimoto S, Kusumoto K, Nakajima Y, Kahita A, Uchimo J, Natori T, Aizawa M: Orthotopic liver transplantation in rats receiving FK506. *Transplant Proc* 21:1064–1065, 1989.

210. Todo S, Podesta L, Chapchap P, et al: Orthotopic liver transplantation in dogs receiving FK506. *Transplant Proc* 19:64 (Suppl), 1987.

211. Ochiai T, Nagata M, Nakajima S, et al: Studies of the effects of FK506 on renal transplantation in beagle dogs. *Transplantation* 44:729, 1987.

212. Todo S, Ueda Y, Demetris AJ, et al: Immune suppression of canine, monkey and baboon allografts by FK506 with special reference to synergism with other drugs and tolerance induction. *Surgery* 104:239, 1988.

213. Starzl TE, Fung J, Jordan M, et al: Kidney transplantation under FK506. *JAMA* 264:63, 1990.

214. Reyes J, Gayawski T, Fung J, Todo S, Alessiani M, Starzl TE: Expressive dysphasia possibly related to FK506 in two liver transplantation recipients. *Transplantation* 50:1043–1044, 1990.

215. Shapiro R, Fung JJ, Jain A: The side effects of FK506 in humans. *Transplant Proc* 22:35, 1990.

216. Starzl TE, Todo S, Fung J: FK506 for liver, kidney and pancreaus transplantation. *Lancet* 2:1000, 1989.

217. Stephen M, Woo J, Hanson NU, Whiting PH, Thomson AW: Immunosuppressive activity, lymphocyte subset analysis and acute toxicity of FK506 in rats. *Transplantation* 47:60–65, 1989.

218. Murase N, Todo S, Lee PH: Heterotopic heart transplantation in the rat receiving FK506 alone or with cyclosporine. *Transplant Proc* 19:71, 1987.

219. Heyworth MF: Clinical experience with anti-lymphocyte serum. *Immunol Rev* 65:79, 1982.

220. Agnew HD: The effect of heterologous anti-lymphocyte serum on the small lymphocyte populations of rats. *J Exp Med* 128:111, 1968.

221. Cosimi AB: Clinical development of orthoclone OKT3. *Transplant Proc* 19:1, 1987.

222. Goldstein G: Overview of the development of orthoclone OKT3: Monoclonal antibody for therapeutic use in transplantation. *Transplant Proc* 19 (Suppl):1, 1987.

223. Ortho Multicenter Transplant Study Group: A randomized clinical trial of OKT3 monoclonal antibody for acute rejection of cadavaric renal transplant *New Engl J Med* 313:337, 1985.

224. Kirkman Rl, Barrett LV, Gaulton GN, et al: Administration of an anti-interleukin-2 receptor monoclonal antibody prolongs cardiac allograft survival in mice. *J Exp Med* 162:358–362, 1985.

225. Junghans RP, Waldman TA, Landotti NF, et al. Anti-Tac-H, a humanized antibody to the interleukin 2 receptor with new features for immunotherapy in malignant and immune disorders. *Cancer Res* 50:1495–1502, 1990.

— 6 —

LIVER TRANSPLANTATION: SELECTION OF PATIENTS FOR REFERRAL

Thomas L. Fabry and Franklin M. Klion

The goal of liver transplantation is to extend life expectancy or at least improve quality of life. Therefore, candidates for transplantation are patients whose prognosis is so poor that transplantation, even with its associated risk factors, will improve survival and quality of life. With critical selection of recipients, improved surgical techniques and advances in immunosuppression one-year survival rates exceed 80%.[1] The prospect of long-term survival for these patients is excellent.[2] Technical factors and surgical skills have become uniform among various institutions; therefore individual success rates primarily depend on appropriate selection of patients[3,4] and the correct timing of liver transplantation.

Survival is also based on the type and severity of the liver disease. Although the severity of chronic, far-advanced liver disease is difficult to evaluate, cholestatic liver disease is usually associated with a lower surgical risk than hepatocellular disease. On the other hand, survival from fulminant hepatic failure depends on other factors; therefore, selection for transplantation must be considered separately from chronic, end-stage liver disease.

Proper timing of referral for liver transplantation prevents premature surgical mortality in patients with stable end-stage liver disease and minimizes surgical risks for patients with far-advanced disease.[5,6] In this context, two aspects of risk factors should be considered: (1) whether transplant is the most appropriate treatment at this stage of the liver disease and (2) whether the psychological and other medical factors are such that the quality of life will be high and surgical risk low. Chapter 7 will cover exclusion of those patients whose risk factors outweigh potential gains.

The remainder of this chapter deals with the selection of patients for referral based on symptomatology and etiology of the liver disease. This evaluation is best done by the local physician before referral to the transplant center.

CHRONIC LIVER DISEASE

All patients with end-stage liver disease are potential candidates for orthotopic liver transplantation. Ideally patients should be identified before the onset of significant or multiple complications that signal the terminal stage. The selection of a liver transplant recipient depends on criteria based on multiple factors, such as the state of the liver disease, the patient's general medical, psychological condition, and age.

In addition to the clinical evaluation, deteriorating laboratory values, especially elevation of bilirubin and prothrombin time, signal acceleration of disease and urgent need for liver transplant. Referral of patients for liver transplantation ultimately depends on clinical judgment based on symptoms and laboratory tests.

Accumulating experience with the results of orthotopic liver transplantation has led to the development of general and disease specific criteria for indications as well as contraindications. Regional centers, like the New York Center for Liver Transplantation (NYCLT), are instruments in developing and re-evaluating standards for patient selection and quality assessment. These and related topics are discussed by Rogut and Rueger in Chapter 3.

When the patient is selected, ongoing care should be provided at the local level. Some input from the transplant center is needed, since acceptance for liver transplantation will significantly modify care. This is discussed in Chapter 10.

GENERAL CRITERIA FOR REFERRAL TO TRANSPLANT CENTER

Several algorithms and formulas have been developed, based on symptoms and laboratory values, to predict prognosis and help with the timing of liver transplantation. Most of these models relate to cholestatic liver disease, such as primary biliary cirrhosis[6,7] and sclerosing cholangitis,[8] which have a more prolonged and predictable course. The Mayo formula developed for primary biliary cirrhosis for example predicts the probability of survival based on age, bilirubin, albumin, prothrombin time, and fluid retention, without requiring the results of a liver biopsy.[7] None have proven to be satisfactory, because they are not predictive for the individual patient. In the absence of an accurate formula the physician must rely on other parameters. Table 6-1.

Complications such as ascites, variceal bleeding, fatigue, wasting, encephalopathy, and worsening laboratory tests of synthetic function reflect a rapidly

TABLE 6-1. General Criteria for Patient Selection

Refractory ascites
Uncontrolled variceal bleeding
Unmanageable encephalopathy
Wasting
Fatigue interfering with normal daily activities
Hypoxemia secondary to liver disease
Hepatorenal syndrome

deteriorating clinical state and are independent of etiology. The inability to manage these specific signs and symptoms with conventional treatment prompts consideration of liver transplantation.

Signs and Symptoms

Ascites

Ascites is not an indication itself for liver transplantation. The onset of ascites is a poor prognostic sign, even though appropriate medical treatment is frequently successful in controlling fluid retention. Diagnostic paracentesis should be performed in all patients who present with new onset ascites to exclude infection and neoplasia. A 1000 ml of ascitic fluid can safely be removed and is adequate for diagnostic purposes.

Ascites should be treated when it results in respiratory compromise or disabling fatigue from the increased work necessary to carry the large volume. The presence of an abdominal hernia is also an indication for treatment.

Dietary Management of Ascites: Salt and Water. The patient's daily fluid intake should be limited to 1000 mL (~32 oz). Further restriction may be necessary, but 750 mL is the practical limit. Salt intake must be carefully monitored and restricted to 500–750 mg of sodium. To achieve patient compliance we provide

TABLE 6-2. General Guidelines for Patient Compliance

NAME

1. Your maximum daily protein allowance is ____
2. Your total daily sodium allowance is ____
3. You may drink only____ oz, total liquids.

GENERAL RULES

1. No food is to be eaten unless found in food lists.
2. Total daily protein intake is to be divided into three equal portions.
   IMPORTANT: All portions should be accurately weighed at home or prepackaged by butcher. 1 oz = 7 gr protein.
3. No soups or carbonated beverages.
4. Do not add salt or salt substitutes.
5. Read all food labels carefully to determine protein and salt contents.

general guidelines (Table 6–2) and a list of allowed foods (Appendix D). Patients should keep a daily log of their weights to motivate and improve compliance.

Diuretic Use. When salt and fluid management alone is ineffective diuretic therapy is added.

Loop diuretics (furosemide, ethacrinic acid, bumetanide) are best suited for the patients with severe liver disease because they are least likely to cause elevation of renal vein ammonia, are short-acting, and are dose-dependent. Small, frequent, but inadequate doses that do not produce diuresis are inefficient and dangerous because they may cause hypokalemia and decreased renal perfusion. Therefore if diuresis is not achieved with the initial dose, dosage should be doubled stepwise until a 2–3-lb weight loss per day is achieved. Diuretics can be administered daily or on alternate-day regimens; multiple daily doses are never indicated. Spironolactone, an aldosterone antagonist, is useful to augment diuresis and prevent hypokalemia. Since the inhibition is competitive, large doses, up to 400 mg per day in divided doses may be necessary. Tender gynecomastia in men and nausea are infrequent side effects which necessitate the discontinuation of the drug.

In patients with normal renal function we start with furosemide 40 mg 3 times a week and 25–50 mg of spironolactone 4 times a day (qid). The dose of furosemide is doubled until adequate diuresis is achieved. Sodium, potassium, BUN, and creatinine levels should be monitored frequently. Hyponatremia frequently reflects non-compliance of fluid restriction. Hyperkalemia and deteriorating renal function necessitates reduction in diuretics and consideration of alternative treatments. Azotemia can also be secondary to infection or bleeding and should be dealt with appropriately. When the ascitic fluid is a simple transudate treatment with dietary management and diuretics is usually all that is necessary.

Therapeutic Paracentesis. In patients who are either refractory or intolerant of diuretic therapy, large-volume and repeated paracentesis is an alternative.[9] Up to 20 L per week can be safely removed. Concurrent administration 25–50 gm of serum albumin intravenously may prevent decreased renal function, hemodynamic instability, hyponatremia, and hyperkalemia.[10]

Peripheral edema has no protective effect against hyponatremia or renal insufficiency caused by paracentesis. Ascitic fluid is rich in protein and repeated paracentesis may result in further nutritional depletion therefore return of ascitic fluid into the vascular space may be desirable. This can be accomplished by the use of peritoneal–venous shunts.

Use of Peritoneal–Venous Shunts. Peritoneal–venous shunts enhance diuresis and may improve renal function and nutrition. Infection, bleeding, disseminated intravascular coagulation (DIC), and congestive heart failure are potential short-term complications. Long-standing shunts can complicate hepatic transplant surgery, because they become encased in fibrin and are difficult to remove without significant bleeding. Peritoneal–venous shunts are useful for the short-term management of refractory ascites with the expectation that transplantation will be performed in the near future.

Complications of Ascites. Spontaneous bacterial peritonitis (SBP) is an absolute short-term contraindication for orthotopic liver transplantation; however, after 5–10 days of effective antibiotic treatment transplantation can be performed. Currently, a third-generation cephalosporin is the treatment of choice, since gram-negative organism or mixed infections are frequent. Aminoglycoside use in a cirrhotic patient is associated with an increased incidence of renal failure and should be avoided. Since a single episode of SBP signals a poor prognosis, the patient should be referred for liver transplantation. Recurrent episodes of peritonitis require prompt transplantation.

An abdominal hernia in the presence of tense ascites is life-threatening because of possible rupture or infection. Medical or surgical control of ascites is indicated, followed by repair of the hernia. Unfortunately the surgery is associated with high morbidity and recurrence. Refractory ascites indicates deteriorating liver function and the need for liver transplantation.

Gastrointestinal Bleeding

Bleeding in far-advanced cirrhosis is life-threatening. Hypotension from blood loss results in extensive liver necrosis secondary to ischemia. The protein load resulting from the blood in the gastrointestinal tract usually precipitates encephalopathy, which further accelerates deterioration. Bleeding episodes frequently lead to the hepato-renal syndrome. Major sources of bleeding are varices, portal gastropathy, peptic ulcer, and occasionally hemorrhoids or rectal varices. An accurate endoscopic diagnosis is mandatory for appropriate treatment.

Peptic ulcer disease frequently complicates end-stage liver disease.[11] However, it is not an indication for selection or accelerated timing of liver transplantation. It should be treated with antiacid or H2 blocker therapy. Some clinicians prefer to use famotidine, because there are reports of hepatic dysfunction resulting from cimetidine or ranitidine use. The indications for endoscopic intervention of bleeding peptic ulcer in the cirrhotic patient are the same as in the general population. Invasive endoscopic treatment with heater probe, bicap, or injection is effective.

Portal gastropathy is a source of persistent, recurrent bleeding.[12] It can be managed with transfusions, but can be cured only by gastric resection[13] or laser treatment. If extensive gastric surgery is performed, there is an added risk to subsequent liver transplant. Transplantation with resolution of portal hypertension is also curative.

Esophageal variceal bleeding in an otherwise asymptomatic patient is not an indication for transplantation. Acute bleeding due to esophageal variceal hemorrhage can be controlled with sclerotherapy or rubber-band ligation. Variceal bleeding recurs frequently, especially early in the course of endoscopic treatment. Uncontrolled variceal bleeding after appropriate endoscopic treatment needs portal decompression. Surgically mesocaval or distal splenorenal shunts may be used to temporize awaiting a donor and will not complicate transplantation. Radiologically placed transjugular intrahepatic portosystemic shunt[13a] can be used as an alternative to surgical decompression. Because of the complications of bleeding, prophylactic pretransplant sclerotherapy has been advocated by some workers[14] who have shown a decrease in number of bleeding episodes and morbidity. Gastric varices, without an esophageal component are not amenable to sclerotherapy; they require either surgical decompression or transplantation.

Hemorrhoids are an infrequent source of bleeding, and we avoid surgical intervention, unless bleeding cannot be controlled.

Hepatocerebral Syndrome and Hepatic Encephalopathy

Encepalopathy and chronic hepatocerebral disorders have to be distinguished from organic disease and chronic neuropsychiatric disorders. The latter two will not improve after transplantation. Acute encephalopathy frequently is precipitated by hypokalemia, azotemia, or drugs with GABA (γ aminobutyric acid) agonist activity.[15] Once hypokalemia and/or azotemia has been corrected and encephalopathy still does not respond to a strict, protein-restricted diet, lactulose, and/or neomycin, liver transplantation is indicated. Chronic hepatocerebral disorders may also be reversed by transplantation.[16]

Similarly, patients who develop severe psychiatric impairment as a sequelae to their liver disease, must be distinguished from endogenous psychiatric disorders. In the absence of objective criteria, psychiatric illness as a sole indication for liver transplantation is controversial and consultation with an experienced psychiatrist familar with liver disease is imperative before referral (see the discussion in Chapter 8).

Hypoxemia

Portal hypertension can cause arterial desaturation resulting in severe pulmonary disability.[16a] The hepatopulmonary syndrome is caused by arterial desaturation either by A-V shunting or V-Q mismatch.[16b,c] If breathing 100% oxygen corrects the hypoxemia it is due to A-V shunting and will probably be corrected by transplantation.[17-19] If transplantation is not performed before the pulmonary disease becomes advanced, the surgical risk is very high and the patient may not survive the long (2–3 weeks) period before shunting is reversed.[20] Intrapulmonary shunting associated with PBC may be reversed by transplantation.[21,21a]

Patients with pulmonary hypertension are at high risk and evaluation, including lung biopsy, is necessary to exclude other potentially treatable lesions. Most of these patients will require combined liver and lung transplants.[22,23]

Fatigue

Overwhelming fatigue may force early retirement and may be severe enough to interfere with activities of daily living. Usually there are other symptoms to satisfy the criteria for transplantation, but occasionally fatigue is the only symptom of underlying liver disease. Under these circumstances a detailed psychiatric evaluation is required to be sure that other factors beside liver disease are not operative. This is best done by an experienced psychiatrist. The decision to transplant such a patient is difficult since objective criteria for outcome are lacking (see Chapter 8).

Wasting

Wasting occurs earlier in parenchymal liver disease and is a preterminal state in cholestatic disease. As life is prolonged with better control of bleeding, ascites, and infection, wasting is becoming a more frequent signal of terminal disease. However, wasting still is a seldom applied criterion for liver transplantation partly because of the lack of an objective measure. When wasting becomes extreme, transplantation is no longer feasible because of the increased operative and post-operative complications.

No index of malnutrition (albumin, prothrombin time, anergy, absolute lymphocyte count) has proven to be a prognostic factor for the success of the transplantation.[24] Our feeling is that patients with progressive malnutrition, even in the absence of other criteria should be referred for transplantation, since the severity of this problem usually is underestimated.

Laboratory Tests

Laboratory test results are not per se considered as criteria for selection of patients for transplantation, but are important to collaborate clinical judgment and to fine-tune timing for transplantation. Rising bilirubin, falling albumin and elevation of prothrombin time are all poor prognostic features of end-stage liver disease.

Bilirubin

Of all laboratory tests, elevated bilirubin (>10 mg%) appears to be the best indicator of very advanced liver disease and poor prognosis, especially in patients with cholestatic syndromes.[25]

Albumin and Prothrombin Time

Albumin values, measures by serum protein electrophoresis, and prothrombin time are good indicators of the synthetic function of the liver. Transient deterioration may be due to infection, bleeding, or decreased nutritional intake. Albumin levels <2.5 mg/dL and prothrombin time 5 sec over control, if not corrected by vitamin K, are characteristic of advanced hepatocellular injury. No improvement can be expected and early selection for transplantation is advisable.

Pancytopenia

Hypersplenism with pancytopenia is rarely symptomatic and need not be treated. Splenectomy is contraindicated, not only because it often elevates portal pressure but is an additional operative risk to hepatic transplantation. Hypersplenism should not influence the decision to transplant the patient. Orthotopic liver transplantation corrects this condition.[26]

Renal Function

Chronic, end-stage renal disease is not a contraindication to liver transplantation, provided simultaneous renal transplantation is feasible.[27] Kidney biopsy is sometimes necessary to distinguish functional renal failure secondary to liver disease (hepatorenal syndrome) from primary renal disease and predict the potential for the reversibility. Transient deterioration may be due to infection or bleeding. Hepatorenal syndrome, previously considered fatal, can be successfully treated with transplantation.[28-30]

DISEASE-SPECIFIC CRITERIA FOR REFERRAL TO THE TRANSPLANT CENTER

The general criteria discussed above for transplantation are often modified, depending on the etiology of the liver disease.

Cholestatic Liver Disease

Primary Biliary Cirrhosis

Probability of survival of a patient with primary biliary cirrhosis can be calculated from a formula developed by workers at the Mayo Clinic.[7] As formulated, it does not directly indicate the appropriate timing for transplantation; however, an abrupt change in the value of the risk factor calculated from this formula predicts a poor prognosis and supports a change in the management of the patient, i.e., liver transplantation.[31] As a rule of thumb,[25] if the bilirubin rises to >10 mg/dL, the disease is in its terminal stage and mortality can be expected within 2 years in the majority of the patients.

Osteoporosis is particularly severe in primary biliary cirrhosis.[32] If pain is unmanageable or vertebral collapse occurs, transplantation is indicated. Pretransplant (calcitonin and/or bisphosphonate) therapy should be considered. We discuss treatment in Chapter 14 pp 201–202.

Primary Sclerosing Cholangitis

Primary sclerosing cholangitis is an insidiously progressive disease, characterized by recurrent episodes of cholangitis, progressive jaundice, and in the late stages cirrhosis. Patients with primary sclerosing cholangitis form a clinically homogenous group irrespective of whether they have inflammatory bowel disease (including Crohn's disease). Most patients have involvement both of the intra- and extrahepatic biliary system. Intrahepatic duct destruction only (15% of cases) does not change the clinical course.[33] Since no effective treatment is available, most patients will require liver transplantation. Low-risk patients have a 95% surgical survival, opposed to patients in poor condition, where surgical mortality is high. Because of the predictable clinical course and favorable surgical prospects for patients transplanted while they are still in good condition, early referral for transplantation is indicated.[34,34a] Radical surgical procedures to correct biliary obstruction should be avoided, so subsequent transplantation is not compromised. Individual strictures may be balloon-dilated and stents placed for longer areas of narrowing. ERCP with brushing is mandatory to exclude cholangiocarcinoma, an infrequent and incurable complication of primary sclerosing cholangitis. Patients with universal ulcerative colitis are at high risk (5%) for primary sclerosing cholangitis.[35] Activity of ulcerative colitis does not affect the severity of the cholangitis and does not influence acceptance for transplantation. Liver transplantation takes precedence over colectomy for inflammatory bowel disease unless toxic dilatation, perforation, or other surgical emergency occurs. In our experience the control of colitis with immunosuppression post-transplant is facilitated.[35a]

Congenital Biliary Disease

The symptomatic form of congenital biliary disease, presenting in childhood, is a heterogenous group of conditions, called Alagille's syndrome (arteriohepatic dysplasia). They are characterized by hypoplastic intralobular bile ducts and a cholestatic syndrome. Cardiac abnormalities are common, and may be a contraindication to surgery.[36] Patients who reach adulthood may develop a severe cholestatic picture and hepatocellular carcinoma. In common with other cholestatic diseases, transplantation should be considered when jaundice is persistent and progressive, and there is evidence of hepatic decompensation manifested by ascites, encephalopathy, or both.

A nonsyndromatic form of congenital biliary disease has recently been described[37] in adults, which may progress to severe or even fatal liver failure. Since this disorder progresses so rapidly to death, transplantation should be considered as soon as the diagnosis is made.

Biliary atresia is discussed by Benkov and Rosch (Chapter 16).

Polycystic Liver Disease

Adult polycystic liver disease is a rare and usually asymptomatic disorder of the liver parenchyma. It usually presents with abdominal pain or swelling, without liver function compromise. Individual cysts of the liver can be resected, but unroofing of the cysts is not recommended, since many will continue to secrete fluid and lead to unmanageable ascites.[38,38a] The polycystic liver may grow to large size, but transplantation is indicated only when infection or malignant transformation intervenes.

Life expectancy may be shortened if kidney disease is present as well. In these cases morbidity and mortality are almost always due to the associated kidney disease. Combined hepatic and renal transplantation should be considered.

Parenchymal Liver Disease

Autoimmune Hepatitis

Chronic autoimmune hepatitis usually progresses to cirrhosis with or without steroid and/or immunosuppression therapy. Cirrhosis and chronic hepatitis occur independently of each other. Early in the course of the disease symptoms depend on the state of the chronic hepatitis, but ultimately the prognosis depends on the complications of cirrhosis. Steroid treatment is effective for symptoms of chronic hepatitis only. Cirrhosis may be present for long periods of time before becoming symptomatic.

The major causes of death in these patients are infection, variceal bleeding, and encephalopathy: these symptoms form the basis for selection of patients for transplantation. Laboratory values are not particularly useful, especially in patients on corticosteroid treatment.

Chronic Hepatitis B

Hepatitis and cirrhosis usually coexist. When the prognosis is poor, because of end-stage cirrhosis, management will depend on the activity of hepatitis B. Three groups of patients have to be distinguished:

1. Cirrhotic patients with hepatitis B surface antibody only.
2. Cirrhotic carriers, i.e., patients with positive surface antigen, but without active hepatitis or viral replication.
3. Patients with active hepatitis, i.e., when both the surface and e antigens are positive or hepatitis B virus DNA (HBV-DNA) is detectable in the serum, indicating ongoing viral replication.

With the exception of patients who are surface-antibody-positive (group 1), hepatitis B frequently recurs after transplantation because of residual virus remaining in mononuclear and other cells.[39] The prognosis is better when the e antigen is negative or the HBV-DNA titer is at low levels.[40,41] This high rate of recurrence results in increased short- and long-term mortality. At the present time no therapy has been proved effective to prevent recurrence. Clinical trials with alpha (α) interferon, active and passive immunization and newer antiviral agents must be continued,[42] and these patients should be transplanted only in controlled clinical trials. Transplantation should not be denied to patients with chronic B hepatitis and end-stage cirrhosis because in a significant number of cases hepatitis B does not recur.[43] Concomitant infection with hepatitis D virus decreases the severity of recurrent hepatitis B.[41]

Chronic Hepatitis C

Confirmation of infection with the hepatitis C virus is based on detection of the serum antibody to the virus and histologic examination of the liver. Currently available commercial tests [enzyme-linked immunoabsorbant assay (ELISA)] for serum antibody to hepatitis C virus may not become positive for 6 months after infection. Newer tests based on structural viral protein (RIBA II) are more specific. Polymerase chain reaction (PCR) is the most accurate and specific means for establishing the diagnosis and may indicate ongoing viral replication.

Approximately 50% of the patients with non-A, non-B hepatitis are positive for hepatitis C. Of the patients with suspect alcoholic liver disease, 30% are also positive for hepatitis C. Some of these patients have hepatitis C on liver biopsy.

Hepatitis C may recur after liver transplantation, and like pretransplant hepatitis C may be indolent, with only minimal increase in enzymes, but may lead to chronic disease and need for retransplantation. The exact frequency of recurrence is not known because of paucity of data, but may be as high as 17%.[44,45]

Cryptogenic Cirrhosis

In a small percentage of the patients no etiology of the liver disease can be established. These patients represent mainly non-B, non-C disease or a missed case of metabolic liver disease (see below). Occasionally these patients are confused with drug-induced liver disease. In these cases a liver biopsy is helpful (also discussed below).

Metabolic Liver Disease

Wilson's Disease

Most patients with Wilson's disease present in childhood or as young adults. Detailed discussion is given by Benkov and Rosch in Chapter 16. Effective treatment is available and transplantation may not become necessary until late in the course of the disease. Sternlieb[46] describes three groups of patients who should be transplanted:

1. Cirrhotic patients who fail to respond to therapy after 2–3 months of treatment.
2. Those patients, who are well controlled, but discontinue medications, resulting in a rapid declining course.
3. Fulminant hepatic failure (discussed on p. 96).

Alpha-1 Antitrypsin Deficiency

Alpha-1 antitrypsin deficiency may present as end-stage cirrhosis in patients up to 60 years of age. At diagnosis pulmonary disease is present in about 60% of cases but is frequently mild. Serum protein electrophoresis for detection of decreased α-1 globulin, is a good screening test. Phenotyping and quantitative determination of α-1-antitrypsin are more specific. Liver biopsy is confirmative. Positive family history is not necessary for the diagnosis. Hepatocellular carcinoma is a complication of this disease and should be sought for prior to transplantation. Indications for transplantation depend on the complications of cirrhosis, but it should be performed before advancing pulmonary disease precludes successful transplantation.[47]

Galactosemia

Galactosemia[48] is a rare cause of "cryptogenic cirrhosis" in adults up to 50 years of age. A history of neonatal cholestasis should increase the index of suspicion. Liver biopsy is helpful in establishing the diagnosis.

Protoporphyria

Onset of liver disease in porphyria is followed by a rapidly declining clinical course,[49,50] and for this reason transplantation should be considered once the diagnosis is established.

Chronic Alcoholic Liver Disease

Ethical and moral considerations should not prevent patients with alcoholic liver disease from receiving liver transplants. However, some reluctance to transplant alcoholic patients is justified because of the potential risk for recidivism and the consequent lack of compliance with medical treatment posttransplantation.[51,52] Current data[53] suggest that these problems affect about 10% of the transplantees. In view of the shortage of funds and donor livers, some transplant physicians feel priority should be given to patients without these additional risk factors. The issue is further complicated, because of abstinent patients even with well-established alcoholic cirrhosis frequently do well without any treatment.[53a] Early mortality may be slightly higher in alcoholics because of postoperative infections, but long-term survival do not appear to be different from a medically similar group of nonalcoholic cirrhotic patients. In conclusion, alcoholic liver disease, per se, is not a contraindication for transplantation.[54]

Drug-Induced Liver Disease

Hepatic dysfunction secondary to drug therapy is difficult to diagnose. Chronic active hepatitis and cirrhosis resulting from methotrexate[55] or amiodorone ingestion have distinctive histologic features. Damage from other drugs, such as α-methyldopa, mimic chronic active hepatitis. Combinations of drugs, such as valproic acid combined with a psychotropic agent, have been reported to cause cirrhosis that is difficult to categorize. Several of these patients have required transplantation.

These patients usually have a protracted course and waiting for muscle wasting or other late manifestations of the disease results in higher surgical risks. Since no treatment is available, these patients should be transplanted while they are still in good general medical and nutritional condition. Early transplantation is especially indicated when amiodorone or disulfiram is the etiologic agent, because either one may involve multiple organs.

Nonhepatic Causes of Portal Hypertension

Trauma

Trauma and surgical misadventures are unusual causes for liver transplantation. The patients are frequently young in generally good medical condition,[56,57] and the prognosis is excellent.

Budd-Chiari Syndrome and Other Vascular Causes

Determination of the etiology of the Budd-Chiari syndrome is important, because of differences in pre- and posttransplant management and prognosis. Myeloproliferative disorders and oral birth-control medications are now the most common cause of the Budd-Chiari syndrome. Congential webs of the vena cava and hepatic veins are less frequent.[58] A shunt decompression procedure may be the treatment of choice early in the course, when liver cell injury, as determined by liver biopsy, is not extensive. Transplantation is necessary, when extensive centrolobar hemorrhagic necrosis is present and synthetic function deteriorates.[59,60] Patients with Budd-Chiari syndrome secondary to myeloproliferative disease should be transplanted and anticoagulated after transplantation. Successful transplantation, however, depends on the good control of the underlying disease prior to transplantation.

Hemangiomas, even though they can become giant and deforming, are not indications for liver transplantation. Transplantation becomes necessary if the hemangioma becomes infected and cannot be resected.

Neoplastic Diseases

Hepatocellular carcinomas, when <5 cm in diameter, can be transplanted with low surgical mortality and good one-year survival. Before transplantation, extra-hepatic metastasis has to be excluded by imaging techniques. But occasionally the hepatoma recurs, mostly in an extra-hepatic location. Survival is especially good, when the hepatocellular carcinoma is found incidentally during the course of transplantation for nonmalignant disease.[62] Patients transplanted for primary hepatocellular carcinoma in non-cirrhotic livers have a better survival than patients with malignancy and cirrhosis.[62a]

Certain tumors, such as the lamellar type of hepatocellular carcinoma, are more amenable to transplantation, since they are slow-growing and metastasize late. Medium-term (2–5 years) survival therefore is increased over hepatocellular carcinoma, but long-term survival is not. Cholangiocarcinomas and Klatskin tumors are not indications for transplantation because of the poor survival.[63]

Vascular neoplasms, epithelioid hemangioendothelioma, and angiosarcoma are usually multicentric and therefore curable only by transplantation. Surgical experience is limited, but the possibility of cure or at least prolongation of life justifies transplantation. Long-term follow-up for these patients is as yet not available.

Metastatic carcinoma is not an indication for transplantation, except in patients with a neuroendocrine tumor (carcinoid, glucagonoma, etc). They benefit from transplantations, since the symptoms, due to the high levels of circulating hormones, are reduced. These tumors are generally slow growing, but it is still unclear whether survival is prolonged.[64]

Other Systemic Diseases

Sarcoidosis rarely leads to cirrhosis. End-stage liver involvement usually manifests itself in variceal bleeding, which is difficult to control with sclerotherapy.

Schistosomiasis produces portal hypertension, without cirrhosis or significant hepatic dysfunction. Rarely there may be progressive fibrosis, after successful portal decompression, resulting in liver failure. Liver biopsy is necessary to assess the degree of liver injury and the need for liver transplantation. Liver transplantation may then become the definitive treatment.

CONSIDERATION OF RISK FACTORS BEFORE REFERRAL FOR TRANSPLANTATION

If specific indications for liver transplantation are present, the final decision for transplantation is made after a rigorous medical, social, and psychological evaluation at the transplant center. Some of these patients are clearly not suitable candidates because of risk factors. A simple screening at the local level by the referring physician is helpful. In the following we discuss some of the risk factors that should be considered before referral to the transplant center.

Alcohol and Substance Abuse

Abstinence is an absolute requirement for referral. This is not only a moral issue, but necessary to ensure compliance with post-transplant medication and to avoid adverse drug interactions. To further assure compliance most transplant centers require enrollment in an active support group, like Alcoholics Anonymous (AA), in addition to strong support by family or by close friend before evaluation for transplantation.

Cardiac evaluation is essential to exclude significant cardiomyopathy prior to referral. A history of bacterial endocarditis without valvular heart disease is not a contraindication, but with valvular damage, the prognosis is so poor that liver transplantation is not indicated.

Nonhepatic Neoplastic Disease

If the patient is in good general medical condition and the life expectancy from the malignancy is at least 5 years, transplantation can be considered. In patients with treated breast, colon, and other solid neoplasm, when the prognosis is relatively good, transplantation is acceptable. Immune suppression post-transplant does not affect the cancer adversely. Patients receiving chemotherapy should not be transplanted. Patients with lymphomas, both Hodgkin's and non-Hodgkin's, are acceptable candidates, if the disease is under control and the patient is not receiving chemotherapy.

Pregnancy

In our opinion pregnancy itself is not a contraindication to transplantation. A patient transplanted intrapartum for fulminant hepatic failure delivered a healthy baby.[81]

General Medical Condition

Nutrition

Malnutrition is an underestimated and poorly studied risk factor for transplantation. Shaw et al.,[65] in their risk analysis include nutrition as an added risk factor but they provide no objective measure of nutrition. The Mayo Clinic workers also found no clear correlation between success of liver transplantation and nutritional status in their first 100 patients.[24] Referral should not be withheld because of poor nutritional status.

Anergy, a late sequela of nutritional depletion, considered by some workers to correlate with a poor surgical prognosis, is also not a contraindication for referral for liver transplantation. More data from controlled studies are essential in this area.

Age

Advanced age itself is not an absolute contraindication to transplantation. There is no strict age limit. In 1983 patients over 50 years were excluded; currently patients over 70 are candidates, if there are no other contraindications. Age does raise economic, ethical, and moral issues. Surgical morbidity and mortality increases with age. Older patients also have more limited posttransplant life expectancy.

Infancy also possesses certain technical and ethical issues, as discussed by Benkov and Rosch in Chapter 16.

Complicating Systemic Diseases

Cardiac

Coronary heart disease, if corrected by bypass surgery or angioplasty, is not a contraindication for transplantation provided left ventricular function is good. Patients with severe valvular heart disease complicated by severe pulmonary hypertension or alcoholic cardiomyopathy are not candidates for transplantation at this time. They may become candidates for cluster operations. Aortic stenosis must be evaluated carefully, since patients with severe stenosis or poor left ventricular function cannot tolerate transplantation.

Pulmonary Disease

Patients with healed pulmonary tuberculosis are acceptable candidates, but active disease must be treated for at least 3 months before transplantation, and continued up to 1 year, if possible.

Patients with severe, progressive primary lung disease, whose pulmonary functions are irreversibly compromised, should be excluded from referral.

Functional lung disease (e.g., asthma) and lung disease secondary to liver failure (hepatopulmonary syndrome, respiration compromised by ascites or muscle wasting) does not prohibit referral and subsequent transplantation. Pneumonectomy, provided the function of the remaining lung is not compromised and the patient is functional, does not influence the outcome of transplantation. We accept patients with asbestosis as transplant candidates.

Chronic Infectious Diseases

Suppurative infectious diseases are absolute contraindications for transplantation. This includes osteomyelitis, sinusitis, gingivitis, and all abscesses. These patients must have received therapy and show no active inflammation before referral.

Individuals who are infected with the HIV virus are not acceptable candidates. Patients transplanted with HIV infection had a markedly decreased life expectancy, with AIDS being the leading cause of death. Immunosuppression seems to accelerate the transition of HIV infection to AIDS.[66]

Treated and stable syphilis and lyme disease patients can be referred for transplantation. Serologic evidence of previous exposure to cytomegalovirus, herpes (HSV I and II; VZ), Epstein-Barr virus or other viral illness may complicate the posttransplant picture, but does not exclude referral. Thus patients with genital herpes can be referred.

Other infections such as chronic fungal disease may exacerbate under immunosuppression and prohibit transplantation.

Rheumatic Diseases

Patients with uncomplicated connective tissue diseases (systemic lupus, scleroderma, etc.) can be transplanted without increased complications. If their disease is complicated by renal insufficiency, combined hepatic and renal transplantation is possible. Scleroderma with gastrointestinal pulmonary involvement may cause significant perioperative complications. Such candidates are an extremely high risk.

Endocrine Disorders

Diabetes, adrenal disorders, and thyroid disease are not contraindications. Patients with osteoporosis, whether it is a complication of cholestatic liver disease or postmenopausal, can be referred for transplantation. If the pretransplant evaluation shows severe osteoporosis, treatment should be initiated.

Gastrointestinal Diseases

Patients with primary sclerosing cholangitis secondary to ulcerative colitis are at risk for development of colon cancer. Transplantation is indicated in the absence of dysplasia on colonoscopic biopsies. It is an open question whether these patients, committed to an unending course of immunosuppression, should undergo prophylactic colectomy[67] before (or after) transplantation.

Current immunosuppressive drugs are fat-soluble and require pancreatic enzymes for absorption from the gut. Chronic pancreatitis therefore may be considered as a relative contraindication, depending on extent of disability and malabsorption. This has not been substantiated in the literature. In our experience this has not been a problem in alcoholic patients.

Rectal and perianal fistulae have to be treated prior to transplantation.

Urologic Disorders

Urinary retention should be corrected before referral. A permanent indwelling catheter is not acceptable in a transplant candidate, but conversion to a suprapubic cytostomy may allow transplantation and prostatectomy, if indicated, may be performed at a later date.

Bleeding Disorders

Hemophilia has reportedly been corrected by transplantation.[68,69] Platelet disorders and von Willebrandt's disease may require replacement therapy during surgery, but do not appear to affect mortality.

Previous Abdominal Surgery

Long-standing portacaval shunts and peritoneojugular shunts increase surgical morbidity due to blood loss and extended operative time needed for lysis of adhesions and surgical exposure, but transplantation is still feasible.[70] Biliary tract complications were increased in patients with previous portosystemic shunt, but overall mortality rate was not effected.[70a] Right-upper-quadrant surgery (cholecystectomy and previous gastric surgery) increases surgical mortality to only a slight extent.

Communication Barriers

A language barrier can be overcome by help from family members or multilingual staff. Blind or deaf patients can also be transplanted with appropriate support.

ACUTE HEPATIC FAILURE

Acute hepatic failure is defined as hepatic dysfunction with encephalopathy and/or coagulopathy less than 6 months after the onset of liver disease. This group of hepatitides has been arbitrarily subdivided into fulminant (< 2 weeks), subfulminant (2–12 weeks), and late-onset (12 weeks to 6 months).[71] These subdivisions have little clinical usefulness in referral, selection, and prognosis.

Although worldwide experience in transplantation of patients with acute liver failure is limited, it is generally accepted that the age of the patient and the etiology of the liver disease are the most important prognostic factors for survival. A rapidly shrinking liver, progressive encephalopathy, and prothrombin time > 20 secs are harbingers of a poor prognosis.[72,73] Even considering these factors survival is still unpredictable, and many patients are transplanted who might recover with medical management. On the other hand, procrastination with the transplantation increases surgical mortality in patients with fulminant disease. Recently factor V levels were proposed to use as a prognostic indicator in acute liver failure. Usually below 50% the prognosis is poor.

Once the decision to proceed with transplantation is made prognosis may ultimately depend on the availability of a donor organ. For these reasons, a patient who develops encephalopathy or coagulopathy soon after the onset of symptoms of hepatic failure should be referred immediately to a transplant center.

Patients with fulminant hepatitis A and B have a fair (A 67%; B 39%) survival, without transplantation.[74] The prognosis is less favorable with drug-induced fulminant liver failure (halothane 12%, acetaminophen 52%) and hepatitis non-A, non-B (20%).

VIRAL HEPATITIS

Most of our experience with transplantation for fulminant liver failure is derived from patients with viral hepatitis. One-year survival is upward of 60%.[75,76] Hepatitis A, although infrequently fatal, comprises a significant portion of patients transplanted for fulminant hepatitis. Transplantation is curative.

Hepatitis B can also acutely proceed to fulminant hepatic failure. Recurrence of hepatitis B after transplantation for fulminant disease is less common than for chronic hepatitis B. This may be due to the lack of incorporation of the hepatitis B virus in the human genome early in the course of infection.

Patients presenting with acute hepatitis, with negative serology for hepatitis A and B, are best classified as hepatitis non-A non-B, rather than making the tentative diagnosis of hepatitis C. Test for the antigen to hepatitis C virus is negative in early infection. Further, there is conflicting evidence that cases considered to be non-A, non-B are actually hepatitis C.[77] The diagnosis of acute hepatitis C, can be made with the polymerase chain reaction (PCR) using liver tissue. This, however, is rarely available prior to transplantation.

Hepatitis C also may recur after transplantation for acute disease. (See Chapter 14).

Drug-Induced and Toxic Hepatitis

Acute toxic and drug-induced hepatitis frequently can be managed medically. The severity of liver dysfunction may not correlate with ultimate survival, especially in acetaminophen toxicity, where early supportive medical therapy and the use of acetylcystine is extremely successful.

The liver failure of severe mushroom poisoning manifests as coagulopathy, with little encephalopathy. In the circumstance the coagulopathy alone should herald the need for transplantation.[78,79]

Patients with acute alcoholic hepatitis should not be transplanted because of the coexistence of toxic multisystem involvement of acute alcohol intoxication. Evaluation of significant liver injury is difficult, and prognosis is uncertain in the patient presenting with acute alcoholic hepatitis. Following resolution of the acute alcoholic injury, reevaluation may be considered.

Wilson's Disease

Wilson's disease must be considered in the differential diagnosis of any young (< 35 years of age) patient presenting with acute hepatic failure. Sternlieb[46] suggests that these patients frequently have transaminase and alkaline phosphatase values that are disproportionately low relative to the severity of the liver disease and have a Coombs-negative hemolytic anemia. Since this is a life-threatening presentation in an otherwise healthy individual, early consideration for liver transplantation is indicated. Most cases are diagnosed by low to low normal ceruloplasmin levels and/or the presence of Kaiser-Fleisher rings. If both of these tests are normal, an elevated 24-hr urinary copper level can establish the diagnosis. In addition to orthotopic liver transplantation heterotopic transplantation has been performed[80] in a case of fulminant hepatic failure when a liver with matched blood type could not be obtained.

Acute Fatty Liver of Pregnancy

Fatty liver of pregnancy commonly responds to aggressive supportive measures and early delivery of the fetus. Ockner et al.[82] suggests that patients not responding to this regimen are candidates for orthotopic liver transplantation, based on their experience with a single case.

REFERENCES

1. Roberts JP, Forsmark C, Lake JR, Ascher NL: Liver transplantation today. *Ann Rev Med* 40:287–303, 1989.
2. Wall WJ: Liver transplantation: current concepts. *Can Med Assoc J* 139:21–28, 1988.
3. Rydning A, Schrumpf E, Abdelnoor M, Elgjo K, Jenssen E: Factors of prognostic importance in primary biliary cirrhosis. *Scand J Gastroenterol* 25:119–126, 1990.
4. Markus BH, Dickson ER, Grambsch PM, et al: Efficiency of liver transplantation in patients with primary biliary cirrhosis. *New Engl J Med* 320:1709–1713, 1989.
5. Lautz HU, Pichlmayr R: Special aspects of timing of liver transplantation in patients with liver cirrhosis. *Baillieres Clin Gastroenterol* 3:743–756, 1989.
6. Neuberger J, Altman DG, Polson R, et al: Prognosis after liver transplantation for primary biliary cirrhosis. *Transplantation* 48:444–447, 1989.
7. Dickson ER, Grambsch PM, Fleming TR, Fisher LD, Langworthy A: Prognosis in primary biliary cirrhosis: model for decision making. *Hepatology* 10:1–7, 1989.
8. Wiesner RH, Grambsch PM, Dickson ER, et al: Primary sclerosing cholangitis: natural history, prognostic factors and survival analysis. *Hepatology* 10:430–436, 1989.
9. Kellerman PS, Linas SL: Large volume paracentesis in treatment of ascites. *Ann Int Med* 112:889–891, 1990.
10. Gines P, Tito L, Arroyo V, et al: Randomized comparative study of therapeutic paracentesis with and without albumin in cirrhosis. *Gastroenterology* 94:1493–1502, 1988.
11. Rabinovitz M, Schade RR, Dindzans V, Van Thiel DH, Gavaler JS: Prevalence of duodenal ulcer in cirrhotic males referred for liver transplantation. Does the etiology of cirrhosis make a difference? *Dig Dis Sci* 35:321–326, 1990.
12. DeWeert T, Gostout CJ, Wiesner RH: Congestive gastropathy and other upper endoscopic findings in 81 consecutive patients undergoing orthotopic liver transplantation. *Am J Gastroenterol* 85:573–576, 1990.
13. Jabbari M, Cherry R, Lough JO: Gastric antral vascular ectasia: the "watermelon" stomach. *Gastroenterology* 1165–1170, 1986.

13a. Ring EJ, Lake JR, Roberts JP, Gordon RL, et al: Using transjugular intrahepatic portosystemic shunts to control variceal bleeding before liver transplantation. *Ann Int Med* 116:304–309, 1992.

14. Garrett KO, Reilly JJ, Jr, Schade RR, Van Thiel DH: Bleeding esophageal varices: treatment by sclerotherapy and liver transplantation. *Surgery* 104:819–823, 1988.

15. Basile AS, Hughes RD, Harrison PM, et al: Elevated brain concentrations of 1,4-benzodiazepines in fulminant hepatic failure. *New Engl J Med* 325:473–478, 1991.
16. Powell EE, Pender MP, Chalk JB, et al: Improvement in chronic hepatocerebral degeneration following liver transplantation. *Gastroenterology* 98:1079–1082, 1990.
16a. Eriksson LS: Hypoxemia in patients with liver cirrhosis. *Acta Gastroenterol Belg* 53:209–215, 1990.
16b. Eriksson LS, Soderman C, Ericzon BG, Eleborg L, Wahren J, Hedenstierna G: Normalization of ventilation/perfusion relationships after liver transplantation in patients with decompensated cirrhosis: evidence for a hepatopulmonary syndrome. *Hepatology* 12:1350–1357, 1990.
16c. Eriksson LS, Soderman C, Ericzon BG, Eleborg L, Hedenstierna G, Wahren J: Hypoxemia cured by liver transplantation. *Transplant Proc* 22:172–173, 1990.
17. Krowka MJ, Cortese DA: Pulmonary aspects of liver disease and liver transplantation. *Clin Chest Med* 10:593–616, 1989.
18. Krowka MJ, Cortese DA: Hepatopulmonary syndrome: an evolving perspective in the era of liver transplantation comment. *Hepatology* 11:138–142, 1990.
19. Hockerstedt K, Ericzon BG, Eriksson LS, et al: Survival after liver transplantation for primary biliary cirrhosis: use of prognostic indices for comparison with medical treatment. *Transplant Proc* 22:1499–1500, 1990.
20. Mews CF, Dorney SF, Sheil AG, Forbes DA, Hill RE: Failure of liver transplantation in Wilson's disease with pulmonary arteriovenous shunting. *J Pediatr Gastroenterol Nutr* 10:230–233, 1990.
21. Stoller JK, Moodie D, Schiavone WA, et al: Reduction of intrapulmonary shunt and resolution of digital clubbing associated with primary biliary cirrhosis after liver transplantation; see comments. *Hepatology* 11:54–58, 1990.
21a. Eriksson LS: Is intrapulmonary arteriovenous shunting and hypoxemia a contraindication for liver transplantation? *Hepatology* 14:575–576, 1991.
22. Wallwork J, Williams R, Calne RY: Transplantation of liver, heart, and lungs for primary biliary cirrhosis and primary pulmonary hypertension. *Lancet* 2:182–185, 1987.
23. Harjula AL, Baldwin JC, Oyer PE, Stinson EB, Shumway NE: Recipient selection for heart-lung transplantation. *Scand J Thorac Cardiovasc Surg* 22:193–196, 1988.
24. DiCecco SR, Wieners EJ, Wiesner RH, Southorn PA, Plevak DJ, Krom RA: Assessment of nutritional status of patients with end-stage liver disease undergoing liver transplantation. *Mayo Clin Proc* 64:95–102, 1989.
25. Shapiro JM, Smith H, Schaffner F: Serum bilirubin: a prognostic factor in primary bilary cirrhosis. *Gut* 20:137–142, 1979.
26. Duquesnoy RJ: Cellular aspects of intragraft immunity in liver transplantation. *Transplant Proc* 21:3629–3630, 1989.
27. Gonwa TA, Nery JR, Husberg BS, Klintmalm GB: Simultaneous liver and renal transplantation in man. *Transplantation* 46:690–693, 1988.
28. Punukollu RC, Gopalswamy N: The hepatorenal syndrome. *Med Clin N Am* 74: 933–943, 1990.
29. Wood RP, Ellis D, Starzl TE: The reversal of the hepatorenal syndrome in four pediatric patients following successful orthotopic liver transplantation. *Ann Surg* 205:415–419, 1987.
30. Gonwa TA, Poplawski S, Paulsen W, et al: Hepatorenal syndrome and orthotopic liver transplantation. *Transplant Proc* 21:2419–2420, 1989.

31. Klion FM, Fabry TL, Palmer M, Schaffner F: Prediction of survival of patient with primary biliary cirrhosis. *Gastroenterology* 102:310–313, 1992.

32. Maddrey WC: Bone disease in patients with primary biliary cirrhosis. *Prog Liver Dis* 9:537–554, 1990.

33. Ludwig J, LaRusso NF, Wiesner RH: The syndrome of primary sclerosing cholangitis. *Prog Liver Dis* 9:555–566, 1990.

34. Langnas AN, Grazi GL, Stratta RJ, et al: Primary sclerosing cholangitis: the emerging role for liver transplantation. *Am J Gastroenterol* 85:1136–1141, 1990.

34a. Rosen CB, Nagorney DM, Wiesner RH, Coffey RJ, Jr, LaRusso NF: Cholangiocarcinoma complicating primary sclerosing cholangitis. *Ann Surg* 213:21–25, 1991.

35. Olsson R, Danielsson A, Jarnerot G, et al: Prevalence of primary sclerosing cholangitis in patients with ulcerative colitis. *Gastroenterology* 100:1319–1323, 1991.

35a. Hudes B, Klion FK, Fabry TL, et al: Course of inflammatory bowel disease of the colon after hepatic transplantation. In press.

36. Alagille D, Estrada A, Hadchouel M, et al: Syndromic paucity of interlobular bile ducts (Alagille's syndrome or atrio-hepatic dysplasia, review of 80 cases). *J Pediatr* 110:195–200, 1987.

37. Zafrani ES, Metreau JM, Douvin C, Larrey D, et al: Idiopathic biliary ductopenia in adults, a report of five cases. *Gastroenterology* 99:1823–1828, 1990.

38. Starzl TE, Reyes J, Tzakis A, Mieles L, Todo S, Gordon R: Liver transplantation for polycystic liver disease. *Arch Surg* 125:575–577, 1990.

38a. Vauthey JN, Maddern GJ, Blumgart LH: Adult polycystic disease of the liver. *Br J Surg* 78:524–527, 1991.

39. Feray C, Zignego AL, Samuel D, et al: Persistent hepatitis B virus infection of mononuclear blood cells without concomitant liver infection. The liver transplantation model. *Transplantation* 49:1155–1158, 1990.

40. Demetris AJ, Todo S, Van Thiel DH, et al: Evolution of hepatitis B virus liver disease after hepatic replacement. Practical and theoretical considerations. *Am J Pathol* 137:667–676, 1990.

41. O'Grady JG, Williams R: Liver transplantation for viral hepatitis. *Br Med Bull* 46:481–491, 1990.

42. Todu S, Demetris AJ, Van Thiel D, Teperman L, Fung JJ, Starzl TE: Orthotopic liver transplantation for patients with hepatitis B virus-related liver disease. *Hepatology* 13:619–626, 1991.

43. Lake JR, Wright TL: Liver transplantation for patients with hepatitis B: What have we learned from our results? *Hepatology* 13:796–799, 1991.

44. Hart J, Busuttil RW, Lewin KJ: Disease recurrence following liver transplantation. *Am J Surg Pathol* 14(Suppl 1):79–91, 1990.

45. Martin P, Munoz SJ, DiBisceglia AM, et al: Recurrence of hepatitis C virus infection after orthotopic liver transplant. *Hepatology* 13:719–721, 1991.

46. Sternlieb I: Wilson's disease: indications for liver transplantation. *Hepatology* 4: 15S–17S, 1984.

47. Esquivel CO, Marino IR, Fioravanti V, Van Thiel DH: Liver transplantation for metabolic disease of the liver. *Gastroenterol Clin N Am* 17:167–175, 1988.

48. Otto G, Herfarth C, Senninger N, Feist G, Post S, Gmelin K: Hepatic transplantation in galactosemia. *Transplantation* 47:902–903, 1989.

49. Samuel D, Boboc B, Bernuau J, Bismuth H, Benhamou JP: Liver transplantation

for protoporphyria. Evidence for the predominant role of the erythropoietic tissue in protoporphyrin overproduction. *Gastroenterology* 95:816–819, 1988.

50. Bloomer JR, Weimer MK, Bossenmaier IC, Snover DC, Payne WD, Ascher NL: Liver transplantation in a patient with protoporphyria. *Gastroenterology* 97:188–194, 1989.

51. Moss AH, Siegler M: Should alcoholics compete equally for liver transplantation? *JAMA* 265:1295–1298, 1991.

52. Cohen C, Benjamin N: Alcoholics and liver transplantation. *JAMA* 265:1299–1302, 1991.

53. Van Thiel DH, Gavaler JS, Tarter RE, et al: Liver transplantation for alcoholic liver disease: a consideration of reasons for and against. *Alcoholism (NY)* 13:181–184, 1989.

53a. Bird G: The practical business of treatment. Can't treat, won't treat? Alcoholic liver disease. *Br J Addict* 86:695–700, 1991.

54. Kumar S, Stauber RE, Gavaler JS, et al: Orthotopic liver transplantation for alcoholic liver disease. *Hepatology* 11:159–164, 1990.

55. Gilbert SC, Klintmalm G, Menter A, Silverman A: Methotrexate-induced cirrhosis requiring liver transplantation in three patients with psoriasis. A word of caution in light of the expanding use of this "steroid-sparing" agent. *Arch Intern Med* 150:889–891, 1990.

56. Esquivel CO, Bernardos A, Makowka L, Iwatsuki S, Gordon RD, Starzl TE: Liver replacement after massive hepatic trauma. *J Trauma* 27:800–802, 1987.

57. Angstadt J, Jarrell B, Carabasi A, et al: Liver transplantation following severe liver trauma. *Transplantation* 46:321–322, 1988.

58. Klein AS, Cameron JL: Diagnosis and management of the Budd-Chiari syndrome. *Am J Surg* 160:128–133, 1990.

59. Oldhafer KJ, Ringe B, Wittekind C, Pichlmayr R: Budd-Chiari syndrome: portacaval shunt and subsequent liver transplantation. *Surgery* 107:471–474, 1990.

60. Halff G, Todo S, Tzakis AG, Gordon RD, Starzl TE: Liver transplantation for the Budd-Chiari syndrome. *Ann Surg* 211:43–49, 1990.

61. O'Grady JG, Polson RJ, Rolles K, Calne RY, Williams R: Liver transplantation for malignant disease. Results in 93 consecutive patients. *Ann Surg* 207:373–379, 1988.

62. Penn I: Hepatic transplantation for primary and metastatic malignancies of the liver. *Surgery* 110:726–734, 1991.

62a. Ismail T, Angrisani L, Gunson BK, et al: Primary hepatic malignancy: the role of liver transplantation. *Br J Surg* 77:983–987, 1990.

63. Wolff H, Ridwelski K, Lorf T: Surgical treatment of malignant tumor of the hepatic duct junction. *Zentralb Chir* 115:1–14, 1990.

64. Alsina AE, Bartus S, Hull D, Rosson R, Schweizer RT: Liver transplant for metastatic neuroendocrine tumor. *J Clin Gastroenterol* 12:533–537, 1990.

65. Shaw BW, Jr, Wood RP, Stratta RJ, Pillen TJ, Langnas AN: Stratifying the causes of death in liver transplant recipients. An approach to improving survival. *Arch Surg* 124:895–900, 1989.

66. Tzakis AG, Cooper MH, Dummer JS, Ragni M, Ward JW, Starzl TE: Transplantation in HIV+ patients. *Transplantation* 49:354–358, 1990.

67. Higashi H, Yanaga K, Marsh JW, Tzakis A, Kakizoe S, Starzl TE: Development of colon cancer after liver transplantation for primary sclerosing cholangitis associated with ulcerative colitis. *Hepatology* 11:477–480, 1990.

68. Bontempo FA, Lewis JH, Gorenc TJ, et al: Liver transplantation in hemophilia A. *Blood* 69:1721–1724, 1987.

69. Delorme MA, Adams PC, Grant D, Ghent CN, Walker IR, Wall WJ: Orthotopic liver transplantation in a patient with combined hemophilia A and B. *Am J Hematol* 33:136–138, 1990.

70. Abramson SJ, Berdon WE, Altman RP, Amodio JB, Levy J: Biliary atresia and noncardiac polysplenic syndrome: US and surgical considerations. *Radiology* 163: 377–379, 1987.

70a. AbouJaoude MM, Grant DR, Ghent CN, Mimeault RE, Wall WJ: Effect of portasystemic shunts on subsequent transplantation of the liver. *Surg Gynecol Obstet* 172:215–219, 1991.

71. O'Grady JG, Alexander GJ, Thick M, Potter D, Calne RY, Williams R: Outcome of orthotopic liver transplantation in the aetiological and clinical variants of acute liver failure. *Q J Med* 68:817–824, 1988.

72. O'Grady JG, Alexander GJ, Hayllar KM, Williams R: Early indicators of prognosis in fulminant hepatic failure. *Gastroenterology* 97:439–445, 1989.

73. Emond JC, Aran PP, Whitington PF, Broelsch CE, Baker AL: Liver transplantation in the management of fulminant hepatic failure. *Gastroenterology* 96:1583–1588, 1989.

74. O'Grady JG, Gimson AE, O'Brien CJ, Pucknell A, Hughes RD, Williams R: Controlled trials of charcoal hemoperfusion and prognostic factors in fulminant hepatic failure. *Gastroenterology* 94:1186–1192, 1988.

75. Schafer DF, Shaw BW, Jr: Fulminant hepatic failure and orthotopic liver transplantation. *Semin Liver Dis* 9:189–194, 1989.

76. Van de Stadt J, Gelin M, Bourgeois N, De Prez C, Adler M, Lambilliotte JP: Liver transplantation for fulminant and subacute viral hepatic failure in adults. *Transplant Proc* 22:1505–1508, 1990.

77. Read AE, Donegan E, Lake J, et al: Hepatitis C in patients undergoing liver transplantation. *Ann Intern Med* 114:282–284, 1991.

78. Klein AS, Hart J, Brems JJ, Goldstein L, Lewin K, Busuttil RW: Amanita poisoning: treatment and the role of liver transplantation. *Am J Med* 86:187–193, 1989.

79. Pinson CW, Daya MR, Benner KG, et al: Liver transplantation for severe Amanita phalloides mushroom poisoning. *Am J Surg* 159:493–499, 1990.

80. Stamppfl DA, Munoz SJ, Moritz MJ, et al: Heterotropic liver transplantation for fulminant Wilson's disease. *Gastroenterology* 99:1834–1836, 1990.

81. Fair JA, Klein S, Feng T, Merritt WT, Burdick JF: Intrapartum orthotopic liver transplantation with successful outcome of pregnancy. *Transplantation* 50:534–535, 1990.

82. Ockner SA, Brunt EM, Cohn SM, Krul ES, Hanto DW, Peters MS: Fulminant hepatic failure caused by fatty liver of pregnancy treated by orthotopic liver transplantation. *Hepatology* 11:59–64, 1990.

— 7 —

PREOPERATIVE MEDICAL EVALUATION OF THE PROSPECTIVE RECIPIENT

Franklin M. Klion and Thomas L. Fabry

Once the decision is made that liver transplantation is indicated and no obvious medical or psychological contraindications are present, a more detailed evaluation is performed at the coordinated facilities of the transplant center, following a strict protocol. Evaluation of specific organ systems assess the patient's ability to undergo surgery and guides in posttransplant management (Table 7-1). Psychological and social evaluations are conducted simultaneously with the same goals. The latter two evaluations are the subject of the next two chapters.

INFORMATION FOR ORGAN MATCHING AND TRANSPLANT SURGERY

Anatomic information is needed for organ matching and technical help with the surgery. The patient's height, weight, and liver volume [estimated by computerized axial tomographic (CAT) scanning] determine the maximum acceptable size for the donor organ. Tissue matching for liver transplantation, unlike that for kidney transplantation, requires blood group determination only.

Hepatic transplantation requires suitable portal venous channels. Segmental thrombosis of the portal and other mesenteric veins may technically complicate transplantation, but is not an absolute contraindication. The portal venous system and the inferior vena cava, therefore, have to be evaluated by duplex ultrasonography.[1,2] This will confirm the diagnosis of portal hypertension and dem-

TABLE 7-1. Components of transplant candidate medical evaluation

1. Anatomic
   size
   blood type
   bile ducts and venous channels
2. Etiologic
   Nature of liver disease
   Complications of liver disease
3. Co-existing medical diseases.
   cardiac
   pulmonary
   renal
   hematologic
   infectious
   gastroenterologic
   neoplastic
   metabolic

onstrates portal and splenic vein patency and direction of bloodflow.[3] If the results are ambiguous, more invasive angiographic or venographic studies are required.[4,5] Magnetic resonance imaging (MRI) angiography has been demonstrated to yield comparable results and may replace these invasive techniques.[6] Endoscopic retrograde cholangiopancreatography (ERCP) or percutaneous transhepatic cholangiogram (PTC) insures that the bile ducts are normal and can be used for anastomoses.

Patients who have no evidence of previous cytomegalovirus (CMV) infection (seronegative for CMV) usually receive their liver from a CMV-negative donor. Seronegative kidney transplant recipients who received organs from a seropositive donor had a 36% incidence of clinical CMV disease.[7] Similarly, donor organ seropositivity was the major risk factor for the development of cytomegalovirus infection in seronegative liver transplant recipients.[8-10]

LIVER AND BILIARY SYSTEM

The liver and biliary systems are evaluated to confirm the etiology of the liver disease and to exclude concomitant neoplasia. The etiology is important since many pre- and postoperative therapeutic decisions are dependent on the nature of the liver disease, including recurrence of disease after transplantation.

To clarify the etiology we routinely obtain the following serologic markers and related tests: hepatitis B—surface antigen and antibody, e antigen and antibody, core antibody, hepatitis B virus DNA; hepatitis C antibody (the screening ELISA assay should be confirmed by the more specific RIBA 2 test); antinuclear antibody (ANA), antimitochondrial antibody (AMA), anti-smooth-muscle antibody (ASMA), antibodies to Epstein-Barr virus (EBV); and cytomegalovirus (CMV), α-fetoprotein (AFP), and carcinoembryonic antigen (CEA).

Liver biopsy may be required when the etiology is unclear, such as in an alcoholic patient, who has hepatitis C antibodies or in the Budd-Chiari syndrome. If severe coagulopathy is present, a transvenous, jugular biopsy is performed. Polymerase chain reaction (PCR) test of the liver biopsy is especially useful to confirm hepatitis C, when hepatitis C antibody is not present, such as in acute hepatitis C.

Hepatocellular carcinoma complicates many cases of cirrhosis, including primary biliary cirrhosis and other cholestatic liver diseases. A CAT scan is always necessary to exclude tumor, since AFP is neither a sensitive nor a specific test for hepatocellular carcinoma.[11] MRI is able to detect smaller lesions; it can be used, therefore, to both refine and confirm the diagnosis. CAT scan during arterial portography is the most sensitive imaging technique for hepatic masses,[12] but is not widely available. Any solid space-occupying lesion should be biopsied under CT or sonographic guidance. Primary hepatocellular carcinomas <5 cm in diameter do not constitute a contraindication for transplant[13] if there is no evidence of metastasis.

Cholangiocarcinoma, an infrequent complication of sclerosing cholangitis, is not cured by transplantation. Diagnosis is difficult and often missed, even when biliary tract brush biopsies are performed during ERCP. Carcinoembryonic antigen, a marker for cholangiocarcinoma, occasionally uncovers an unsuspected lesion. Survival is poor and therefore is a contraindication.[14,15] Cholangiocarcinoma, when found incidentally in the resected specimen posttransplantation, also has a poor prognosis.[16] Only the occasional patient with localized disease benefits from transplantation, and survival of up to 2 years has been reported.[17] If transplantation is considered, then the extent of the disease must be defined by visualization of the duct by cholangiography (either transhepatic or endoscopic), sonography, and CAT scan.[18] Occasionally angiography is necessary.

In summary, final *clearance* for liver transplantation requires a CT scan to determine liver volume and detect intrahepatic lesions. A color Doppler (duplex) ultrasound study evaluates the portal and splenic venous systems. ERCP and/or transhepatic cholangiogram ensures that the bile ducts are normal and may be used for bile duct anastomoses. MRI, angiography, or venography are occasionally required to confirm or exclude the findings from other diagnostic techniques.

CARDIAC EVALUATION

The dramatic hemodynamic stresses that occur during transplantation, especially when the new liver is revascularized,[19] are well tolerated by most patients. However, to reduce operative cardiac morbidity and mortality, any patient who may have difficulty tolerating this stress has to be identified preoperatively.

Preoperative cardiac evaluation is obtained for all patients with cardiac symptoms, an abnormal cardiac examination, or multiple risk factors. Valvular heart disease, especially aortic stenosis, significantly increases the operative risk. We routinely perform a cardiac evaluation on all patients over 60 years of age. Patients who are older than 50 years and have a single risk factor, such as history of smoking, family history of heart disease, diabetes, or hypertension, will require the same tests.

All patients with alcoholic liver disease require studies of left ventricular functions to exclude cardiomyopathy. Similarly, patients with systemic diseases that are frequently associated with cardiac involvement, such as hemochromatosis, lupus erythematosus, and sarcoidosis, also require a detailed evaluation.

We request an exercise test and studies of left ventricular function, such as an echocardiogram or a gated blood pool. The standard treadmill test is acceptable, but if the patient has an abnormal electrocardiogram, left bundle branch block, left ventricular hypertrophy, or ST-T changes, a thallium treadmill test should also be performed. The persantin thallium test is reserved for patients who cannot adequately exercise because of ascites or generalized weakness.

PULMONARY EVALUATION

Abnormalities in pulmonary function are frequently present in patients with chronic liver disease. About 50% of nonsmokers and 75% of smokers had diffusion impairment. Widened alveolar-arterial oxygen gradient and ventilatory restriction is also frequent (45 and 25% of patients, respectively).[20] Both autoimmune liver disease and PBC are frequently associated with interstitial fibrosis and pulmonary hypertension.

Patients with possible lung disease require pulmonary function tests (PFTs). Blood gases are required in those patients who have hypoxemia secondary to shunting or PFTs that show evidence of impairment of diffusion capacity or obstructive disease. If arterial oxgen tension is <80 mmHg, and is not corrected by 100% O_2 breathing, further evaluation is necessary with lung biopsy and image intensified echo angiography.[21] Patients with primary pulmonary hypertension should have a lung biopsy in addition to cardiac catheterization to exclude vasculitis.

RENAL EVALUATION

Creatinine alone is an adequate indicator of satisfactory renal function in uncomplicated cases. In general, a serum creatinine >3 mg/dL is a contraindication for transplantation because of increased operative mortality.[22] In addition, a flat plate of the abdomen can be helpful, since small kidneys may suggest chronic renal disease. Patients with end-stage liver and kidney disease should be evaluated for simultaneous transplantation of both organs.[23]

Hepatorenal syndrome is thought to be reversible by transplantation;[24-26] therefore, higher creatinine levels are acceptable. Intrinsic renal disease may masquerade as hepatorenal syndrome. In these cases renal biopsy may be required to confirm the diagnosis.

CHRONIC INFECTIOUS DISEASES

PPD testing for tuberculosis is routinely performed. Individuals who are suspected of having tuberculosis on clinical or historical grounds have to be evaluated with cultures, including bone marrow, sputum, and ascitic fluid. BCG vaccination, common in many countries, results in positive PPD tests. Patients with active tuberculosis or proven recent convertors should be treated for tuberculosis for 12 months prior to transplant. If transplantation cannot be postponed, at least 2 months of therapy is considered adequate. Postoperatively all PPD positive patients (except those with BCG vaccinations), with or without active disease, will require treatment.

Chronic suppurative infections, such as osteomyelitis, infected stasis dermatitis, decubitus ulcer, and perirectal disease, should be controlled fully before transplantation. This may require antibiotic treatment and possible surgical intervention.

If the VDRL is positive and syphilis is confirmed by testing for antibody, treatment with antibiotics must be completed before transplant. Patients who have antibodies to human immunodeficiency virus (HIV) are excluded from transplantation in most centers, even in the absence of AIDS.[27,28]

Titers for markers of viral infections, CMV, EBV, toxoplasma, and varicella are obtained to help with the diagnosis of possible posttransplant complications, but no treatment is necessary before transplantation.

Fungal infections are treated before transplantation.

IMMUNITY TO INFECTIOUS DISEASES

Immunity to measles, mumps, and rubella is checked by determining serum levels of antibodies. If the candidate is not immune, vaccination has to be carried out with one dose of MMR vaccine. All patients receive recombinant vaccine for hepatitis B and pneumococcus. We also recommend polio (Salk, inactivated virus), diphtheria, and tetanus boosters. We are concerned about the live virus (Sabine) vaccine, because it causes postinoculation viral shedding which may be harmful to the other, immunosuppressed patients.

HEMATOLOGIC EVALUATION

There is a great individual variation in abnormalities of coagulation in patients with far advanced liver disease.[29] Decreased synthesis of factors II, V, VII, IX, and X and fibrinogen, and increase in fibrinolysis due to decreased synthesis of fibrinolysin inhibitors, occur with thrombocytopenia and platelet dysfunction. Disseminated intravascular coagulation, a late complication, is secondary to bleeding and is rarely a clinical problem prior to transplantation.

Where there are no special hematologic complications, PT, PTT, and platelet count are used as primary screening procedures and should be repeated immediately before surgery. If these tests are abnormal, more specific determinations, such as levels of factors V and VII, may be performed. These specific abnormalities are treated just before transplantation.

In special cases, such as the Budd-Chiari syndrome, hematologic consultation is always needed to evaluate those factors that determine the balance of clotting and fibrinolysis. Bone marrow biopsy, tests of platelet aggregation, determination of proteins S and C, cardiolipin, and bleeding time are required.

GASTROENTEROLOGIC EVALUATION

Endoscopic abnormalities are frequent in pretransplant patients. DeWeert et al.[30] found that 91% of their patients had an abnormal upper gastrointestinal endoscopy, with esophageal varices being the most common finding. Portal gastropathy was also frequent, followed by gastric varices, esophagitis, gastric ulcers, duodenal ulcer, and postsclerotherapy complications.

The etiology of any previous upper gastrointestinal bleeding should be confirmed. If esophageal varices are the source of the bleeding, sclerotherapy should be initiated or continued. Gastric varices do not respond to sclerotherapy, and attempts to sclerose them have frequently led to significant complications of bleeding and ulceration. Portal gastropathy is not treatable endoscopically, but it rarely causes life-threatening bleeding. Active peptic ulcer disease is not a contraindication for transplantation.

Patients with ulcerative colitis should have a recent surveillance colonoscopy to define activity and rule out neoplasia. Small-bowel x-rays are obtained for patients with perirectal disease to exclude granulomatous bowel disease.

Since posttransplant absorption of immunosuppressants is crucial for survival, suspicion of pancreatic and other malabsorption syndromes should be evaluated with fecal fat determinations and a D-xylose absorption test. If treatment is available for the cause of malnutriton, it should be initiated. If the malabsorption is not treatable, the immunosuppression regimen is modified. Many attempts were made to correlate nutritional status with the outcome of transplantation,[31] but nutritional evaluation has not generally been proven important.

CANCER SCREENING

Cancer screening is performed in all patients unless it was done recently. This includes all of the tests recommended by the American Cancer society; pap smear and mammogram for applicable age groups. In addition we recommend that a colonoscopy is performed in all persons who either have a positive fecal occult blood test or are age 45 or over.

SPECIAL CONSIDERATIONS FOR PRIMARY BILIARY CIRRHOSIS PATIENTS

Patients with PBC have increased incidence of breast cancer, and should be evaluated with mammography. If neoplasia is detected, transplantation must be delayed until definite therapy is completed.

Osteoporosis is frequent in PBC patients and is accelerated in the posttransplant period due to steroid therapy.[32] Since posttransplant fractures are related to the preexisting osteoporosis, a pretransplant evaluation should be performed and therapy initiated.

REFERENCES

1. Morton MJ, James EM, Wiesner RH, Krom RA: Applications of duplex ultrasonography in the liver transplant patient. *Mayo Clin Proc* 65:360–372, 1990.
2. Longley DG, Skolnick ML, Zajko AB, Bron KM: Duplex Doppler sonography in the evaluation of adult patients before and after liver transplantation. *Am J Roentgenol* 151:687–696, 1988.
3. Johansen K, Paun M: Duplex ultrasonography of the portal vein. *Surg Clin Am* 70:181–190, 1990.
4. Coire CI, Qizilbash AH, Castelli MF: Hepatic adenomata in type Ia glycogen storage disease. *Arch Pathol Lab Med* 111:166–169, 1987.
5. Langer R, Langer M, Neuhaus P, Scholz A, Felix R: Angiographic diagnosis in liver transplantation. I: Evaluation before transplantation. *Digitale-Bilddiagn* 10:62–66, 1990.
6. Finn JP, Edelman RR, Jenkins RL, et al: Liver transplantation: MR angiography with surgical validation. *Radiology* 179:265–269, 1991.
7. Weir MR, Henry ML, Blackmore M, et al: Incidence and morbidity of cytomegalovirus disease associated with a seronegative recipient receiving seropositive donor-specific transfusion and living-related donor transplantation. A multicenter evaluation. *Transplantation* 45:111–116, 1988.
8. Gorensek MJ, Carey WD, Vogt D, Goormastic M: A multivariate analysis of risk factors for cytomegalovirus infection in liver-transplant recipients. *Gastroenterology* 98:1326–1332, 1990.
9. Singh N, Dummer JS, Kusne S, et al: Infections with cytomegalovirus and other herpesviruses in 121 liver transplant recipients: transmission by donated organ and the effect of OKT3 antibodies. *J Infect Dis* 158:124–131, 1988.
10. Stratta RJ, Shaefer MS, Markin RS, et al: Clinical patterns of cytomegalovirus disease after liver transplantation. *Arch Surg* 124:1443–9, 1989.
11. Andorno E, Salizzoni M, Schieroni R, de Hemptinne B: Role of serum alphafetoprotein in pre- and post-orthotopic liver transplantation (OLT) for malignant disease. *J Nucl Med Allied Sci* 33:132–134, 1989.
12. Heiken JP, Weyman PJ, Lee JK, et al: Detection of focal hepatic masses: prospective evaluation with CT, delayed CT, CT during arterial portography, and MR imaging. *Radiology* 171:47–51, 1989.
13. Polson RJ, O'Grady JG, Williams R: Liver transplantation in the treatment of hepatic malignancy. *Baillieres Clin Gastroenterol* 1:171–182, 1987.
14. Ringe B, Wittekind C, Bechstein WO, Bunzendahl H, Pichlmayr R: The role of liver transplantation in hepatobiliary malignancy. A retrospective analysis of 95 patients with particular regard to tumor stage and recurrence. *Ann Surg* 209:88–98, 1989.
15. Ismail T, Angrisani L, Gunson BK, et al: Primary hepatic malignancy: the role of liver transplantation. *Br J Surg* 77:983–987, 1990.
16. Herbener T, Zajko AB, Koneru B, Bron KM, Campbell WL: Recurrent cholangiocarcinoma in the biliary tree after liver transplantation. *Radiology* 169:641–642, 1988.
17. Stieber AC, Marino IR, Iwatsuki S, Starzl TE: Cholangiocarcinoma in sclerosing cholangitis. The role of liver transplantation. *Int Surg* 74:1–3, 1989.

18. Wolff H, Ridwelski K, Lorf T: Surgical treatment of malignant tumor of the hepatic duct junction. *Zentralb Chir* 115:1–14, 1990.
19. Kalpokas M, Bookallil M, Sheil AG, Rickard KA: Physiological changes during liver transplantation. *Anaesth Intensive Care* 17:24–30, 1989.
20. Hourani JM, Bellamy PE, Tashkin DP, Batra P, Simmons MS: Pulmonary dysfunction in advanced liver disease: frequent occurrence of an abnormal diffusing capacity. *Am J Med* 90:693–700, 1991.
21. Krowka MJ, Tajik AJ, Dickson ER, Wiesner RH, Cortese DA: Intrapulmonary vascular dilatations (IPVD) in liver transplant candidates. Screening by two-dimensional contrast-enhanced echocardiography. *Chest* 97:1165–1170, 1990.
22. McCauley J, Van Thiel DH, Starzl TE, Puschett JB: Acute and chronic renal failure in liver transplantation. *Nephron* 55:121–128, 1990.
23. Gonwa TA, Nery JR, Husberg BS, Klintmalm GB: Simultaneous liver and renal transplantation in man. *Transplantation* 46:690–693, 1988.
24. Punukollu RC, Gopalswamy N: The hepatorenal syndrome. *Med Clin Am* 74:933–943, 1990.
25. Wood RP, Ellis D, Starzl TE: The reversal of the hepatorenal syndrome in four pediatric patients following successful orthotopic liver transplantation. *Ann Surg* 205:415–419, 1987.
26. Gonwa TA, Poplawski S, Paulsen W, et al: Hepatorenal syndrome and orthotopic liver transplantation. *Transplant Proc* 21:2419–2420, 1989.
27. Tzakis AG, Cooper MH, Dummer JS, Ragni M, Ward JW, Starzl TE: Transplantation in HIV+ patients. *Transplantation* 49:354–358, 1990.
28. Dummer JS, Erb S, Breinig MK, et al: Infection with human immunodeficiency virus in the Pittsburgh transplant population. A study of 583 donors and 1043 recipients, 1981–1986. *Transplantation* 47:134–140, 1989.
29. Ritter DM, Owen CA, Jr, Bowie EJ, et al: Evaluation of preoperative hematology-coagulation screening in liver transplantation. *Mayo Clin Proc* 64:216–223, 1989.
30. DeWeert TM, Gostout CJ, Wiesner RH: Congestive gastropathy and other upper endoscopic findings in 81 consecutive patients undergoing orthotopic liver transplantation. *Am J Gastroenterol* 85:573–576, 1990.
31. DiCecco SR, Wieners EJ, Wiesner RH, Southorn PA, Plevak DJ, Krom RA: Assessment of nutritional status of patients with end-stage liver disease undergoing liver transplantation. *Mayo Clin Proc* 64:95–102, 1989.
32. Maddrey WC: Bone disease in patients with primary biliary cirrhosis. *Prog Liver Dis* 9:537–554, 1990.

— 8 —

PSYCHIATRIC EVALUATION OF THE LIVER TRANSPLANT CANDIDATE

Stephen Snyder

For years, organ transplant teams have called on psychiatrists to assess the psychological health of candidates for organ transplantation.[1] One reason for the request is to help decide whether a given patient should be refused surgery "on psychological grounds," or is in need of psychiatric treatment in order to become an acceptable candidate. However, there are no clear guidelines regarding how such decisions should be made,[1] and there is remarkably little systematic research which might inform the clinical process.

Patients referred for psychiatric clearance pretransplantation commonly assume that the purpose of the evaluation is "to see whether I can stand the stress of the surgery." In fact, concerns about the perioperative period are relatively unimportant to the evaluating psychiatrist; a good general hospital psychiatrist can manage most acute difficulties occurring during the initial hospitalization. Instead, the psychiatrist's major concern is the potential for successful long-term medical management following transplantation. In our experience, it is useful to consider whether (1) any mental disorder is present that might interfere with treatment, (2) the general level of psychological function or any specific personality traits might be problematic, and (3) the home environment is adequate.

Mental disorders constitute a broad range. The most commonly seen DSM-III-R disorders in liver transplantation candidates may be the *organic mental disorders,* (delirium, dementia, etc.), *adjustment disorders,* and *substance-use disorders* (including alcohol dependence and abuse; see below).[2,3] Other relatively common mental disorders, which are occasionally present in transplantation candidates, include *schizophrenia, mood disorders* (major depression, bipolar disorder, and their variants) and *anxiety disorders* (such as panic disorder, obsessive–compulsive disorder, and posttraumatic stress disorder), as well as a variety of others, including the so-called personality disorders (e.g., borderline, antisocial, schizotypal personality disorder).[2] A detailed presentation of these various disorders is beyond the scope of this chapter. The medical clinician should recall, however, that psychiatric diagnosis is an uncertain art, and that errors are common even in the best of hands. The clinician should be wary of accepting psychiatric diagnoses to which patients may have been assigned by previous physicians.

Diagnosis of a mental disorder should not by itself disqualify a patient from transplantation. However, a careful assessment should be performed of the impact of the psychiatric disorder on the patient's level of psychological function. How has the patient dealt with the mental illness? Has the patient been able to obtain effective treatment and to comply with prescribed medication? Has the patient been able to preserve social and work function, and to keep the interest and affection of family and friends who can be of assistance posttransplant? Again, it is not the disorder itself, but the effect of the disorder on the patient's level of psychological function that is of concern. Two case examples of "dual-diagnosis" individuals with bipolar disorder and alcohol dependence should serve to illustrate this point:

Case 1: A nearby hospital sought to transfer a 51-year-old man with alcoholic cirrhosis and bipolar disorder for liver transplantation evaluation. He was intubated and markedly encephalopathic and could give no history. History was obtained by telephone from his private psychiatrist. Although the patient has responded in the past to lithium, his compliance had been poor, and he had had numerous mood episodes. Several times he had sought inpatient alcohol rehabilitation, but after discharge had always resumed drinking. He had been abstinent from alcohol since becoming ill 9 months previously. He was currently on disability and had been living with a girlfriend, with little other family involvement. In view of his history of poor impulse control and the difficult course of his bipolar disorder and alcohol dependence, he was judged not acceptable for transplantation, and transfer was denied.

Case 2: A 41-year old woman with alcoholic cirrhosis and bipolar disorder was referred for outpatient evaluation for liver transplantation. She had had an initial manic episode at age 31, and went on to have several more before becoming compliant with lithium at the age of 34. Since then, she had been seeing a private psychiatrist weekly and had been able to avoid further hospitalizations. Her psychiatrist was contacted, and confirmed that her compliance had been excellent. Since 34, she attended AA (Alcoholics Anonymous) 5 times per week. She had worked full time before adopting her 4-year-old daughter. She was currently living apart from her husband, and said she was considering divorce. The patient lived alone. The daughter was in the husband's care. Although the patient's bipolar disorder and alcohol dependence both appeared to be under control, concern was expressed to the patient about the stability of her home situation and adequacy of supports. She responded by bringing to her next visit several of her close friends and AA associates, all of whom pledged their support and commitment to her medical treatment. She was judged acceptable for transplantation.

A review of the patient's past behavior in work and social life will usually indicate whether there are any difficulties that might stand in the way of the candidate's being a successful transplant patient. Attributes necessary for successful function in health as well as in sickness include the following:

> *Self-care and planning:* Is the patient able to hold a job, pay rent, and take care of basic personal needs, or is he relatively helpless in these matters?
>
> *Communications skills:* Can the patient understand instructions and communicate difficulties when they occur?
>
> *Frustration tolerance:* Does the individual have the patience necessary to handle prolonged physical discomfort, or does he become easily enraged and seek impulsive solutions [such as demanding to sign out against medical advice (AMA), or substance abuse]?
>
> *Object constancy:* Can the patient tolerate the stress of frustrating experiences with staff (e.g., physician error or staff turnovers) and still preserve the treatment alliance, or does he become overwhelmed with anger, possibly expressed self-destructively (e.g., in medication noncompliance or other hostile–masochistic behavior)?
>
> *Honesty and responsibility:* Can the patient be trusted? Or is there a history of criminal behavior, lying, or avoidance of responsibility? (As in the DSM-III-R "antisocial personality disorder,"which has been identified in heart transplantation as a predictor of postoperative management difficulty.[4])

In our experience, maladaptive personality traits are likely to be a burden to the patient's family, to other supporting individuals, and to the transplantation staff. The decision to transplant a difficult patient should be made with the most information possible concerning areas of potential difficulty, and should involve preparatory discussion with the patient's family or other support network who will be called on to share the burden.

Another crucial ingredient for successful long-term medical management posttransplantation is the patient's home environment. Most patients are relatively disabled for many weeks following discharge. Ideally, there should be a stable home with concerned, involved helpers, to handle the additional stress. Patients occasionally present for evaluation with difficult home situations, such as chronic family fighting, divorce in progress, rebellious or drug-using children, or even domestic violence. Often patients' unspoken expectation is that once they receive the new organ they will be able to deal more effectively with the troublesome situation at home. We often tell such patients, "Imagine that you will be bringing a baby home," to emphasize that transplantation will at least initially bring with it further obligations and burdens rather than being a release from such burdens. Patients should attempt to settle acute family issues prior to transplantation.

A crisis situation is presented by the patient with fulminant hepatic failure due to a suicide attempt. The patient may be densely encephalopathic by the time the evaluation occurs. One such case admitted to our service was a schizophrenic woman in her 30s who presented in hepatic coma following acetaminophen ingestion. She had a history of serious suicide attempts every few years, but in between functioned at a stable level in a sheltered work situation and had been living on her own with close family contact. Most importantly, her family expressed a great willingness to be involved with her care. It was estimated, on the basis of her previous pattern, that if she survived she would be likely to recover from her acute psychiatric episode and have several years of reasonable function, although she would be likely to attempt suicide again. The decision was made to perform liver transplantation. However, she expired before this could be arranged.

ALCOHOLISM

A steady increase in alcoholic patients referred for liver transplantation has been noted in recent years,[5-8] and the issue of whether alcoholics should receive liver transplants has been hotly debated.[9-12] In 1988, Starzl and coworkers demonstrated a reasonable outcome in a cohort of 41 alcoholic cirrhosis patients transplanted since the introduction of cyclosporin.[7] The case for the feasibility of transplantation for alcoholic cirrhosis has since then been further strengthened by an additional report from the Pittsburgh group, in which a total of 73 alcoholic patients transplanted since 1982 were studied.[8] The calculated one-year survival rate was 74%, comparable to that for patients transplanted for nonalcoholic hepatocellular disease.[8] The evidence so far seems to be that a group of appropriately selected patients with alcoholic cirrhosis can achieve an outcome in terms of survival and quality of life equivalent to that of nonalcoholic patients with hepatocellular disease. Several questions of importance to transplantation of the alcoholic patient, though, remain largely unexplored. These include the issue of what are appropriate selection criteria for alcoholic patients, and when and how to provide alcoholism treatment.

Return to drinking has been shown to occur in some alcoholic patients after transplantation.[7,8,13] Kumar and coworkers, in their 1991 series of 73 patients transplanted for alcoholic liver disease, reported that 6 out of 52 patients surviving an average of 25 $\pm$ 9 months had returned to drinking, as assessed by telephone interviews with the patients, their spouses, and their physicians.[8] In 2 of 6 cases, patient and spouse both denied drinking but the physician had reason to believe that alcohol was being consumed. In all cases, consumption was estimated as "social" or as "moderate" (not more than three drinks per week). Of the 21 patients who had died after transplantation, one died of rejection in the setting of medication noncompliance and alcohol use.[8] In a British study, 18 patients surviving for at least 3 months after liver transplantation for alcoholic cirrhosis were evaluated. Four of the 18 patients (22.2%) showed "laboratory and clinical evidence of a return to heavy drinking."[13] Considering the above studies together, it appears that some recidivism is expectable posttransplantation, given the current state of sophistication in selecting alcoholic liver transplant candidates. The recidivism rate at any given center would be expected to vary depending on demographic characteristics of the applicant pool, selection criteria used, length of follow-up, and intensity of the rehabilitation effort.

There are no universally agreed-on criteria as to which alcoholic patients should be accepted or rejected for transplantation. Selection criteria may vary between centers, and none has been subjected to systematic study. The most controversial of possible selective criteria may be that of a "minimum period of abstinence" pretransplantation. Both the Pittsburgh group[7] and the University of Michigan group[5,6] have rejected the use of a minimum period of abstinence. However, Kumar and coworkers at Pittsburgh report that return to drinking was more common in patients abstinent less than 6 months than in those abstinent for longer periods.[8] Bird and coworkers in Britain found that 3 of 4 known recidivists posttransplant had been among those "not abstinent at the time of the transplant operation."[13] Although decreased survival for patients abstinent <6 months before transplantation has not been demonstrated,[8] results from the Pittsburgh and British groups are suggestive that nonabstinent and <6-months-abstinent patients are at higher risk for postoperative drinking. (Anecdotally, a particularly high-risk case is represented by the encephalopathic alcoholic patient for whom transplantation is sought by others, and whose own motivation may turn out to be poor. Two such cases reported by Starzl and coworkers ended in death, due at least in part to drinking and/or medication noncompliance.[7])

There are no general guidelines for when and how to provide alcoholism treatment for transplantation candidates or recipients. Starzl and coworkers have claimed that transplantation itself represents "the ultimate sobering experience."[7] However, with the accumulation of evidence that some alcoholic patients do in fact return to drinking after transplantation,[7,8,13] it seems that alcoholism treatment is indicated for at least selected patients. Our own thinking has been that transplantation may help promote abstinence only in patients whose character and supports are sufficient to help them translate fear into effective change. Not all patients are able to do this. Some demonstrate life patterns that are clearly self-destructive and that may be unchanged after transplantation (unpublished observations).

EVALUATION OF THE ALCOHOLIC CANDIDATE FOR LIVER TRANSPLANTATION

At the Mount Sinai Medical Center in New York City, our approach has been based, with certain modifications, on the work of Beresford and coworkers at the University of Michigan.[5,6] Evaluation is done on a case-by-case basis, along lines similar to those set out by the Michigan group,[6] with attention to (1) the alcohol-related psychiatric diagnosis, (2) the acceptance of this diagnosis by the patient and family, and (3) the degree of social stability and presence of certain other factors that have been shown to predict long-term abstinence in alcoholics.[6,14,15] An effort is made, where the risk of relapse or of treatment noncompliance is judged to be unacceptably high, to work with the applicants to strengthen their candidacy through alcohol rehabilitation and/or lifestyle change, and to reject candidates only if they are unwilling or unable to follow the team's recommendations.

Alcohol History and Diagnosis

An alcohol history is obtained, ideally with the patient and family together, in order to confirm a diagnosis of alcohol dependence or abuse. The DSM-III-R nomenclature of the American Psychiatric Association defines *alcohol dependence* in terms of inability to control drinking alcohol and a characteristic pattern of effects of drinking on the individual's life.[2] To qualify for the diagnosis of alcohol dependence, there must be at least one month for which the patient meets at least three out of nine specific criteria. These criteria cover such points as lack of control over the amount of alcohol consumed; interference with role responsibilities; alcohol consumption despite adverse consequences, tolerance and withdrawal; and a pattern wherein alcohol use dominates one's life to the detriment or exclusion of other interests. It is to be noted that the quantity one drinks does not define whether one meets the criteria for alcohol dependence. It is rather the presence of addictive signs and symptoms that makes the diagnosis.

Certain patients may consume significant quantities of alcohol and yet not show the pattern of addictive behavior required for the diagnosis of alcohol dependence. For these latter patients, the term "alcohol abuse" is used. These individuals show heavy but controlled use of alcohol, with some adverse consequences (the DSM-III-R lists specifically what qualifies as an adverse consequence), but without the addictive signs and symptoms of alcohol dependence.[2] It has been claimed that alcohol abuse is a more favorable prognostic category in terms of potential for achieving stable remission than is alcohol dependence.[6]

Although duration of abstinence does appear relevant to the risk of post-transplantation drinking,[8,13] we do *not* feel that patients who are only recently abstinent should be automatically excluded from consideration for transplantation. We do, however, generally require applicants who have been abstinent for <6 month to begin alcohol rehabilitation before transplantation can be considered. Referral is usually made to a local alcoholism treatment facility.

Acceptance by Patient and Family of the Alcohol-Related Psychiatric Diagnosis

In the case of alcohol dependence, we require the patient and family to be able not only to state a recognition of the diagnosis, but also to be able to demonstrate a knowledge of what this means, including the ongoing risk of relapse, the danger of rationalization and self-deception, and the necessity of continuous commitment to remission. In cases where there is denial of some of the implications of the diagnosis, or where the patient appears ignorant of the alcoholism concept, we require that the patient begin alcohol rehabilitation.

Social Stability and Other Predictive Factors

Following Beresford et al.,[6] we evaluate the current living situation with respect to the presence of a steady job, a stable residence, and the presence of a spouse or stable partner at home. In addition, four factors shown to be predictive of long-term remission are assessed: (1) a substitute dependency such as a hobby or Alcoholics Anonymous, (2) understanding of specific negative consequences of drinking, (3) discovery of an activity or interest that provides hope or self-esteem, and (4) an acceptance relationship.[6,14,15] Where these various attributes are significantly lacking [e.g., unemployed man living alone and idle in a SRO (single-room-occupancy) hotel since being evicted by his wife 3 months ago for alcohol-related behavior problems], a frank discussion is held with the applicant in which it is emphasized that relapse occurs commonly under such conditions and that the team requires a more adequate situation in order to ensure a good outcome. Social work involvement is frequently sought at this point to assist in whatever changes can be made.

In our opinion, various other features of the applicant's history or presenting behavior may have a bearing on the suitability for transplantation, and on whether to require alcohol rehabilitation before transplantation can be considered. These include a history of failed alcohol treatment and dependence on or abuse of multiple substances (e.g., alcohol and cocaine), "dual diagnosis" wherein alcoholism coexists with another mental disorder (as in cases 1 and 2 above), conflicting stories from family members concerning recent use, and hostile or uncooperative behavior by the patient during the evaluation. The patient's response to the team's recommendation of alcohol rehabilitation is also important: rationalizations and excuses are to be noted and confronted. One looks for the patient to demonstrate an ability to strive to initiate and maintain a commitment to alcoholism treatment.

A difficult situation occurs when a patient who may have been recently drinking presents encephalopathic or comatose and is in need of immediate transplantation. The evaluation in such cases relies on the interview with family members and previous medical-care providers. In cases such as case 1 above, transplantation may be contraindicated. In other cases, where social factors (such as job and family stability) are optimal and the family seems especially capable and committed, the team may elect to assume the risk and to proceed with transplantation.

OTHER SUBSTANCE-USE DISORDERS

No guidelines exist that might cover the tremendous range of situations posed by liver transplant patients with substance use disorders involving substances other than alcohol. Common sense, skepticism, and good psychiatric consultation are required. At the one extreme are individuals in midlife with stable careers and families, who during adolescence were briefly dependent on heroin or cocaine, and who have since been free of all addictive behavior for a decade or two. We have accepted such patients for transplantation without requiring additional drug rehabilitation. At the other extreme is the recent user in whom substance dependence is associated with considerable impairment of social and vocational life. We require many months of intensive drug rehabilitation before such an individual can be considered for transplantation. The long-term outcome in such cases is not known.

In our experience, methadone use is not a contraindication to liver transplantation, and continuing involvement in a methadone treatment program may be a positive factor in promoting recovery. However, we have seen patients in methadone treatment who abuse or are dependent on other substances such as alcohol and cocaine, and where this has gone undetected by the methadone program.

REFERENCES

1. House RM, Trzepacz PT, Thompson TL: Psychiatric consultation to organ transplant services. In Tasmàn A, Goldfinger SM, Kaufmann CA: *American Psychiatric Press Review of Psychiatry*, Vol. 9, pp 515–536, Washington, DC, American Psychiatric Press, 1990.
2. American Psychiatric Association: *Diagnostic and Statistical Manual*, 3d ed., rev. Washington, DC, American Psychiatric Association, 1987.
3. Trzepacz PT, Brenner R, VanThiel DH, et al: Psychopathology in heart transplant candidates. *J Heart Transplant* 7:223–226, 1988.
4. Frierson RL, Lippmann SB: Heart transplant candidates rejected on psychiatric indications. *Psychosomatics* 28:347–355, 1987.
5. Lucey MR, Merion RM, Henley KS, et al: Selection of patients with alcoholic liver disease for orthotopic liver transplantation. *Hepatology* 10:572 (abstr), 1989.
6. Beresford TP, Turcott JG, Merion R, et al: A rational approach to liver transplantation for the alcoholic patient. *Psychosomatics* 31:241–254, 1990.
7. Starzl TE, Van Thiel D, Tzakis AG, et al: Orthotopic liver transplantation for alcoholic cirrhosis. *JAMA* 260:2542–2544, 1988.
8. Kumar S, Stauber RE, Gavaler JS, et al: Orthotopic liver transplantation for alcoholic liver disease. *Hepatology* 11:159–164, 1990.
9. Moss AH, Siegler M: Should alcoholics compete equally for liver transplantation:? *JAMA* 265:1295–1298, 1991.
10. Cohen C, Benjamin M: Alcoholics and liver transplantation. *JAMA* 265:1299–1301, 1991.
11. Atterbury CE: The alcoholic in the lifeboat: Should drinkers be candidates for liver transplantation? *J Clin Gastroenterol* 8:1–4, 1986.
12. Flavin DK, Niven RG, Kelsey JE: Alcoholism and orthotopic liver transplantation. *JAMA* 259:1546–1547, 1988.
13. Bird GLA, O'Grady JG, Harvey FAH, et al: Life transplantation in patients with alcoholic cirrhosis: selection criteria and rates of survival and relapse. *Br Med J* 301:15–17, 1990.
14. Vaillant GE, Clark W, Cyrus C, et al: Prospective study of alcoholism treatment: eight year followup. *Am J Med* 75:455–463, 1983.
15. Vaillant GE: *The Natural History of Alcoholism*. Cambridge, MA, Harvard University Press, 1983.

—9—

SOCIAL EVALUATION OF THE TRANSPLANT CANDIDATE

Juan Prieto

Liver transplantation is the only definitive treatment of end-stage liver disease. The majority of the patients are adults over 40 years of age with many different types of liver disease. Most of the patients have been sick for years and view transplant as a miracle. However, as patients realize the delicate nature of a transplant and its risks, they become appropriately fearful and begin to question the anticipated quality of life postoperatively.

The liver transplant program at The Mount Sinai Medical Center in New York City has performed over 300 liver transplants and evaluates approximately 10 new candidates weekly. The evaluation process is a complex one involving many different disciplines. On the completion of the evaluation, the data and results are examined carefully and a recommendation is made for or against transplantation. During this period, most patients are anxious and fearful of the committee's decision. As mentioned previously, liver transplant, in many cases, is the only cure to their end-stage liver disease, and this is known to most patients. One can imagine the impact that this 2–3 week evaluation has on the lives of the patients and the relief that patients feel on acceptance of their candidacy. However, this relief progressively diminishes as the waiting time for transplant increases and the deterioration of their condition accelerates. Moreover, as the prospect of transplantation becomes a reality, their concerns about family, employment, leisure, and life as a whole become magnified.

The initial psychosocial evaluation occurs during the patient's first visit to the clinic. However, the assessment is an ongoing process that is dictated by the changes in the candidate's lifestyle and medical condition. The social worker will follow the transplant patient from the evaluation period for suitability for transplant and make psychosocial assessments of the patients and family's social, financial, and environmental supports.

A careful psychosocial evaluation can allow for the development of the patient's and family's coping skills. This assessment enables data to be analyzed and synthesized into a working plan. One must look closely at the nature of the patient's concerns and problems and the role they and others play in the evaluation process. The social worker should carefully seek out the patient's (1) strengths, deficiencies, and limitations; (2) personality assets; (3) motivation to resolve problems, (4) resources available to resolve problems; and (5) the environmental factors that contribute to the patient's concerns and problems that need further investigation.

In order to formulate potential areas of intervention, a careful assessment should commence with a complete evaluation of the patient's history, including medical and family backgrounds. This is the starting place of a knowledge base for formulating potential strategies of intervention. The social worker should carefully examine and investigate the patient and family history for alcohol, drug use, and psychiatric illness. Attention should also be focused on the patient's cultural and ethnic background.

Information about the patient is obtained through different ports. The examination of a background or face sheet prepared by the patient, verbal reports of the patient, direct observation of nonverbal behavior, interaction between spouse, friends, or other family members are some of the way information is gathered. Collateral information from friends, physicians, and nurses adds to the fund of information. The multiple sources of information eliminate any bias that the patient alone may present, especially if the patient's liver disease is complicated by encephalopathy. It is of vital importance that the information obtained is as accurate as possible and that a trust develops between patient and staff. Every patient must be thoroughly evaluated so that unfortunate events resulting from misunderstandings are avoided in the pre- and postoperative period.

Appreciating the patient's and family's history is important in determining interventional techniques and assists in determining the patient's motivation and compliance. Language barriers can distort the information, and cultural and ethnic biases must be taken into account to make valid judgments. The patient and family must understand the nature of the candidate's illness and, if it is related to alcohol or drug use, must be aware that compliance will be an issue relevant to their acceptance as a candidate.

A complete family history can also serve to explore strengths and weaknesses in both families and patients. The level of potential support is defined and helps the worker assist patients in developing coping strategies. One should also pay attention to the work history of the patient and family. This serves as a guideline in determining insurance concerns as well as anticipating future issues such as disability, loss of income, and returning to employment.

As one examines patients' knowledge and perception of their medical condition, one appreciates that those who have a clear understanding are usually fearful of the prognosis. Additional education and support is required for those who have only limited understanding of their condition. The reaction of their illness usually fluctuates given the length of illness. Their feelings are normally one of hopelessness and fear. Many of the patients we see have been ill for many years and the type of medical treatment they have received has not been successful. Patients become discouraged and in many instances pessimistic about their future.

At this point one should explore the motivation and strength of the patient. A careful analysis allows the worker to tap the patient's strengths effectively. Most patients unknowingly have developed certain strengths and coping skills that have assisted in their continued struggle with their illness. A skilled social worker's assessment should identify these strengths and skills. Those strengths that they bring to coping need to be supported. The development of their defense mechanisms and coping skills help the team develop appropriate levels of interventions and help in the tapping of key figures in the patients supportive structure.

During the assessment process, the social worker needs to investigate the patient and family's perception of the transplant. One must allow the patient to openly engage in the discussion of future expectations and how they view themselves 1–5 years postoperatively. This assists the worker in determining the patient's level of optimism and motivation. One's perception of one's future is an important piece of the assessment in that it allows one to discuss some of one's fears with the worker as well. Many patients at this stage are concerned about the well-being of their family and will discuss issues of death, disability, sexual performance and financial hardships. The underlying theme that these fears symbolize is that of maintaining identity and dignity as an independent human being who is capable of working, living, and accomplishing life's goals. The ability to verbalize these fears and plan strategies for coping with possible losses is often helpful providing the patient and family with a game plan. The discussion of negative issues and helping the patient and family to plan for the worst allows them to see that most issues can be dealt with. It is important not to give false hope, but instead to allow the ventilation of their fears. Moreover, it again allows for the formulation of strengths that can be very useful in the future.

These discussions help patients verbalize anticipated problems. It also allows for discussing future expectations of the physical effects of the transplant. This stage usually helps the patient and family discuss personal concerns such as pain (physical and emotional) more openly. The information and understanding that the patients and families have can now be assessed. Continued education and information allays the patient's and family's anxiety and should be repeated, reinforced, and clarified. The members of the team need to be consistent and provide the same general information. Each discipline concentrates on a different aspect of the patient's social and emotional needs.

Motivation should be discussed with the patients. The level of motivation present helps one determine the effects of psychosocial stresses and how a social worker can effectively assist patients with their strengths. The assessment process can also serve as a means of observing levels of depression in patients. Moreover, issues of compliance can evolve as one assesses a patient's motivation. For example, lack of motivation is a clear sign of depression; therefore, assessing the motivation of patients is extremely important in locating potential difficulties. The anxiety and fear of transplantation, in many cases, obstructs the patient's strength and coping skills. Evaluating the level of motivation can help assist the social worker in bringing out coping skills of which the patient may not have been aware. Patients who lack motivation may pose compliance problems in the future. However, a careful assessment must look at what may be causing the lack of motivation (depression, fear, lack of information, etc.). Finally, a patient's motivation to live serves as a major coping skill. In an alcoholic patient this can greatly reinforce abstinence from alcohol. Therefore, assessing compliance is critical.

Investigating past and present problems requires an interdisciplinary approach to establish the patient's past behavior patterns. Speaking to a patient's physician, employer, and family is crucial in predicting their compliance. Families play an integral part in a patient's coping process both pre- and postoperatively, and a strong supportive network helps improve a patient's compliance. It also assists the interviewer in making a thorough assessment and improving the quality of future interventions. Moreover, as patients become sicker, one must rely on the input of family. Noncompliant patterns can be changed by the social worker; for instance, the alcoholic can be referred for rehabilitation.

One must carefully determine the level of noncompliance and the future implications it will have on the patient, staff, and society. The scarcity of organs makes this prediction important. The staff has a responsibility not only to the patients, but also to society. A patient's noncompliance with medications, alcohol, and postoperative care can have a detrimental effect on their prognosis. Noncompliance has not only medical but ethical ramifications.

Family relationships and roles are evaluated closely since understanding how families function can help to increase the staff's effectiveness in dealing with the difficulties the patient faces. It is the responsibility of the staff to make contact with the families and seek strengths to use in the helping process. The assessment of family roles examines the patient's available emotional support. Who will assist the patient if on discharge from the hospital that person cannot meet the normal activities of daily living (ADLs)? The role of family members needs to be identified, and those family members need to be aware of potential difficulties. Family members are also faced with difficulties, especially stress, which makes their emotional and physical health in need of attention. Further evaluation is needed to identify individuals to support the family members. Otherwise, who will be there to assist the patient in need of support?

Finally, the financial responsibility of a family needs special attention. Questions of disability, employment, insurance, and the roles of family members or friends who can financially assist with these important needs should be explored carefully.

Insurance concerns become a very important part of the evaluation process. A social worker's evaluation needs to include all of the above and also the long-term ramifications of their health insurance policy. One must not only inquire about what type of health insurance the patients have, but also what the particular policy covers. Even a policy that seems to provide adequate coverage, may pose important issues to be concerned with in the future. One must research any time limits that an insurance policy may have. In many cases, insurance coverage have limits on the time a patient can be out of work and continue to be covered. Many health insurance policies have maximum limits in their coverage and other exclusions (e.g., no medication or outpatient coverage). In some cases, lack of satisfactory medical insurance may prevent the patient from receiving adequate posttransplant care. Most patients are unable to meet the cost of the necessary medications and outpatient care out of their own funds. Moreover, if the patient cannot qualify for government assistance due to their rigid guidelines, the ability to receive a transplant becomes impossible. Without good outpatient follow up care and the crucial medications required, a patient cannot expect to survive postoperatively.

Some recently issued life insurance policies may cover transplantation and to a certain extent posttransplant medical care as well. Other issues of great importance in a resource assessment include availability of housing and the ability to afford rent or mortgage payments with a reduced income if the patient becomes less productive or disabled postoperatively. One should therefore investigate financial resources and supports as well as community and environmental resources available to assist the patient pre- and postoperatively. The utilization of volunteer services of previous liver transplant patients is particularly beneficial. Moreover, support groups provide an essential part in coping with the transplant process. This outreach plan helps patients realize that they can be independent functioning individuals and not a lifelong burden to their families and society.

REFERENCES

1. Williams JW, Vera S, Evans LS: Socioeconomic aspects of hepatic transplantation. *Am J Gastroenterol* 82:1115–1119, 1987.
2. Heyink J, Tymstra T, Slooff MJ, Klompmaker I: Liver transplantation—psychosocial problems following the operation. *Transplantation* 49:1018–1019, 1990.
3. Schweizer RT, Rovelli M, Palmeri, D, Vossler E, Hull D, Bartus S: Noncompliance in organ transplant recipients. *Transplantation* 49:374–377, 1990.
4. Tarter RE, Erb S, Biller PA, Switala J, Van Thiel DH: The quality of life following liver transplantation: a preliminary report. *Gastroenterol Clin N Am* 17:207–217, 1988.
5. Kober B, Kuchler T, Boelsch C, Kremer B, Henne Bruns D: A psychological support concept and quality of life research in a liver transplantation program: an interdisciplinary multicenter study. *Psychother-Psychosom* 54:117–131, 1990.

—10—

MEDICAL AND SURGICAL MANAGEMENT OF THE CANDIDATE FOR LIVER TRANSPLANTATION

Eliezer Katz and Audrey H. Schwersenz

The relative shortage of donor livers has made the term "waiting list" a reality in the daily life of the patient with end-stage liver disease who has been accepted as a candidate for liver transplantation.

In our experience of 250 patients, the mean waiting time between placement on the waiting list and liver transplantation ranges from 3 to 6 months, depending on the blood type of the patient. The amount of time spent on the waiting list is in part dependent on the patient's clinical stability. Deterioration and occasionally improvement in the patient's clinical condition are important considerations for the transplant center in defining the urgency for transplant and making appropriate changes in status.

Continuous deterioration in clinical status, however, is usually the rule in patients with cirrhosis, regardless of the etiology of their liver disease. Mortality (10–15%) and morbidity on the waiting list is therefore the unfortunate experience of all large transplant centers.

The main factor that can reduce waiting list mortality is an increase in the availability of donor livers. While the donor "pool" has been increased somewhat by the use of relatively new techniques, such as living-related donors and reduced-sized grafts, there is no indication that a significant change will occur in the near future.

Given this reality close follow-up, a high index of alertness to any changes in the patient's condition that might alter that person's waiting list status, knowledge and ability to treat the unique complications of end-stage liver disease in the patient awaiting transplant, and close communication with the transplant center are imperative to reduce the morbidity and mortality on the waiting list.

This chapter covers the practical aspects of management in the pretransplant period. Treatment options are discussed that take into account the forthcoming transplant. Emphasis is placed on changes in the patient's clinical condition that may alter that individual's waiting list status. In addition changes in the patient's general medical condition are monitored to ensure that the patient is still a candidate for liver transplantation.

GASTROINTESTINAL BLEEDING IN THE CIRRHOTIC PATIENT

Although the major bleeding complications in the patient with end-stage liver disease are due to portal hypertension, gastrointestinal bleeding from other sources may occur as well. Bleeding is exacerbated by the underlying coagulopathy in these patients, due to hypersplenism and impaired hepatic synthesis of clotting factors. This section discusses the management of both variceal and nonvariceal gastrointestinal hemorrhage in the transplant candidate, both of which carry significant morbidity and mortality.

Variceal Bleeding

Varices are collateral vessels that form in an effort to decompress the portal system. These portosystemic communications occur at multiple sites. *Esophageal varices* have the highest predilection for bleeding; in part this is due to their location in the lamina propria, which provides weak stromal support.[4] Bleeding from a varix occurs when the portal pressure >12 mmHg,[5] and therefore may be precipitated by rapid blood volume expansion or angiography.[6,7] *Gastric varices* are generally classified into two distinct groups: *junctional* (gastroesophageal), which are basically continuations of esophageal varices; and *isolated,* which are usually fundal in location but may occur anywhere in the stomach.[8,9] Fundal varices are difficult to identify endoscopically because they are camouflaged by the surrounding gastric folds. Bleeding from gastric varices is less frequent than esophageal varices but can be more torrential and carries a higher mortality.[10] *Intestinal varices* may occur anywhere along the GI tract as a consequence of portal hypertension. These varices rarely bleed, but are very difficult to control without surgical intervention when they do.[11] Bleeding from *stomal varices* is an unusual but well-recognized complication of portal hypertension in patients who have intestinal stomas.[12-14] These include patients with sclerosing cholangitis and ulcerative colitis who have undergone colectomy, or infants who have had Kasai procedures for biliary atresia including exteriorization of the jejunal loop. Mortality from bleeding is 3–4%[15] which is considerably lower than the mortality from gastroesophageal hemorrhage. Bluish discoloration of the skin at the site of the stoma and an ileostomy caput medusae are rarely seen, but herald the presence of such varices.[14] The majority of patients (74%) will have esophageal varices as well.[16] Local trauma and spontaneous erosion usually precipitate hemorrhage.[1,17] *Hemorrhoidal varices* are common in these patients, as part of the venous portosystemic shunting system.[18]

Management of Bleeding Esophageal Varices

The rupture of esophageal varices is perhaps one of the most dramatic complications of portal hypertension. Approximately one-third of all patients with established esophageal varices will bleed, and the mortality after each episode of variceal hemorrhage can be as high as 50%.[1-3] A nonsurgical approach is paramount in the treatment of variceal hemorrhage in the pretransplant patient. In some centers failure to respond to medical management may be an indication for urgent transplantation.

Endoscopic sclerotherapy is the safest and most effective treatment modality for actively bleeding varices or esophageal varices that have recently bled.[19] It can be performed locally, without transferring the patient to the transplant center. Nevertheless, the transplant center should be notified so that the patient's status can be updated. If sclerotherapy is successful in controlling the initial bleeding event, it should be repeated a week later and continued at 4-week intervals,[24,25] with the goal of obliterating the esophageal varices completely.

Although new endoscopic approaches to the treatment of esophageal varices exist, such as rubber-band ligation[26] and laser therapy,[27] we feel that experience is limited with these techniques in the management of the acutely bleeding transplant candidate at the current time.

Beta blockade using propranolol or nadolol (which is not metabolized in the liver) seems to have some effect in preventing recurrences of bleeding from esophageal varices, via reduction in gastroesophageal collateral blood flow. It may be effective for prevention of initial bleeding episodes as well.[28] It should *not* be used at the time of an acute bleed since its effects may diminish the patient's ability to tolerate acute blood loss. *Vasopressin* is an appropriate pharmacologic treatment for the acutely bleeding patient who has not responded to sclerotherapy.[29] It can be given at infusion rate of 0.2–0.8 unit/min or as a bolus (20 units over 20 min). Combined use with a *nitroglycerin* infusion of 40–400 μg/min may ameliorate some of the deleterious effects of the drug (limb ischemia, myocardial ischemia, bowel necrosis).[30,30a] *Somatostatin* has been shown to decrease portal blood flow and lower portal pressure via splanchnic vasoconstriction with minimal side effects, but its clinical usefulness is not yet established.[30a] *Antacid therapies* have not been shown to reduce the incidence of bleeding from variceal hemorrhage.[31]

If a combination of pharmacological therapy and sclerotherapy fails to control bleeding, then *balloon tamponade* using a Sengstaken-Blakemore tube should be applied, and the transplant center must be notified emergently. Tamponade stops bleeding in about 78% of cases.[32-34] Since this method has no long-term therapeutic effect and has a high rebleeding rate (42%),[32-34] it should be used only to stabilize the patient while arranging immediate transfer to the transplant center. Tamponade carries a high complication rate, including aspiration, ulceration, airway obstruction, and esophageal rupture.[35,36] Airway protection should be strongly considered in patients needing this type of therapy. Once transferred the patient will be put on the UNOS stat list for transplantation, and will usually receive a transplant within 48 hr.[37]

For an acutely bleeding patient who is retractory to medical management and not hemodynamically stable for safe transfer, surgical treatment of the acute variceal bleeding may be the only option. The specific method used generally will not affect the ability to perform liver transplantation. The relatively short time interval between the two operations should eliminate the technical difficulties that usually are encountered when performing a transplant in a patient who previously underwent elective surgical treatment for variceal bleeding.[38] The surgical approach to bleeding esophageal varices is based on two different principles: portosystemic shunting and devascularization. *Decompression of the portal system* via portosystemic shunting results in a decrease in portal pressure and therefore a decrease in the flow and pressure in the esophageal venous collaterals. Operations based on this principal include the classic portocaval shunt, the mesocaval shunt, and the more recent splenorenal (proximal and distal) shunt. The *portocaval shunt* can be used in the acute setting, although the dissection of the hilum of the liver in these patients can be difficult and bloody. The *H-mesocaval shunt* is easier to perform, effectively controls the bleeding, and is preferred to the portocaval shunt.[38,39] The *splenorenal shunts,* distal or proximal, are also effective for decompressing the portal system. These operations require optimal conditions and more time than are usually present in the acute situation, but they can be used. Of the two, the distal splenorenal is more physiologic and does not require splenectomy. *Devascularization of the venous system* that feeds the esophageal varices will also control acute variceal bleeding.[40] This is best accomplished by *transection of the esophagus,* with ligation of the short gastric vessels as well as the coronary vein. Sugiura has described this operation in detail.[41]

Recently, a new invasive radiologic shunting technique was developed as an alternative to the various surgical methods.[42] This technique consists of percutaneous catherization of the right hepatic vein through the jugular vein. Using a needle, a connection is established between a hepatic vein and a portal vein and a large stent is introduced that establishes an *intrahepatic portosystemic shunt.* So far, a fairly high early success rate has been reported (>90%), although the follow-up period is short (9 months). If these results are confirmed in further clinical trials, then it may be the treatment of choice for uncontrolled variceal bleeding in the patient awaiting liver transplantation. Since this method is nonsurgical and entirely intrahepatic, it will create no difficulties in performing the planned liver transplant surgery.

Elective surgical treatment for variceal bleeding has its place in the patient who is *not* considered a candidate for liver transplantation, but has no role in the patient who is on the active list awaiting liver transplantation.[43,44] Not only do these operations create problems for future liver transplantation, but these patients, who generally have Child's B or C liver disease, suffer a morbidity and mortality from the surgical treatment of variceal hemorrhage that far exceeds the morbidity and mortality from liver transplantation.[43,44]

Management of Gastric Variceal Hemorrhage

While junctional gastric varices may be amenable to endoscopic sclerotherapy, fundal varices are not, and bleeding from these varices may require the same approach applied to variceal bleeding uncontrolled by sclerotherapy.[45] Balloon tamponade can be used for junctional varices; success is higher with the Linton-Nachalas tube compared with the Sengstaken-Blakemore tube.[46] Bleeding from either class of gastric varices carries a higher morbidity and mortality[8] than does hemorrhage from esophageal varices. Therefore, uncontrolled bleeding of gastric varices needs to be approached aggressively by either emergency transplantation or a surgical shunting procedure followed by liver transplantation.

Management of Stomal and Hemorrhoidal Varices

Few nonsurgical treatment options are successful in treating bleeding stomal varices. Sclerotherapy has been performed, but it requires multiple injections and carries a high incidence of rebleeding.[47] Percutaneous transhepatic embolization of varices has been the most successful at controlling bleeding[48] and may provide the best nonsurgical option in the pre–liver transplant patient. If these approaches are unsuccessful, then the transplant center should be notified emergently so that the patient can be transferred to undergo urgent liver transplant. Surgical approaches, such as bowel resection, variceal ligation, stomal revision, and portosystemic shunting, should not be attempted prior to discussion with the transplant team. Liver transplantation is probably the best surgical option.

Whenever liver transplantation is performed on a patient with a history of stomal bleeding, exploration of the abdomen at the time of transplant is mandatory in an attempt to localize the site of the varices and to free and divide any adhesions that may contribute to the development of the varices. In our experience, a patient with stomal varices continued to bleed in the immediate post-transplant period. At exploration an adhesion band was found that was obstructing the drainage of a large varix.

Elective surgical treatment for hemorrhoidal varices should not be performed on patients on the waiting list for liver transplantation. In rare cases of significant bleeding, limited procedures should be used for control of the bleeding. Usually this type of bleeding is easily controlled, and will not affect the status of the patient.

Nonvariceal Gastrointestinal Hemorrhage

Not all episodes of gastrointestinal bleeding are due to varices. Nonvariceal upper GI hemorrhage is a significant source of morbidity in cirrhotic patients, although mortality is rare. A esophagogastroduodenoscopy is indicated in all cirrhotic patients with upper GI bleeding even if there is a known history of esophageal varices to exclude gastritis, portal gastropathy, esophageal tears, or duodenal ulcers.

Portal hypertensive gastropathy or congestive gastropathy is now recognized as a distinct entity in patients with portal hypertension[49] and is a significant source of upper GI bleeding in cirrhotic patients but is rarely associated with mortality.[50] The pathophysiology is poorly understood. A typical "mosaic pattern" is seen on endoscopy, consisting of erythematous areas outlined by a subtle yellowish network, or diffuse hyperemia or "red spots" if the gastropathy is more severe.[51] These changes are more frequently seen in the fundus, but may be seen in the antrum as well. The histology usually shows dilatation of the capillaries and venous congestion in the gastric mucosa.[52] There may be an associated mucositis, due to increased susceptibility of the mucosa to injury from noxious agents, such as aspirin, bile, acid, and alcohol.[53-55] Helicobacter Pylori infection is not associated with this lesion.[56] There is no specific medical treatment for portal hypertensive gastropathy; however, propranolol appears to be successful in preventing or reducing rebleeding episodes,[50] and H_2 antagonists probably protect against the mucosal inflammation. Gastrectomy, the definitive treatment for congestive gastropathy, should not be used in a patient awaiting liver transplantation.

Duodenal ulcers occur 10 times more commonly in patients with cirrhosis than their age-matched counterparts, perhaps because of failure to metabolize circulating gastrointestinal hormones.[57] H_2 blockers can be used in these patients to prevent the significant bleeding that may occur. Again, avoidance of surgical intervention is recommended, although persistent and severe bleeding may require surgical control followed by prompt liver transplantation. Other sources of bleeding, such as *Mallory-Weiss tears,* or *acute gastritis,* should alert the medical team to the possibility of alcohol recidivism in the patient with alcoholic cirrhosis. *Erosive esophagitis* due to gastroesophageal reflux disease in the cirrhotic patient with ascites may be responsible for a small percentage of bleeding episodes. Lower gastrointestinal hemorrhage may also be an important cause of morbidity in the cirrhotic patient. Patients with autoimmune hepatitis and sclerosing cholangitis may have preexisting inflammatory bowel disease; *colitis* activity may appear worse due to the presence of coagulopathy. "*Portal colopathy*" has recently been reported.[58] It is similar to portal gastropathy, and presumably shares the same pathophysiologic mechanism.

In summary, variceal hemorrhage is a life-threatening event in the cirrhotic patient. Esophageal varices are the most likely to rupture, but they are amenable to some nonsurgical remedies, including endoscopic sclerotherapy. Variceal hemorrhage that is not controlled with supportive measures or sclerotherapy may indicate the urgent need for liver transplantation. Surgical approaches should not be attempted without discussion with the transplant team, since mortality is high and ability to perform successful transplantation subsequently is reduced. In certain instances, a temporizing surgical procedure may be required to control bleeding, while awaiting an appropriate organ donor.

Nonvariceal gastrointestinal bleeding can also be a significant source of morbidity for the patient with end-stage liver disease because of the coexistence of coagulopathy and thrombocytopenia. Nonvariceal hemorrhage is rarely an indication to raise the priority of the patient on the waiting list. However, in cases of persistent bleeding not responsive to medical management and supportive care, liver transplantation should be considered before attempting other surgical procedures.

ASCITES AND HERNIAS

The management of ascites and electrolyte abnormalities in the pre–liver transplant patient can be both challenging and frustrating for the medical team. Overaggressive removal of fluid may lead to hyponatremia, hypovolemia, and renal failure. On the other hand, fluid overload is often a complication of medical management, when volume expansion is needed to treat other conditions such as sepsis or hemorrhage. Intractable ascites may predispose to complications and can become an indication to reevaluate the patient for earlier transplantation.

Portal hypertension, hypoalbuminemia, and sodium retention all contribute to the development of ascites in the patient with end-stage liver disease.[59,60] Hypoalbuminemia may be due to decreased synthetic function of the failing liver, poor nutrition, or both.[60] A sodium-retentive state is usually present in cirrhotic patients despite the presence of hyponatremia. Controversy still exists as to whether the sodium retention is a primary event or due to a decrease in "effective" plasma volume[61] or increased aldosterone[62,63] activity.

The presence of mild ascites is not necessarily an indication for treatment, especially as it is nearly impossible to eliminate all of the ascitic fluid and treatment carries inherent risks. Treatment is indicated when massive ascites leads to respiratory difficulty or severe discomfort or anorexia. The increased intraabdominal pressure caused by ascites may cause intractable gastroesophageal reflux, but this does not increase the risk of hemorrhage from esophageal varices.[63,64] Abdominal wall hernias may develop as a complication of severe ascites; rupture of an umbilical hernia is an unusual complication.[65]

Management of Ascites

The goal of the medical management of ascites in the pretransplant period is to temporize, since transplantation will eliminate the ascites. In addition to salt and water restriction, *diuretic therapy* should be aimed at reducing fluid overload without compromising systemic blood pressure or causing severe electrolyte abnormalities and renal failure. A reduction of fluid by one pound per day is a relatively safe goal[67] in the hospitalized patient.

Ascites and fluid overload in the hospital may sometimes be iatrogenic. Efforts should be made to reduce the free water given with medications. In addition, many systemic antibiotics have a high sodium content, and this should be considered when attempting salt restriction in the patient. Severe water restriction is reserved for profound hyponatremia.[66]

Refractory ascites may be due to noncompliance, or failure to provide adequate diuretics. Effective diuretic therapy can be determined by measuring the urine Na:K (sodium/potassium) ratio, which should be >1.[72]

Paracentesis is an effective technique for eliminating excess salt and water from the patient with massive ascites who has failed diuretic therapy. Coagulopathy is *not* a contraindication to paracentesis, as the risk of bleeding is only 1%.[68] Large-volume paracentesis (4–6 L of ascitic fluid per day) has recently regained popularity but should always be accompanied by albumin infusion (at a dose of 40 g after each paracentesis) to maintain circulating blood volume.[69] Because of the scarcity and expense of albumin, other plasma volume expanders, such as Dextran-70[70] and hemaccel,[71] have been tried with success, but with some evidence of compromise of systemic vascular resistance.

As mentioned briefly, even the most modest approaches to ascites management are fraught with potential hazards. The most serious risk posed by overaggressive diuresis or large-volume paracentesis is the precipitation of hepatorenal syndrome or hepatic encephalopathy,[72] due to the large compartmental shifts of fluid, the decrease in intravascular volume, and the alteration in electrolyte composition. Less dramatic complications include malnutrition from excessive dietary restrictions; electrolyte disturbances such as hypokalemia, hyponatremia, and hypocalcemia; and the risk of introducing peritoneal infection during paracentesis, rendering the patient temporarily ineligible for transplantation.

Peritoneovenous shunting also carries a high mortality (10–18%),[73,74] and these shunting procedures probably have few advantages over large-volume paracentesis.[75] For this reason, the patient on the waiting list with intractable ascites should be considered first for earlier transplant, rather than a surgical procedure.

Portosystemic shunting for ascites is almost never justified in the pretransplant patient because of the high morbidity and mortality that ensues. Nevertheless, there are exceptions to this rule. Patients who have intractable ascites disproportionate to the degree of liver dysfunction (e.g., patients with Budd-Chiari Syndrome) in whom transplantation may be quite a few months away may benefit from a shunting procedure.

Surgical Management of Abdominal Wall Hernias in Patients with Ascites

Abdominal wall hernias, commonly umbilical or incisional, occur frequently in patients with end-stage liver disease and tense ascites. Reducing the quantity of ascites via optimal medical management will reduce the intraabdominal pressure, and hopefully halt the progression of the fascial defect.

As a rule, *elective repair* of an abdominal wall hernia should not be performed in a patient who is on the waiting list for liver transplantation. We usually find that repair of the hernia during transplant surgery is feasible. If not, the hernia can be repaired electively during the posttransplant period, when the procedure is safer and simpler due to the correction of the coagulopathy and disappearance of the ascites.

Emergency hernia repair is indicated when there is breakdown of the skin covering the hernial sac with leakage of ascites, or if the hernia becomes incarcerated. In these cases the patient should be taken to the operating room following correction of the coagulopathy. The anesthesia team must be prepared to replace the large volume of ascitic fluid that is rapidly drained when the peritoneum is opened. All the ascites must be drained to prevent high intraabdomianl pressure in the postoperative period.

After the hernial sac is resected and its contents (if they exist) are put back into the peritoneal cavity, the fascial defect is repaired. Patients who have had tense ascites usually have a very elastic abdominal wall, allowing the fascial defect to be closed with no tension. We choose to close the defect in these cases with interrupted "Mayo" sutures[76] using Proline #0. The skin above the hernia, especially in umbilical hernias, should be excised because it is usually infected or necrotic. The wound usually closes without problems. We recommend the use of perioperative antibiotics and the resumption of medical management of the ascites.

In our experience there has been no significant morbidity or mortality following repair of abdominal wall hernias in this patient population; nor has there been recurrence of the hernia or leakage of ascites through the repair. Since portal vein thrombosis can be a hidden but serious complication of emergency hernia repair or any other emergency abdominal procedure, a Doppler ultrasound to determine portal blood flow should be obtained after the procedure.

Although not experienced in our patient population, repair of an umbilical hernia in a cirrhotic patient can precipitate acute bleeding of esophageal varices[77] due to disruption of periumbilical venous collaterals, with resulting increase in pressure in other venous collaterals.

INFECTIONS RELATED TO END STAGE LIVER DISEASE

Patients with cirrhosis, especially when complicated by ascites, are in a relatively immunocompromised state long before transplantation due to loss of a large percentage of their reticuloendothelial system and decreased production of antibacterial "proteins."[78-81] A significant fraction of fatalities in cirrhotics are due to infections.[82,83] In the cirrhotic patient, invasive procedures such as colonoscopy, endoscopic sclerotherapy, and dental procedures will lead to bacteremia, but sepsis is rare. The use of broad-spectrum prophylactic antibiotics is not recommended for most patients.

The major infectious complications of end-stage liver disease are spontaneous bacterial peritonitis and cholangitis.

Spontaneous Bacterial Peritonitis

Spontaneous bacterial peritonitis (SBP) is a leading cause of morbidity in the patient with end-stage liver disease, and mortality from SBP may be as high as 50–80%.[85-87] Early diagnosis and treatment is critical, since the presence of infection will render the patient unsuitable for transplantation.

Cirrhotic patients are at particular risk for peritonitis, not just because they are relatively immunocompromised but also because ascitic fluid is a good culture medium. Portosystemic collateral blood vessels shunt bacteria away from the liver's large reticuloendothelial system, and phagocytic activity may be impaired in the cirrhotic patient.[78,79] Also, ascitic fluid contains less complement and reduced opsonic activity compared to normal peritoneal fluid.[80,81]

The presenting signs of fever, chills, elevated white blood cell count, decreased bowel sounds, and abdominal tenderness with rebound are classical[88] but inconsistent. Peritonitis must be suspected in any cirrhotic patient with fever alone, sudden deterioration in liver function, abdominal pain, or new onset of encephalopathy.[87] When SBP is suspected, the diagnosis must be rapidly confirmed by paracentesis, and is defined by the presence of a fluid neutrophil count

>250 mm^{-3}.[87,89] The fluid may not appear turbid. Measurements of protein and glucose are rarely helpful, although protein levels do tend to be lower in SBP.[90] A gram stain will help to establish the etiologic agent in one-third of the cases.[82] Cultures of fluid are positive in only 65% of cases,[91] but the yield may improve if 5 mL of fluid is inoculated into broth.[87] The most common offending organisms are the streptococcus species (pneumococcus) or gram-negative bacilli.[87] Anaerobic infections are extremely rare.[92]

Once suspected, and after fluid and blood is obtained for culture, empiric antibiotic therapy should be started immediately. Aminoglycosides should not be used because of their enhanced nephrotoxicity in the cirrhotic patient.[84] Aztreonam[86] is effective but requires concomitant use of an antibiotic directed at gram-positive organisms until a pathogen is isolated. The third-generation cephalosporin *cefotaxime* appears to have the most efficacy.[93] Treatment should continue via the parenteral route for 5–10 days, although a full treatment course *is not* necessary to resume the patient's activity on the waiting list. Treatment should proceed even if cultures remain negative.

Prevention of recurrences of SBP can be difficult but may allow the patient a brief infection-free period in which transplantation can be performed. Diuresis to reduce the amount of ascitic fluid may be helpful.[94] Prophylactic antibiotics with trimethoprim/sulfamethoxazole or norfloxacin is effective.[95]

In our experience, as well as others,[74] patients with recurrent episodes of SBP do poorly and should be transplanted as soon as possible, especially since the "window" period between infections is often short. In such cases, after resolution of the active infection (usually within 5–7 days), the patient should be advanced on the waiting list to facilitate transplantation.

Cholangitis

Patients with cirrhosis due to obstructive biliary lesions, such as biliary atresia and primary sclerosing cholangitis (PSC), have an increased susceptibility to bacterial cholangitis.

In adult patients with PSC, treatment of acute episodes of cholangitis should include parenteral antibiotics and, if possible, percutaneous dilatation and drainage of the biliary tree. However, the nature of the pathologic changes in the liver make the success of percutaneous intervention temporary and partial.[96] Surgical treatment of cholangitis in PSC has almost no place in the era of liver transplantation,[97,98] especially if the patient is on the waiting list.

Recurrent episodes of cholangitis, particularly in patients with PSC, are associated with rapid deterioration in clinical status and have a grave prognosis.[74] During treatment of the acute episode, the transplant center should be apprised so that the patient's status on the list can be advanced to promote transplantation.

In our experience, there are rare cases in which severe cholangitis cannot resolve completely with the use of parenteral antibiotics with or without percutaneous drainage procedures. This is usually due to the presence of multiple abscess pockets in the biliary system involving a large part of the liver. Ordinarily, the presence of sepsis or extrahepatic infection is a contraindication to transplantation. In these cases, however, the existence of persistent intrahepatic infection, is an *indication* for liver transplantation. Removal of the infected organ leads to marked improvement in the patient's condition. With postoperative use of appropriate broad-spectrum antibiotics, the infectious complications are usually not significant.

In summary, infections in the cirrhotic patient are life-threatening and may hinder the patient's ability to undergo transplantation. Spontaneous bacterial peritonitis may be a fatal complication of cirrhosis, requiring prompt diagnosis and management. It should be suspected in any patient with new onset of encephalopathy or deteriorating liver function, or when fever, abdominal pain, and decreased bowel sounds are present, and should be treated as soon as suspected. The presence of an active extrahepatic infection may render the patient ineligible for transplantation for the first 5–6 days of treatment. Recurrent SBP, however, is a poor prognostic sign and should prompt earlier transplantation. Recurrent cholangitis is also associated with a grave prognosis and should expedite transplantation. Because it is an intrahepatic process, the presence of ongoing but controlled infection in this case is not an contraindication to transplantation.

HEPATIC ENCEPHALOPATHY AND COMA

Hepatic encephalopathy is a disabling but usually reversible complication of portosystemic shunting. Unlike the encephalopathy of fulminant hepatic failure, the encephalopathy of chronic liver disease tends to be more subacute and amenable to treatment. Nevertheless, encephalopathy can progress to coma. The new onset of encephalopathy in the patient on the waiting list should alert the health care provider to identify and remove precipitating factors. Hepatic encephalopathy must be distinguished from other causes of acute change in mental status, such as neurologic manifestations of Wilson's disease, or acute alcoholism. Refractory encephalopathy is an indication for urgent liver transplantation.

The earliest signs of encephalopathy include reversal of the normal sleep–wake cycle and decreased awareness of the environment.[99-101] Other subtle changes may include depression, increased somnolence, altered speech, and changes in handwriting. Asterixis may or may not be present. Hepatic encephalopathy can be graded to aid clinical objectivity (see Table 10-1). A slow-wave pattern may be evident on EEG, especially over the frontal lobes, and serum ammonia is usually elevated.[99-101] Hepatic encephalopathy may be precipitated by infections such as bacterial peritonitis, gastrointestinal hemorrhage, aggressive diuresis or paracentesis, electrolyte abnormalities such as hypokalemia, use of sedatives (especially benzodiazepines), constipation, and dietary protein.[102]

TABLE 10-1. Stages of Hepatic Encephalopathy

I	Agitation, irritability, impaired calculations
III	Personality changes, memory disturbances, lethargy
III	Delirium, somnolence
IV	Coma

The etiology of hepatic encephalopathy remains undefined. GABA-like substances may exert an influence via benzodiazepine receptor complexes.[103-107]

Treatment of encephalopathy of the patient on waiting list is similar to that of the nontransplant candidate.[108-111] It is aimed at (1) removing any precipitating factors, (2) reducing intestinal flora, and (3) decreasing the gastrointestinal protein load. Adequate calories must be provided to avoid the breakdown of body protein as an energy source. The use of *branched-chain amino acids* to counter the effect of aromatic amino acids has not been promising in clinical trials.[112] *Benzodiazepine receptor antagonists* may eventually be part of the standard treatment for hepatic encephalopathy,[103,113] but until more experience is available, benzodiazepenes should be used cautiously for conscious sedation during endoscopy.

In summary, hepatic encephalopathy is a complication of cirrhosis that may vary in its presentation from subclinical disease to crippling disability to frank coma. The presence of mild encephalopathy is not in itself an indication for urgent transplantation as it generally responds well to medical treatment, such as laxatives, lactulose, neomycin, and restriction of dietary protein. The physician must be attentive to the subtle manifestations of subclinical encephalopathy. The new onset of encephalopathy should promote a vigilant search for triggering event such as GI bleeding, infection, dehydration, constipation, or electrolyte abnormalities. Hepatic encephalopathy is reversible with liver transplantation.

HEPATORENAL SYNDROME

Hepatorenal syndrome (HRS) is the most common cause of renal insufficiency in a patient on the waiting list and indicates urgent need for transplantation of the failing liver. Implicit in the definition of the syndrome is the absence of primary renal pathology. Hepatorenal syndrome should not be the terminal event in the patient awaiting a liver transplant,[114] since it is usually reversible after liver transplantation.[115]

A specific precipitating event is usually not identified, but sepsis must be ruled out. In addition, GI hemorrhage, overaggressive diuresis, the use of IV contrast, and excessive paracentesis without the use of volume expanders, may also trigger the syndrome. The use of aminoglycoside antibiotics and nonsteroidal anti-inflammatory agents may precipitate hepatorenal syndrome as well.[84,119]

Oliguria is the hallmark of HRS, and is accompanied by an increase in BUN and creatinine. Elevations in BUN and creatinine may not reflect the severity of renal dysfunction, since the cirrhotic patient usually has a decreased muscle mass and impaired urea synthesis.[116] Urine sediment is benign, and urine sodium is characteristically $<$20 mEq/L, and often $<$10 mEq/L. There is a high urine/plasma creatinine ratio ($>$30:1). Hyponatremia is common. HRS must be distinguished from other causes of oliguric renal failure, including urinary tract obstruction, prerenal azotemia, and acute tubular necrosis (Table 10-2). Acute tubular necrosis is generally accompanied by elevated urinary sodium concentration and a urine/plasma creatinine ratio of $<$20.[117] Prerenal azotemia is more difficult to distinguish since urinary sodium concentration and creatinine ratios may be similar.

When renal insufficiency develops the patient on the waiting list should be

TABLE 10-2. Distinguishing Hepatorenal Syndrome from Acute Tubular Necrosis

	HRS	*ATN*
Oliguria	Present	Present
Response to volume	None	None
Bun/Cr	Increased	Increased
Urine Na	<10–20 mEq/L	>20 mEq/L
Ucr:Pcr	>30:1	<20:1

Key: HRS—hepatorenal syndrome; ATN—acute tubular necrosis; Ucr—urine creatinine; Pcr—plasma creatinine.

referred to the transplant center for definitive treatment and reevaluation of waiting list standing.

The only known "cure" for hepatorenal syndrome is liver transplantation. However, efforts to halt the progression of renal failure by increasing renal bloodflow have been modestly successful. The most promising treatment is the administration of the synthetic PGE1 analog *misoprostil* in conjunction with plasma volume expansion.[120] We have had favorable results using misoprostil 400 mg po every 6 hr with 25% albumin 12.5 g IV every 12 hr. Other methods to improve renal perfusion without decreasing systemic vascular resistance are promising, and include the use of *ornipressin,* an arginine–vasopressin analog that is still under investigation.[121,122] The use of captopril and saralasin, directed at the renin angiotensin–aldosterone system, has been unsuccessful, probably because of the transient and subtle hypotension that ensues.[123-125] *Dialysis* does not reverse the hepatorenal syndrome but is an important supportive measure when volume overload, pulmonary edema, and hyperkalemia develop and a suitable organ is not yet available for transplantation.[126] Hemodialysis is seldom well tolerated because of hypotension. Peritoneal dialysis is *contraindicated* in patients awaiting liver transplantation because of the risk of introducing infection that will render the patient unsuitable for transplant. Continuous arteriovenous hemoperfusion is probably the best tolerated method.[127] Paracentesis and peritoneovenous shunts are not helpful.

We have had the gratifying experience that the vast majority of our patients with hepatorenal syndrome have achieved full recovery of renal function after liver transplantation. In the most dramatic cases, patients who were anuric for weeks before the transplantation resumed urine output as early as a few hours after reperfusion of the new liver.

NUTRITIONAL SUPPORT OF THE PRE–LIVER TRANSPLANT PATIENT

Malnutrition is an integral part of advanced liver disease.[128] While it is most pronounced in the patient with alcoholic cirrhosis,[129] it may affect any cirrhotic patient. Aggressive nutritional support may improve a patient's Child's score and chances of surviving some of the complications of end-stage liver disease,[130] thereby reducing mortality on the waiting list. In addition, it has been our experience that patients with severe cachexia have higher morbidity and mortality in the posttransplant periods than patients with better nutritional status. Nutritional status therefore must be continually addressed in the patient awaiting liver transplantation.

The cirrhotic patient becomes malnourished for a variety of reasons. Cholestasis leads to *malabsorption of long-chain fats,* including the essential fatty acids, and fat-soluble vitamins.[131] Portal hypertension leads to loss of intestinal lymph,[132,133] which leads to *protein losses,* and further impairs long-chain fat absorption. Protein synthesis is impaired in the cirrhotic patient,[134] and *energy requirements* are usually increased.[131,135,136] *Intake* is usually markedly diminished, as a result of anorexia from severe ascites, fluid restrictions that may inhibit total intake, distaste for food due to severe salt or protein restriction, or depression. In addition, frequent or lengthy hospitalizations and procedures (such as sclerotherapy) or their complications (postsclerotherapy ulcerations and strictures) may contribute to decreased intake.

The objective of nutritional support in the cirrhotic patient is to provide adequate calories without inducing encephalopathy.[137] Indirect calorimetry can be used to estimate energy requirements, but ~2000 kcal/day is usually sufficient for the adult patient.[138] It is important to remember that *failure* to provide adequate energy may *promote* encephalopathy, as muscle protein is being broken down and utilized as an energy source, releasing ammonia. Improved nutrition may raise serum albumin, decrease ascites, increase the liver's capacity for hepatocyte regeneration, or decrease mortality from infections or bleeding episodes,[130,139] and has significant impact on the success of the impending liver transplantation.

Most patients are unable to maintain adequate caloric intake via the oral route, and require some form of supplementation. Enteral nutrition is the preferred way to provide calories,[140] especially since parenteral nutrition carries with it the risk of catheter-related sepsis.[141] A low-protein, low-volume, low-sodium, high-MCT oil formula is best suited for enteral supplementation. No "ideal" formula for the cirrhotic patient is commercially available, but we have had some success using Liposorb™ (Mead-Johnson), which fits many of the criteria mentioned above, and can be used either as an oral supplement or as total enteral nutrition via feeding tube. Formulas are available containing branched-chain amino acids, but these were created with the intention of treating encephalopathy, rather than optimizing nutrition.[142] Branched-chain aminoacids also appear to have an anticatabolic effect on muscle protein.[143] Parenteral nutrition can certainly be used in an inpatient setting when the enteral route cannot be used for prolonged periods of time.

In summary, malnutrition is seen with advanced cirrhosis in almost 100% of cases.[144,145] While there is little the medical team can do to alter the physical manifestations of malnutrition,[130] evidence shows that better nutrition not only improves Child's scores but also increases survival in both the pre- and post-transplant period. Induction of hepatic encephalopathy should not be feared so long as protein intake remains low. We support aggressive use of enteral supplementation in the patient on the waiting list. At the same time, the transplant center should be made aware of the presence of wasting so that efforts can be made to transplant the patient long before severe cachexia ensues.

DRUGS IN END-STAGE LIVER DISEASE

The presence of a failing liver affects the metabolism and clearance of several drugs. Changes in blood levels and toxic effects should be taken in consideration when drugs are being used in the patient on the waiting list for liver transplantation. Many of the medications are not direct hepatotoxins. Nevertheless, their altered pharmacodynamics may magnify their known deleterious effects, or exacerbate the complications of end-stage liver disease.

The pharmacodynamic changes in end-stage liver disease can be grouped into five main categories[146,147] (Table 10-3):

1. *Enhanced free fraction.* Altered protein binding capacity due to impaired protein synthesis, and increased volume of distribution due to ascites (which acts as a reservoir), will result in prolonged half-life of the drugs in this category and will enhance their therapeutic and toxic potential.
2. *Flow-limited hepatic clearance.* Drugs that have a high extraction ratio will accumulate in the circulation due to reduced blood flow through the cirrhotic liver.
3. *Capacity-limited hepatic clearance.* Hepatocellular dysfunction from cirrhosis will lead to impaired enzymatic clearance and thereby increase the systemic bioavailability of the drugs in this category.
4. *Altered renal hemodynamics.* Drugs that have an effect on renal hemodynamics may contribute to the development of hepatorenal syndrome.
5. *Interference with coagulation.* Drugs that have a negative effect on the coagulation cascade and on platelet function may potentiate a coagulopathy.

OTHER MEDICAL CONDITIONS IN THE CIRRHOTIC PATIENT

In selecting a candidate for liver transplantation, medical problems unrelated to the underlying liver disease were evaluated to establish whether the patient is capable of surviving the surgery. After the patient is placed on the waiting list, new extrahepatic illness can occur making the patient an extremely high-risk candidate. The following is a brief list of the conditions that may develop while the patient is on the waiting list and should be given special consideration by the referring physician.

Cardiac Insufficiency

The new onset of angina or the occurrence of a myocardial infarction in a candidate, requires a complete cardiac evaluation and redetermination of candidacy.

TABLE 10-3. Drugs to be Used with Caution in End-Stage Liver Disease

	EFF	*FLHC*	*CLHC*	*ARH*	*IC*
Aminoglycosides	*				
Ampicillin			*		
Aspirin		*			
Cefoperazone	*				*
Cefotetan					*
Ceftriaxone	*				
Chlordiazepoxide			*		
Chlorpromazine			*		
Clindamycin			*		
Diazepam	*		*		
Digitoxin			*		
Diltiazem		*			
Diphenoxylate			*		
Labetalol		*			
Lidocaine		*			
Loperamide			*		
Meperidine		*			
Metoclopramide		*			
Metoprolol		*			
Morphine	*	*			
Moxalactam					*
Nicardipine		*			
Nifedipine		*			
NSAIDs	*		*	*	*
Pentazocine			*		
Phenobarbital			*		
Phenytoin	*		*		
Propranolol		*			
Quinidine	*		*		
Salicylates	*			*	*
Sulfonylureas			*		
Theophylline			*		
Timolol		*			
Tricyclic antidepressants		*			
Valproic acid			*		
Verapamil		*			
Warfarin	*		*		

Key: EFF—enhanced free fraction; FLHC—flow-limited hepatic clearance; CLHC—capacity-limited hepatic clearance; ARH—altered renal hemodynamics; IC—interference with coagulation and/or platelet function; NSAIDs nonsteroidal antiinflammatory drugs.

TABLE 10-4. Clinical Indications for Emergent Transplantation

Uncontrollable variceal hemorrhage
Acute renal failure due to hepatorenal syndrome
Hepatic encephalopathy, stages III and IV

Pulmonary insufficiency

Although pulmonary function tests were part of the pre–liver transplant evaluation, the new development of pulmonary difficulties necessitates repeat performance of the tests. Reversible causes include restrictive lung disease due to massive ascites, or pleural effusions due to a combination of fluid overload and profound hypoalbuminemia. Primary lung diseases such as emphysema are poor prognostic indicators but rarely present after the initial evaluation. Hepatopulmonary syndrome[148] occurs in a small percentage of cirrhotic patients and must be distinguished from primary lung diseases. It is marked by profound hypoxemia, due to arteriovenous shunting in the lung through collaterals. There is also evidence of a diffusion defect, since these patients do respond to high concentrations of inspired oxygen. Since the lesion may reverse with transplantation, its development should prompt higher waiting list status. Nonreversible lesions or progressive deterioration can lead to elimination from candidacy for transplantation.

CONCLUSIONS

Patients with end-stage liver disease who are on the waiting list for liver transplantation walk a tightrope between relative well-being and a progressive downhill course. End-stage liver disease is a dynamic condition, and waiting list status should reflect changes in the patient's clinical situation. The ability to individualize care and to find the right timing for transplantation is a daily challenge for the treating physician and the liver transplant center.

Acute deterioration in a patient's condition can be treated initially by the local physician and hospital facilities. Once stabilization is achieved, transfer to the transplant center is mandatory to enable the transplant team to evaluate the patient and to ensure transplantation without further delay (Table 10-4).

Deterioration of a more chronic nature can usually be managed locally or on an outpatient basis (Table 10-5). The transplant center should be informed so that the patient's waiting list status can be advanced, thereby shortening the time interval to liver transplantation.

As has been discussed in this chapter, the treatment choices for the various complications of end-stage liver disease must be dictated by the imminent transplantation. While treatment options exist that may have a short-term palliative effect, the predominant goal should be the total cure of the underlying liver disease and its complications via liver transplantation. Continuous and detailed communication between the treating physician and the transplant team will help determine the appropriate timing for transplantation and the choice of therapeu-

TABLE 10-5. Clinical Indications to advance the Patient on the Waiting List

Recurrent variceal bleeding
Esophageal
Gastric
Stomal
Hemorrhoidal
Recurrent bacterial peritonitis
Recurrent cholangitis
Intractable ascites
Deterioration in nutritional status (muscle wasting)
Deterioration in liver function tests (elevation in PT and bilirubin, decrease in albumin)

tic interventions for the patient. This will ultimately lead to reduction in mortality and morbidity on the waiting list.

REFERENCES

1. The North Italian Endoscopic Club for the Study and Treatment of Esophageal Varices. Prediction of the first variceal hemorrhage in patients with cirrhosis of the liver and esophageal varices: a prospective multicenter study. *New Engl J Med* 319:983–989, 1988.
2. Gores GJ, Weisner RH, Dickson ER, et al: Prospective evaluation of esophageal varices in primary biliary cirrhosis: development, natural history and influence on survival. *Gastroenterology* 96:1552–1559, 1989.
3. Graham D, Smith JL: The course of patients after variceal hemorrhage. *Gastroenterology* 80:800–809, 1981.
4. Mahl TC, Groszmann RJ: Pathophysiology of portal hypertension and variceal bleeding. *Surg Clin N Am* 70:251–267, 1990.
5. Garcia-Tsao G, Groszmann RJ, Fisher RL, et al: Portal pressure, presence of gastroesophageal varices and variceal bleeding. *Hepatology* 5:1985, 1985.
6. Boyer JL, Chatterjee C, Iber FL, et al: Effect of plasma-volume expansion on portal hypertension. *New Engl J Med* 275:750–755, 1966.
7. Bredfeldt JE, Bosch J, Groszmann RJ: Splanchnic angiography increases portal pressure in portal hypertensive patients (abstract). *Hepatology* 2:684, 1982.
8. Sarin SK, Kumar A: Gastric varices: profile, classification and management. *Am J Gastroenterol* 84:1244–1249, 1989.
9. Korula J, Chin K, Ko Y, et al: Demonstration of two distinct subsets of gastric varices. *Dig Dis Sci* 36:303–309, 1991.
10. Trudeau W, Prindiville T: Endoscopic injection sclerosis in bleeding gastric varices. *Gastrointestinal Endosc* 32:264–268, 1986.
11. Salam AA, Goldman M, Smith D Jr, et al: Gastric, intestinal and gallbladder varices: hemodynamic and therapeutic considerations. *South Med J* 72:402–408, 1979.
12. Eade MN, Williams JA, Cooke UT: Bleeding from an ileostomy caput medusae. *Lancet* 2:166–168, 1969.
13. Graeber GM, Ratner MH, Ackerman NB: Massive hemorrhage from ileostomy and

colostomy stomas due to mucocutaneous varices in patients with coexisting cirrhosis. *Surgery* 79:107–110, 1975.

14. Adson MA, Fulton RE: The ileal stoma and portal hypertension. *Arch Surg* 112:501–504, 1977.
15. Warren WD, Millikan WJ, Henderson JM, et al: Ten years portal hypertensive surgery at Emory: results and new perspectives. *Ann Surg* 195:530–542, 1982.
16. Conte JV, Arcomano TA, Naficy MA, et al: Treatment of bleeding stomal varices. *Dis Colon Rectum* 33:308–314, 1990.
17. Hesterberb R, Stahlknecht CD, Roher HD: Sclerotherapy for massive enterostomy bleeding resulting from portal hypertension. *Dis Colon Rectum* 29:275–277, 1986.
18. Sherlock S (ed): *Diseases of the Liver and Biliary System*, 7th ed, Oxford, Blackwell Scientific Publications, 1985.
19. Larson A, Cohen H, Zweiban B, et al: Acute esophageal variceal sclerotherapy: results of a prospective, randomized controlled trial. *JAMA* 255:497–500, 1986.
20. Schuman BM, Beckman JW, Tedesco FJ, et al: Complications of endoscopic injection sclerotherapy: a review. *Am J Gastroenterol* 82:823–830, 1987.
21. Hunter GC, Steinkirchner T, Burbige EJ, et al: Venous complications of sclerotherapy for esophageal varices. *Am J Surg* 156:497–501, 1988.
22. Sarin SK, Nanda R, Sachdev G, et al: Intravariceal versus paravariceal sclerotherapy: a prospective, controlled, randomized trial. *Gut* 28:657–662, 1987.
23. Silpa ML, Jensen DM, Machido GA, et al: Efficacy and safety of agents for variceal sclerotherapy. *Gastrointest Endosc* 152–153, 1982.
24. Sarin SK, Sachdev G, Nanda R, et al: Comparison of two time schedules for endoscopic sclerotherapy: a prospective, randomized controlled study. *Gut* 27:710–713, 1986.
25. Westaby D, Melia W, Macdougall B, et al: Injection sclerotherapy for esophageal varices: a prospective randomized trial of different treatment schedules. *Gut* 25:129–132, 1984.
26. Stiegmann GV, Sun JH, Hammond WS: Results of experimental endoscopic esophageal varix ligation. *Am Surg* 54:105–108, 1988.
27. Fleischer D: Nd:YAG laser therapy for active esophageal variceal bleeding: a randomized controlled study. *Gastrointest Endosc* 31:4–9, 1985.
28. Olsson R: Beta receptor blocking treatment in portal hypertension. *Scand J Gastroenterol* 25:641–646, 1990.
29. Burnett DA, Rikkers LF: Nonoperative emergency treatment of variceal hemorrhage. *Surg Clin N Am* 2:291–306, 1990.
30. Tsai Y-T, Lay C-S, Lai K-H, et al: Controlled trial of vasopressin plus nitroglycerin versus vasopressin alone in the treatment of bleeding esophageal varices. *Hepatology* 5:406–409, 1986.

30a. Jenkins SA, Baxter JN, Shields R, et al: A prospective, randomized, controlled trial comparing somatostatin and vasopressin in controlling acute variceal hemorrhage. *Br Med J* 290:1275–1276, 1985.

31. MacDougall BRD, Williams R: A controlled clinical trial of cimetidine in the recurrence of variceal hemorrhage: implications about the pathogenesis of hemorrhage. *Hepatology* 3:69–73, 1983.
32. Paquet K-J, Feussner H: Endoscopic sclerosis and esophageal balloon tamponade in acute hemorrhage from esophageal varices: a prospective controlled randomized trial. *Hepatology* 5:580–583, 1985.

33. Novis BH, Duys P, Terblanche J, et al: Fiberoptic endoscopy and the use of the Sengstaken tube in acute gastrointestinal hemorrhage in patients with portal hypertension and varices. *Gut* 17:258–263, 1976.
34. Papadimos D, Kerlin P, Harris OD: Endoscopic sclerotherapy. Lessons from a necropsy study. *Gastrointest Endosc* 32:269–273, 1986.
35. Conn H: Hazards attending the use of esophageal tamponade. *New Engl J Med* 259:701–707, 1958.
36. Conn H, Simpson J: Excessive mortality associated with balloon tamponade of bleeding varices. *JAMA* 202:135–139, 1967.
37. Brems JJ, Hiatt JR, Klein AS, et al: Effect of a prior portasystemic shunt on subsequent liver transplantation. *Ann Surg* 209:51–56, 1989.
38. Wood RP, Shaw BW, Jr, Rikkers LF: Liver transplantation for variceal hemorrhage. *Surg Clin N Am* 70:449–461, 1990.
39. Crass RA, Keeffe EB, Pinson CW: Management of variceal hemorrhage in the potential liver transplant candidate. *Am J Surg* 157:476–478, 1989.
40. Terblanche J: The surgeon's role in the management of portal hypertension. *Ann Surg* 209:381–395, 1989.
41. Sugiura M, Futagawa S: A new technique for treating esophageal varices. *J Thorac Cardiovasc Surg* 66:677, 1973.
42. Zemel G, Katzen B, Becker G, Fallee S and Benenati J. Percutaneous transjugular porto-systemic shunt. *JAMA* 266:390–393, 1991.
43. Rikkers LF: Definitive therapy for variceal bleeding: a personal view. *Am J Surg* 160:80–85, 1990.
44. Bismuth H, Adam R, Mathur S, et al: Options for elective treatment of portal hypertension in cirrhotic patients in the transplantation era. *Am J Surg* 160:105–110, 1990.
45. Sarin SK, Sachdev G, Nanda R, et al: Endoscopic sclerotherapy in the treatment of gastric varices. *Br J Surg* 75:747–750, 1988.
46. Teres J, Cecilia A, Bordas JM, et al: Oesophageal tamponade for bleeding varices. Controlled trial between the Sengstaken Blakemore tube and the Linton Nachalas tube. *Gastroenterology* 75:566–569, 1978.
47. Morgan TR, Feldson SD, Tripp MR: Recurrent stomal bleeding: successful treatment using injection sclerotherapy. *Dis Colon Rectum* 29:269–270, 1985.
48. Samaraweera RN, Feldman L, Widrich WC, et al: Stomal varices: percutaneous transhepatic embolization. *Radiology* 170:779–782, 1989.
49. McCormack TT, Sims J, Eyre-Brooke I, et al: Gastric lesions in portal hypertension: Inflammatory gastritis or congestive gastropathy? *Gut* 26:1226–1232, 1985.
50. Perez-Ayuso RM, Pique JM, Bosch J, et al: Propanolol in prevention of recurrent bleeding from severe portal hypertensive gastropathy in cirrhosis. *Lancet* 337:1431–1434, 1991.
51. Papazian A, Braillon A, Dupas JL, et al: Portal hypertensive gastric mucosa; an endoscopic study. *Gut* 27:1199–1203, 1986.
52. Misra SP, Dwivedi M, Misra V, et al: Endoscopic and histologic appearance of the gastric mucosa in patients with portal hypertension. *Gastrointest Endosc* 36:575–579, 1990.
53. Sarfeh IJ, Tarnawski A, Hajduczek J, et al: Does portal hypertension predispose gastric mucosa to aspirin injury? Histological ultrastructural and functional analysis (abstract). *Gastroenterology* 92:1614, 1987.

54. Sarfeh IJ, Tarnawski A, Maeda R, et al: The gastric mucosa in portal hypertension: effects of topical bile acid. *Scand J Gastroenterol* 92 (Suppl):189–194, 1984.
55. Sarfeh IJ, Tarnawski A, Malki A, et al: Portal hypertension and gastric mucosal injury in rats: effects of alcohol. *Gastroenterology* 84:987–993, 1983.
56. McCormick PA, Sankey EA, Cardin F, et al: Congestive gastropathy and Helicobacter pylori: an endoscopic and morphometric study. *Gut* 52:551–554, 1991.
57. Kirk AP, Dooley JS, Hunt RH: Peptic ulceration in patients with chronic liver disease. *Dig Dis Sci* 25:756, 1980.
58. Kozarek RA, Botoman VA, Bredfeldt JE, et al: Portal colopathy: Prospective study of colonoscopy in patients with portal hypertension. *Gastroenterology* 101:1192–1197, 1991.
59. Gentilini P, Laffi G: Renal functional impairment and sodium retention in liver cirrhosis. *Digestion* 43:1–32, 1989.
60. Atkinson M, Losowsky MS: The mechanism of ascites formation in chronic liver disease. *Q J Med* 30:153–166, 1961.
61. Lieberman FL, Denison EK, Reynolds TB: The relationship of plasma volume, portal hypertension, ascites and renal sodium retention in cirrhosis: the "overflow" theory of ascites formation. *Ann NY Acad Sci* 170:202–208, 1970.
62. Jiminez W, Martinez-Pardo A, Arroyo V, et al: Temporal relationship between hyperaldosteronism, sodium retention and ascites formation in rats with experimental cirrhosis. *Hepatology* 5:245–250, 1985.
63. Bosch J, Arroyo V, Betriu A, et al: Hepatic hemodynamics and the renin-angiotensin-aldosterone system in cirrhosis. *Gastroenterology* 97:1506–1513, 1980.
64. Eckardt VF, Grace ND: Gastroesophageal reflux and bleeding esophageal varices. *Gastroenterology* 76:39–42, 1979.
65. Lemmer JH, Strodel E, Knol JA, et al: Management of spontaneous umbilical hernia disruption in the cirrhotic patient. *Ann Surg* 94:198–201, 1984.
66. Linas SL, Anderson RJ, Miller PD, et al: Rational use of diuretics in cirrhosis. In Epstein M: *The Kidney in Liver Disease*, 2d ed, pp 555–567, New York, Elsevier. 1983.
67. Schiff ER: Treatment of ascites. *Ala J Med Sci* 22:44–49, 1985.
68. Runyon BA: Paracentesis of ascitic fluid: a safe procedure. *Arch Int Med* 146:2259–2261, 1986.
69. Gines P, Tito L, Arroyo V, et al: Randomized comparative study of therapeutic paracentesis with and without albumin in cirrhosis. *Gastroenterology* 94:1493–1502, 1988.
70. Planas R, Gines P, Arroyo V, et al: Dextran-70 versus albumin as plasma expanders in cirrhotic patients with tense ascites treated with total paracentesis. *Gastroenterology* 99:1736–1744, 1990
71. Salerno F, Badalamenti S, Lorenzano E, et al: Randomized comparative study of hemaccel vs. albumin infusion after total paracentesis in cirrhotic patients with refractory ascites. *Hepatology* 13:707–713, 1991.
72. Eggert RC: Spironolactone diuresis in patients with cirrhosis and ascites. *Br Med J* 4:401–403, 1970.
73. Moskovitz M: The peritoneovenous shunt: expectations and reality. *Am J Gastroenterol* 85:917–929, 1990.
74. Dindzans VJ, Schade RR, Van Thiel DH: Medical problems before and after transplantation. *Gastroenterol Clin N Am* 17:19–31, 1988.

75. Gines P, Arroyo V, Vargas V, et al: Paracentesis with intravenous infusion of albumin as compared with peritoneovenous shunting in cirrhosis with refractory ascites. *New Engl J Med* 325:829–835, 1991.

76. Mayo, WJ: Radical cure of umbilical hernia. *JAMA* 48:1842–1844, 1907.

77. Baron HC: Umbilical hernia secondary to cirrhosis of the liver-complications of surgical correction. *New Engl J Med* 263:824, 1960.

78. Cooksley WGE, Powell LW, Halliday KW: Reticuloendothelial phagocytic function in human liver disease and its relationship to hemolysis. *Br J Haematol* 25:147–164, 1973.

79. Lahnborg G, Friman L, Bergham L: Reticuloendothelial function in patients with alcoholic liver cirrhosis. *Scand J Gastroenterol* 16:481–489, 1981.

80. Akalin HE, Laleli Y, Telatar H: Bactericidal and opsonic activity of ascitic fluid from cirrhotic and noncirrhotic patients. *J Infect Dis* 147:1011–1017, 1983.

81. Runyon BA, Morrissey RL, Hoefs JC, et al: Opsonic activity of human ascitic fluid: a potentially important protective mechanism against spontaneous bacterial peritonitis. *Hepatology* 6:396–399, 1986.

82. Cairo JP, Areias ME, Monteiro E, et al: Liver cirrhosis. Clinical experience with 274 unselected cases. *Digestion* 4:223–233, 1971.

83. Sloth K, Juhl E, Tygstrup N: The causes of death in prednisone treated and control patients with cirrhosis. *Scand J Gastroenterol* (Suppl 7):189–193, 1990.

84. Cabrera J, Arroyo V, Ballesta AM, et al: Aminoglycoside nephrotoxicity in cirrhosis: value of urinary B2-microglobulin to discriminate functional renal failure from acute tubular damage. *Gastroenterology* 82:97–105, 1982.

85. Runyon BA: Spontaneous bacterial peritonitis: an explosion of information. *Hepatology* 8:171–175, 1988.

86. Ariza J, Xiol X, Esteve M, et al: Aztreonam vs. cefotaxime in the treatment of gram-negative spontaneous peritonitis in cirrhotic patients. *Hepatology* 14:91–98, 1991.

87. Hoefs JC, Runyon BA: Spontaneous bacterial peritonitis. *Dis Mon* 31–39, 1984.

88. Conn HO: Spontaneous peritonitis and bacteremia in Laennec's cirrhosis caused by enteric organisms. *Ann Int Med* 1964;60:658–80.

89. Jones SR: The absolute granulocyte count in ascites fluid. An aid to the diagnosis of spontaneous bacterial peritonitis. *West J Med* 126:344–346, 1977.

90. Boyer TD, Kahn AM, Reynolds TB: Diagnostic value of ascitic fluid lactic dehydrogenase, protein and WBC levels. *Arch Int Med* 138:1103–1105, 1978.

91. Runyon BA, Hoefs JC: Culture-negative neutrocytic ascites: a variant of spontaneous bacterial peritonitis. *Hepatology* 4:1209–1211, 1984.

92. Targan SR, Chow AW, Guze LB: Role of anaerobic bacteria in spontaneous peritonitis of cirrhosis. Report of two cases and review of the literature. *Am J. Med* 62:397–403, 1977.

93. Felisart H, Rimola A, Arroyo V, et al: Cefotaxime is more effective than ampicillin-tobramycine in cirrhotics with severe infections. *Hepatology* 5:457–462, 1985.

94. Runyon BA, Van Epps DE: Diuresis of cirrhotic ascites increases its opsonic activity and may help prevent spontaneous bacterial peritonitis. *Hepatology* 6:396–399, 1986.

95. Schubert ML, Sanyal AJ, Wong ES: Antibiotic prophylaxis for prevention of spontaneous bacterial peritonitis? *Gastroenterology* 101:550–552, 1991.

96. Skolkin MD, Alspaugh JP, Casarella WJ, Chuang VP, Galambos JT: Sclerosing

cholangitis: palliation with percutaneous cholangioplasty. *Radiology* 170:199–206, 1989.

97. Martin FM, Rossi RL, Nugent FW, et al: Surgical aspects of sclerosing cholangitis. Results in 178 patients. *Ann Surg* 212:551–556, 1990.
98. Thompson JS, Wood RP, Burnett DA, Shaw BW, Jr., Rikkers LF: The role of non-transplant procedures for sclerosing cholangitis. *Am J Surg* 156:505–508, 1988.
99. Gilberstadt SJ, Gilberstadt H, Zieve L, et al: Psychomotor performance defects in cirrhotic patients without overt encephalopathy. *Arch Int Med* 140:519–521, 1980.
100. Gitlin N, Lewis DC, Hinkley L: The diagnosis and prevalence of subclinical hepatic encephalopathy in apparently healthy, ambulant, nonshunted patients with cirrhosis. *J Hepatol* 3:75–82, 1986.
101. Rikkers L, Jenko P, Rudman P, et al: Subclinical hepatic encephalopathy: Detection, prevalence and relationship to nitrogen metabolism. *Gastroenterology* 75:462–469, 1978.
102. Munoz SJ, Maddrey WC: Major complications of acute and chronic liver disease. *Gastroenterol Clin N Am* 17:265–287, 1988.
103. Bassett ML, Muller KD, Skolnick P, et al: Amelioration of hepatic encephalopathy by pharmacological antagonism of the GABA-benzodiazepine receptor complex in a rabbit model of fulminant hepatic failure. *Gastroenterology* 93:1069–1077, 1987.
104. Bansky G, Meier PJ, Riederer E, et al: Reversal of hepatic coma by benzodiazepine antagonist (RO 15-1788). *Lancet* 1:1324–1325, 1985.
105. Baraldi M, Zeneroli ML, Ventura E, et al: Supersensitivity of benzodiazepine receptors in hepatic encephalopathy due to fulminant hepatic failure in the rat: reversal by a benzodiazepine antagonist. *Clin Sci* 67:167–175, 1987.
106. Lavoie J, Giguere JF, Pomier G, et al: Amino acid changes in autopsied brain tissue from cirrhotic patients with hepatic encephalopathy. *J Neurochem* 49:693–697, 1987.
107. Mullen KD, Szauter KM, Galloway PG, et al: CSF of patients with hepatic encephalopathy contains significant benzodiazepine binding activity (abstract). *Hepatol* 7:1103, 1987.
108. Atterbury CE, Maddrey WC, Conn HO: Neomycin-sorbitol and lactulose in the treatment of acute portal-systemic encephalopathy. *Dig Dis Sci* 23:398–406, 1978.
109. Elkington SG, Floch MH, Conn HO: Lactulose in the treatment of chronic portal-systemic encephalopathy: a double blind clinical trial. *New Engl J Med* 281:408–412, 1969.
110. Mortensen PB, Rasmussen HS, Holtug K: Lactulose detoxifies in vitro short-chain fatty acid production in colonic contents induced by blood: implication of hepatic coma. *Gastroenterology* 94:750–754, 1988.
111. Wever FL, Fresard KM, Lally BR: Effects of lactulose and neomycin on urea metabolism in cirrhotic subjects. *Gastroenterology* 82:213–217, 1982.
112. Maddrey WC: Branched chain amino acid therapy in liver disease. *J Am Coll Nutr* 4:639–650, 1985.
113. Grimm G, Lenz K, Kleinburger G, et al: Ro 54-1788 improves coma in 4 out of 5 patients with fulminant hepatic failure; verification of long latency and somatosensory evoked potential. *J Hepatol* 4 (Suppl 1):521, 1987.
114. Ring-Larsen H, Palazzo U: Renal failure in fulminant hepatic failure and terminal cirrhosis: a comparison between incidence, types, and prognosis. *Gut* 22:585–591, 1981.
115. Gonwa TA, Morris CA, Goldstein RM, et al: Long-term survival and renal function

following liver transplantation in patients with and without hepatorenal syndrome: Experience in 300 patients. *Transplantation* 51:428–430, 1991.

116. Rudman D, Difolco TJ, Galambos JT, et al: Maximal rates of urea excretion and synthesis in normal and cirrhotic subjects. *J Clin Invest* 52:2241–2249, 1973.
117. Epstein M: Renal functional abnormalities in cirrhosis: pathophysiology and management. In Zakim D, Boyer TD: *Hepatology: A Textbook of Liver Disease*, p 504, Philadelphia, Saunders, 1990.
118. Skorecki KL, Brenner BM: Body fluid homeostasis in congestive heart failure and cirrhosis with ascites. *Am J Med* 72:323–338, 1982.
119. Epstein M, Berk PD, Hollenberg NK, et al: Renal failure in patients with cirrhosis. *Am J Med* 49:175–185, 1970.
120. Fevery J, Van Cutsem E, Nevens F, et al: Reversal of hepatorenal syndrome in 4 patients by peroral misoprostol (prostaglandin E1 analogue) and albumin administration. *J Hepatol* 11:153–158, 1990.
121. Lenz K, Druml W, Kleinberger G, et al: Enhancement of renal function with ornipressin in a patient with decompensated cirrhosis. *Gut* 26:1385–1386, 1985.
122. Lenz K, Hortnagl H, Druml W, et al: Ornipressin in the treatment of functional renal failure in decompensated liver cirrhosis: effects on renal hemodynamics and atrial natiuretic factor. *Gastroenterology* 101:1060–1067, 1991.
123. Schroeder ET, Anderson GH, Goldman SH, et al: Effect of blockade of angiotensin II on blood pressure, renin and aldosterone in cirrhosis. *Kidney Int* 9:511–519, 1976.
124. Cobden I, Shore A, Wilkinson R, et al: Captopril in the hepatorenal syndrome. *J Clin Gastroenterol* 7:354–360, 1985.
125. Pariente EA, Bataille C, Bercoff E, et al: Acute effects of captopril on systemic and renal hemodynamics and on renal function in cirrhotic patients with ascites. *Gastroenterology* 88:1255–1259, 1985.
126. Wilkinson S, Weston M, Parsons V, et al: Dialysis in the treatment of renal failure in patients with liver disease. *Clin Nephrol* 8:287–292, 1977.
127. Golper TA: Continuous arteriovenous hemofiltration in acute renal failure. *Am J Kidney Dis* 673–686, 1984.
128. Achord J: Malnutrition and the role of nutritional support in alcoholic liver disease. *Am J Gastroenterol* 82:1, 1987.
129. Mendenhall DL, Anderson S, Weesner RE, et al: Protein-calorie malnutrition associated with alcoholic hepatitis. *Am J Med* 76:211–222, 1984.
130. Cabre E, Gonzalez-Huix F, Abad-Lacruz A, et al: Effect of total enteral nutrition on the short-term outcome of severely malnourished cirrhotics. *Gastroenterology* 98:715–720, 1990.
131. Mezey D: Nutritional state in liver disease. Assessment, incidence and mechanisms of malnutrition. In Holm E, Kasper H: *Metabolism and Nutrition in Liver Disease*, pp 5–15, Lancaster, UK, MTP, 1984.
132. Witte CL, Witte MH, Dumont AE, et al: Lymph protein in hepatic cirrhosis and experimental hepatic and portal venous hypertension. *Ann Surg* 168:567–577, 1968.
133. Yablonski ME, Lifson N: Mechanism of production of intestinal secretion by elevated venous pressure. *J Clin Invest* 57:904–915, 1976.
134. O'Keefe SJ, Abraham RR, Davis M, Williams R. Protein turnover in acute and chronic liver disease. *Acta Chir Scand* 507 (Suppl):91–101, 1981.
135. Cerra FB: Hypermetabolism, organ failure, and metabolic support. *Surgery* 101:1–14, 1987.

136. Green JH, Bramley PN, Losowsky MS: Are patients with primary biliary cirrhosis hypermetabolic? A comparison between patients before and after liver transplantation and controls. *Hepatology* 14:464–472, 1991.

137. Fischer JE: Hepatic failure. In Wilmore DW, Brennan MF, Harken AH, et al: *Care of the Surgical Patient: A Publication of the Committee on Pre and Postoperative Care*, pp 1–13, New York, Scientific American Medicine, 1990.

138. Mendenhall CL, Bongiovanni G, Goldberg S, et al: VA cooperative study on alcoholic hepatitis III: changes in protein-calorie malnutrition associated with 30 days of hospitalization with and without enteral nutritional therapy. *JPEN* 9:590–596, 1985.

139. Latifi R, Killam RW, Dudrick SJ: Nutritional support in liver failure. *Surg Clin N Am* 71:567–578, 1991.

140. Heymsfield SB, Bethel RA, Ansley JD, et al: Enteral hyperalimentation: an alternative to central venous hyperalimentation. *Ann Int Med* 90:63–71, 1979.

141. Jones KW, Seltzer MH, Slocum BA, et al: Parenteral nutrition complications in a voluntary hospital. *JPEN* 8:385–390, 1984.

142. Horst D, Grace ND, Conn HO, et al: Comparison of dietary protein with an oral, branched chain-enriched amino acid supplement in chronic portal-systemic encephalopathy: a randomized controlled trial. *Hepatology* 4:279–287, 1984.

143. Marchesini G, Zoli M, Dondi C, et al: Anticatabolic effect of branched-chain amino acid-enriched solutions in patients with liver cirrhosis. *Hepatology* 2:420–425, 1982.

144. Abad A, Cabre E, Gonzalez-Huix F, et al: Influence of the nutritional status in the prognosis and clinical outcome of hospitalized patients with liver cirrhosis. Preliminary report. *J Clin Nutr Gastroenterol* 2:63–68, 1987.

145. Pomar MJ, Bruguera M, Caballeria J, et al: Malnutricion calorico-proteica en pacientes hepaticos hospitalizados. *Gastroenterol Hepatol* 10:434–440, 1987.

146. Somogyi A, Rolan P: Drug disposition and dosing in hepatic disease. *Med J Aust* 145:284–289, 1986.

147. Secor JW, Schenker S: Drug metabolism in patients with liver disease. *Adv Int Med* 32:379–406, 1987.

148. Stoller JK: As the liver goes, so goes the lung (editorial; comment). *Chest* 97:1028–1030, 1990.

—11—

OPERATIVE TECHNIQUES AND STRATEGIES IN LIVER TRANSPLANTATION

Charles M. Miller, Myron E. Schwartz, Sukru Emre, and Cosme Manzarbeitia

Liver transplantation is often claimed to be the most complex and difficult of all general surgical operations.[1] It is of paramount importance that meticulous and delicate surgical technique be utilized throughout the donor and recipient operative procedures.[2] As in any transplant operation, close attention must be constantly given to methods that minimize trauma and ischemia to the organ during procurement and implantation. This chapter will attempt to highlight the important points of both the donor and the recipient operation that allow for the routine and successful transplantation of the liver.

THE DONOR

Prior to a formal discussion of the operative strategies involved in the donor hepatectomy, it is important to have an outline of criteria by which an appropriate liver donor is selected. Although originally age restrictions were placed on liver donors, there is no longer an absolute age limit.[3,4] We have used donors as old as 70 years with excellent results. There is no age restriction, because in contrast to that of the heart, kidney and many other organs, the liver does not suffer appreciable loss of function on the basis of age alone. Additionally, the hepatic arterial supply is almost always spared from the ravages of atherosclerosis and the liver has a dual blood supply, the portal vein, and the hepatic artery.

Many parameters are utilized to determine if a particular donor will be suitable. It is preferable that the donor be hemodynamically stable with a minimal to moderate requirement for pressor agents. Dopamine has not been found to be harmful to the liver, but the use of high-dose epinephrine or other potent visceral vasoconstrictors can cause ischemic damage to the liver and should be avoided.[5] In addition, donors that have suffered prolonged cardiac arrest with $>$ 30-min resuscitation have been found to be less suitable. To assess possible hepatic injury from hypoxia or other causes, serial liver function tests, including ALT, AST, and direct and total bilirubin, are routinely recorded. Elevations in transaminases alone are not a strict contraindication to the use of the liver, especially if serial determinations indicate progressive normalization.[4] An elevated total bilirubin in the presence of a normal direct bilirubin is a common finding and may be more indicative of hemolysis than of poor liver function. Although coagulation parameters are evaluated routinely, an abnormal prothrombin time is more often due to circulating cerebral thromboplastin released by penetrating or blunt brain injury than by hepatic dysfunction.

Before final acceptance of a potential donor liver it is important that serologies for HIV, hepatitis B, hepatitis C, CMV, and VDRL be available for review. A positive HIV test or the presence of hepatitis B surface antigen absolutely contraindicates use of the organ.[5,6] The significance of a positive hepatitis C antibody test is less clear. Organs from hepatitis C positive donors must be used with caution, and many centers are restricting their use to recipients with preexisting hepatitis C antibody or with extremely urgent indications. The presence of a positive VDRL need not contraindicate organ usage; the recipient should be treated with a 10-day course of prophylactic penicillin. Positive CMV serology should be noted by the recipient center, and the recipient, especially if CMV-negative, should receive appropriate prophylaxis.

DONOR SURGICAL TECHNIQUES

Once the donor arrives in the operating room, the anesthesiologist is responsible for maintaining hemodynamic stability and ventilation. This is simply done by ventilating the patient with 100% oxygen, administering a muscle relaxant such as Pavulon and monitoring the central venous pressure, arterial blood pressure, and urine output. Peripheral perfusion should be maintained primarily with appropriate fluid volume replacement and secondarily with pressor agents.

The donor is prepped from the chin to the pubis, and a long midline incision is made from the suprasternal notch to the pubic symphysis, opening the chest and abdomen. The liver is inspected and palpated to ensure that it is soft and that there is no obvious trauma. If the liver is found to be swollen in the face of an elevated central venous pressure, a colloid osmotic agent such as 25% albumin should be given. If the liver becomes softer as a result, indicating congestion rather than hepatic injury as the cause of swelling, the liver may safely be used. A liver that is persistently swollen in the presence of a normal central venous pressure has probably sustained a recent ischemic injury and should be used only with extreme caution.

Once the initial evaluation has been completed, the surgical dissection and removal process is begun. The goal is to remove the liver with its full complement of vascular and biliary structures attached in a rapid and atraumatic fashion.

Over the years this process has been refined and expedited by using en bloc dissection techniques that minimize vasospasm and the possibility for a surgical mishap.[6,7] This approach minimizes manipulation of the liver and its feeding vessels that can produce unrecognized periods of ischemia resulting in eventual poor organ function in the recipient.

A key principle of modern-day procurement technique is that of core cooling accomplished by in situ flushing with cold preservation solution through the aorta and portal vein prior to the removal of the organs.[7,8] To accomplish this, the supraceliac aorta at the level of the diaphragm is dissected and the distal aorta is cannulated. A cannula is also placed via either the splenic vein or the inferior mesenteric vein into the portal vein. The superior mesenteric vein should not be ligated or cannulated, in order to allow continuous portal perfusion of the liver with portal blood until the cold flush is initiated. With this minimal dissection completed, the supraceliac aorta is cross-clamped, and the cold flush initiated. The caval–atrial junction is transected in the chest to assure free venous outflow. When both the heart and the liver are to be procured, the cardiac surgeon may want to clamp the suprahepatic vena cava; in this case, the distal vena cava must be vented. The liver can be seen to blanch immediately. Iced saline slush is poured into the abdomen to provide additional surface cooling of the liver and viscera.

This cooling process is allowed to continue for approximately 5 min during which time the effluent coming from the vena cava becomes virtually blood-free. The liver is then excised en bloc with a large patch of diaphragm. The excised organ must include a long length of vena cava from the caval atrial junction above the liver to the level of the renal veins below. The hepatic and celiac arteries with a small patch of aorta are dissected free by dividing the splenic, left gastric, and gastroduodenal arterial attachments to the viscera. The full length of the portal vein along with a portion of the splenic and superior mesenteric veins is mobilized and removed with the liver. After harvesting of the liver, iliac arteries and veins are procured as a routine procedure for possible utilization as venous or arterial grafts in the recipient.

It is important during this process that the donor surgeon be cognizant of the fact that arterial variations are present in approximately 30% of all organ donors. The left hepatic artery originates from the left gastric artery in 15% of donors and the right hepatic artery arises from the superior mesenteric artery in an additional 12%.[9,10] These variants must be recognized, preserved, and removed en bloc with the liver. Techniques for the reconstruction of these arterial variations have been well worked out,[11,12] so that their presence in the donor should never contraindicate organ utilization.

After excision, the liver is placed in a plastic bag immersed in cold iced saline and reflushed with preservation solution to ensure its even distribution throughout the organ. The biliary system is flushed with preservation solution as well to ensure complete cleansing of caustic bile from the biliary system. This helps avoid autolysis of the biliary epithelium during the preservation period.

With the advent of the University of Wisconsin (UW) solution, cold storage can now be maintained for up to 20 hr with the expectation of prompt function in the recipient,[13] although most centers try to limit the cold-ischemic period to 14–15 hr.

Prior to the use of UW solution there was always a temporal overlap of the donor and recipient operations so as to limit the cold-ischemic interval to ≤ 8 hr. The recipient operation would begin prior to the return of the donor team with the liver. In addition, the recipient hepatectomy was often a rapid and hurried procedure that led to occasional surgical misadventures resulting in hemorrhage, poor organ function, and occasionally death. With the routine use of the UW solution, this hurried approach with its attendant risks has been eliminated. In addition, about 85% of transplants are now performed during the day by a fresh and well-rested surgical team. The recipient operation does not begin prior to the return of the donor team with the liver. This provides the opportunity to perform frozen-section liver biopsy in cases where there is a question about the quality of the donor organ. Only when the liver has received final approval from the recipient surgeon is the patient brought to the operating room and anesthesia initiated.

While anesthesia is being induced, the donor liver is removed from the ice cooler and prepared for implantation on a back bench. The extraneous tissues that accompany organs removed en bloc are trimmed. Arterial reconstruction, if necessary, is performed at this time. The essential principle of arterial reconstruction is to provide a single common inflow vessel so that only one anastomosis need be performed in the recipient. All vessels are then tested for patency and integrity by flushing with sterile preservation solution. The iliac arteries and veins routinely procured at the termination of the donor operation are prepared for use, if necessary, as venous or arterial grafts in the recipient.

RECIPIENT OPERATIVE TECHNIQUE

The basic objective of an orthotopic liver transplant operation is to remove the diseased native organ and then to replace it in exactly the same location with a normal new one. Although simple in concept, this task is made difficult by the strategic location of the liver under the right costal margin and its intimate association with large venous structures, i.e., the portal vein and the inferior vena cava. In addition, portal hypertension, tissue fragility, and coagulation deficiencies associated with end-stage liver disease may make the recipient hepatectomy fraught with the hazard of massive bleeding.[14] These difficulties are magnified even further in patients with prior right-upper-quadrant surgery. Because blood loss can be correlated with subsequent morbidity and mortality, it is imperative that careful attention to the meticulous, gentle handling of tissues and a strict systematic approach to hemostasis be followed throughout the recipient operation.

An expert team of dedicated anesthesiologists is as important for success as the surgical team. Large intravenous catheters are inserted in the upper extremities to allow for rapid fluid volume replacement, a Swan-Ganz catheter is placed for determination of fluid volume status and cardiac output, and a radial arterial line is positioned for continuous blood pressure monitoring and blood gas determinations.

A bilateral subcostal incision with a midline extension to the xiphoid process is routinely used (Fig. 11-1). There is no need to enter the right chest or mediasti-

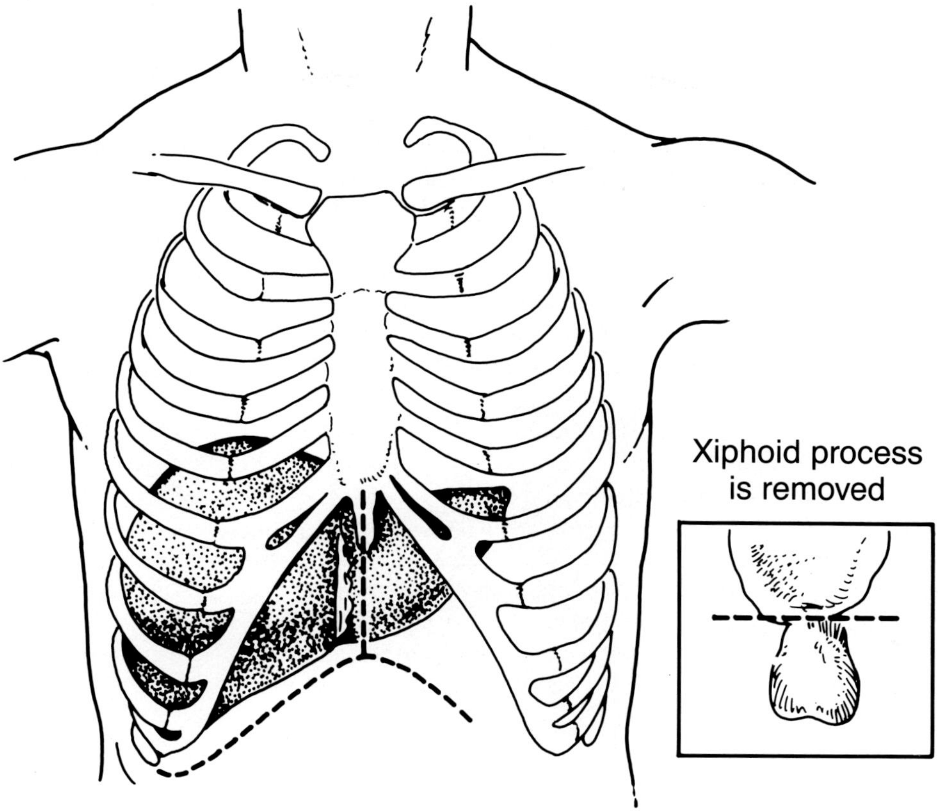

Figure 11-1. Incisions.

num. In addition, small incisions are made exposing the left axillary vein and left saphenous vein that are subsequently cannulated for venovenous bypass which will be described later. Large subcutaneous and intramuscular venous collaterals may be encountered in the abdominal wall that require formal ligation with fine silk. With the abdomen open, the round and falciform ligaments are divided, allowing the placement of a large self-retaining upper abdominal retractor. This device aids greatly in the exposure of the entire liver and, more importantly, the suprahepatic vena cava. There are many ways to proceed, but a sound basic strategy is to start with the hilar dissection (Fig. 11-2) and quickly dearterialize the liver by ligating the right and left hepatic arteries. This step significantly reduces blood loss from raw surfaces of the liver. After the cystic duct is tied and cut, the common hepatic duct is ligated and transected close to the hilum. The only remaining hilar structure is the portal vein surrounded by neurolymphatic connective tissue. The portal vein is carefully cleared from the level of gastroduodenal artery up to its bifurcation. The hepatic artery is now formally dissected, exposing the common hepatic artery to allow for subsequent anastomosis. Venovenous bypass may now be initiated.

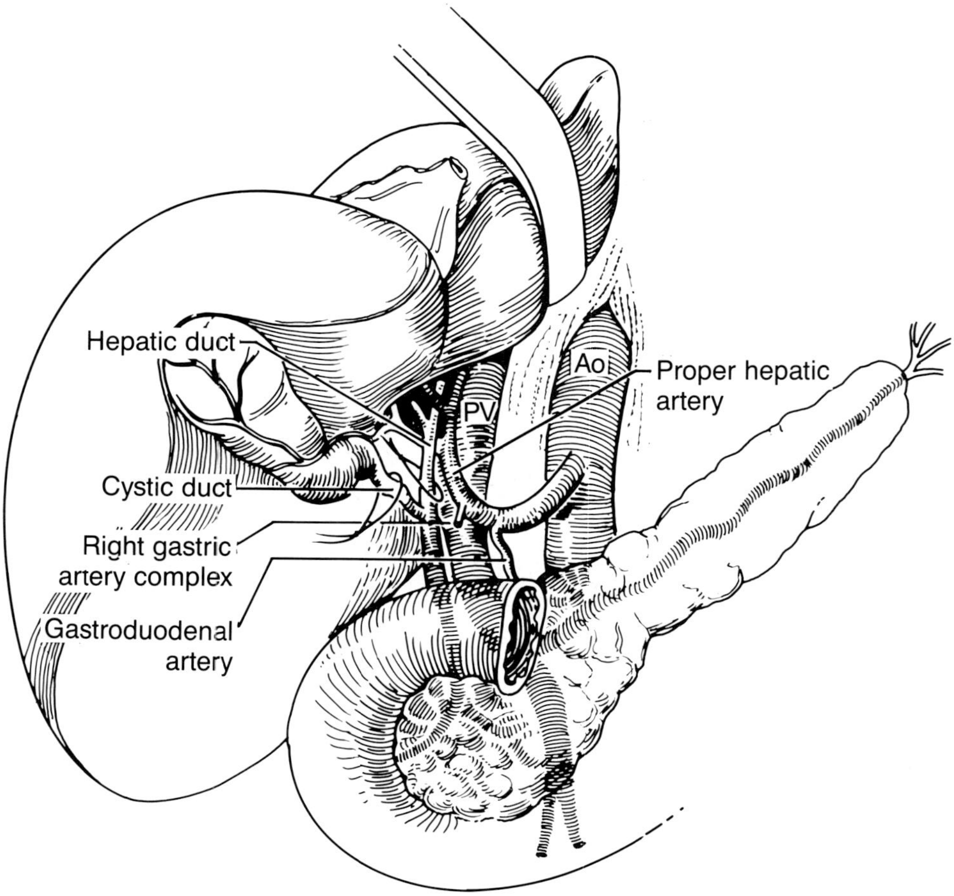

Figure 11-2. Hilar dissection.

Venovenous Bypass

During the anhepatic phase of a liver transplant, the inferior vena cava is occluded. Although most children and some adult patients may tolerate the attendant fall in cardiac output, there may be significant hemodynamic changes. In addition, bleeding as well as damage to the bowel and kidneys may be caused by the unrelieved venous hypertension. In 1983, Griffith et al[15] described the use of a venovenous bypass system using a nonheparinized centrifugal pump that decompressed both the portal and systemic venous systems below the diaphragm by shunting this blood to the superior vena cava via the axillary vein (Fig. 11-3). The venovenous bypass has been widely adopted as standard practice. It is relatively easy to institute, and once in place there is immediate relief of portal hypertension. The liver is completely devascularized, and there is a marked reduction in bleeding. Furthermore, there is no decrease in venous return to the heart when the vena cava is occluded and therefore hemodynamic changes are minimal. For these reasons, the completion of the hepatectomy and

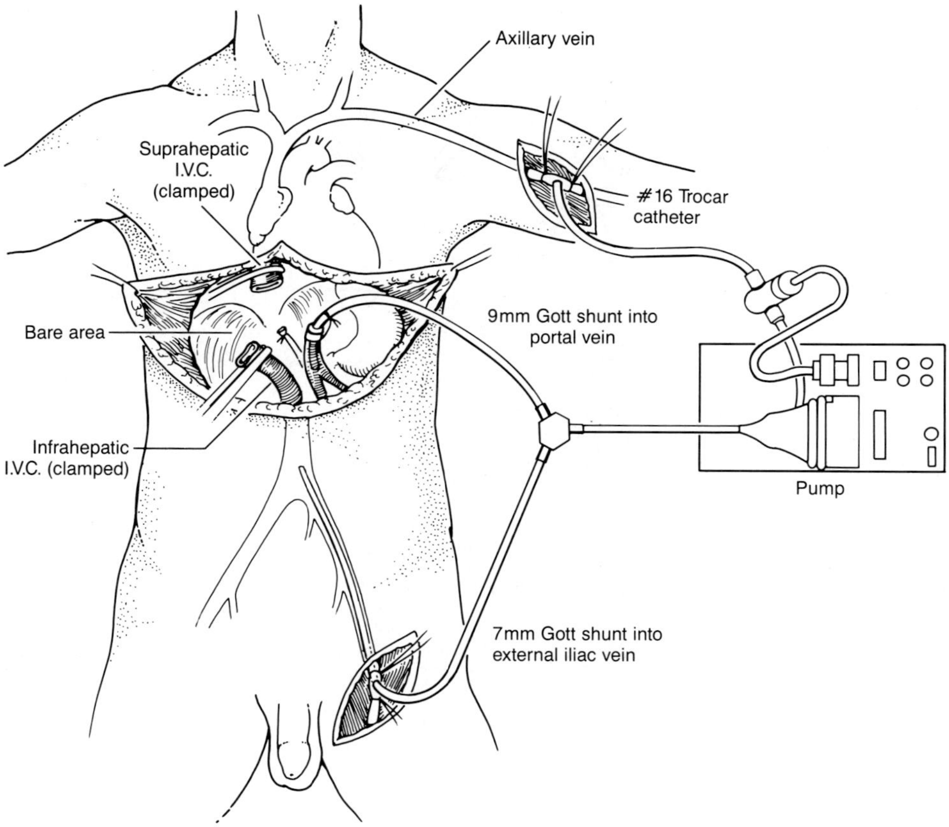

Figure 11-3. Veno-venous bypass.

implantation of the new liver that otherwise must be performed in a very rushed and frenetic manner can now be done in a deliberate and meticulous way that reduces the physiologic stress on the patient and the psychological stress on the surgeon.

Venovenous bypass can be instituted at any point during the hepatectomy operation. The decision when to go on bypass depends on the degree of portal hypertension, the extent of previous surgery with vascularized adhesions, and the degree of bleeding from the raw surface of the liver. In some cases, especially in patients with cholestatic liver disease and no previous surgery, the entire mobilization and dissection of the liver can be done prior to the institution of the venovenous bypass. However, in cases with severe portal hypertension and previous surgery where bleeding is a problem, venovenous bypass should be initiated at the earliest opportunity. The remaining attachments to the liver can then be divided rapidly.

With a bypass instituted and caval clamps applied, the liver is then sharply excised. What remains is an upper caval cuff at the diaphragm that includes the open orifices of the hepatic veins, a lower caval cuff above the renal veins, and the bare area that was behind the right lobe of the liver. The bare area is oversewn for hemostasis, and the vena caval cuff is fashioned for anastomosis (Fig. 11-4).

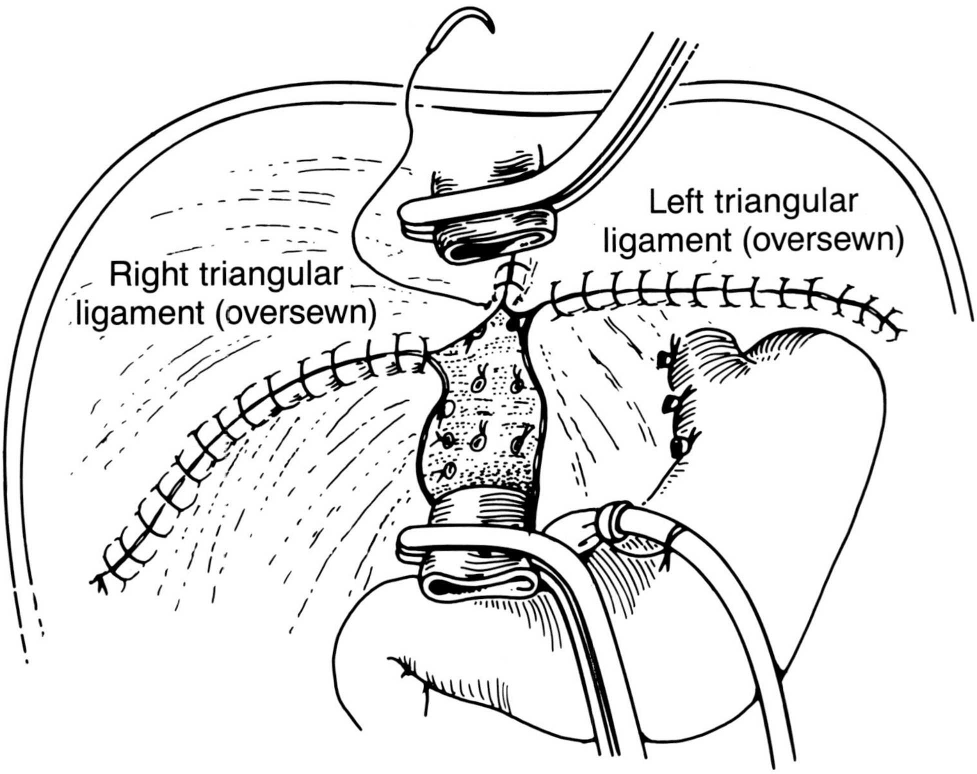

Figure 11-4. Oversewing of bare areas.

The implantation of the liver follows a strict routine. The suprahepatic vena cava is anastomosed first. Although adequate exposure for this anastomosis can be difficult, it is of extreme importance to leave the distance between the upper surface of the liver and the diaphragm extremely short to prevent torsion or kinking of the suprahepatic anastomosis. With this completed, the vena cava is anastomosed below the liver; a venting catheter is left within the cava through the lower caval anastomosis, which is left untied until after reperfusion. The recipient portal vein is now decannulated. The extra lengths of both the donor and recipient portal veins are trimmed and an end-to-end portal anastomosis is performed in a manner that redundancy and kinking is avoided.

Modern preservation solutions have high concentrations of potassium. For this reason, the liver must be flushed free of preservation solution prior to re-opening the circulation. This can be accomplished either by infusion of a crystalloid solution via the portal vein during the infrahepatic vena caval anastomosis or with portal blood subsequent to the portal anastomosis. We now routinely drain through the indwelling cannula in the vena cava the first 500 mL of portal blood reperfusing the liver. In this way, any remaining preservation solution as well as potentially toxic metabolites are removed from the circulation. After this initial reperfusion, the indwelling cannula is removed and the caval clamps are opened, restoring normal flow. A rapid inspection for hemostasis is made, the remaining venovenous bypass cannulae are removed, and attention is turned to the hepatic artery.

HEPATIC ARTERY

Perfect reconstruction of the hepatic artery is essential because, in contrast to native livers that can withstand hepatic artery occlusion, the transplanted liver is devoid of collateral arterial circulation and thus cannot tolerate arterial thrombosis. Hepatic arterial thrombosis in the early postoperative period necessitates retransplantation in approximately 98% of cases.

The important technical points in hepatic artery revascularization are to ensure (1) an adequate inflow vessel, (2) that the handling of this artery is delicate and that the clamps applied to it cause no intimal damage, and (3) that the anastomosis provides perfect intimal approximation and is not stenotic. We have found that the routine use of the common hepatic artery at the level of the gastroduodenal artery usually results in adequate inflow. The anastomosis is performed in an end-to-end fashion, sewing the common hepatic artery to the celiac artery of the donor. We use small, delicate vascular clamps adopted from the neurosurgical experience to minimize or eliminate intimal damage. It is important to leave some redundancy in the hepatic artery as this actually prevents kinking in the postoperative period. To confirm adequacy of the arterial reconstruction, flow is measured with an electromagnetic flowmeter;[16,17] in adults it is, ≥ 200 mL/min at rest. Furthermore, this baseline flow should augment by 30–100% when portal flow is temporarily occluded. If flow is found to be inadequate, the artery is scrutinized to determine the reason and that any problem is corrected.

If there is any doubt as to the adequacy of the inflow, an aortohepatic graft should be used. This is performed by utilizing an iliac artery harvested from the donor. Most commonly, the graft is sewn end-to-side to the aorta at a level just below the renal arteries. It is then tunneled either posterior to the pancreas and into the lesser sac or, as described more recently, anterior to the pancreas and through the transverse mesocolon into the lesser sac.[18] The graft is then sewn end-do-end to the celiac axis of the donor liver. Although aortohepatic grafts are required in only 10% of the cases, they are needed in 25% of retransplantations. They can be life-saving and should not be avoided when there use is deemed necessary (Figs. 11-5 and 11-6).

THE PROBLEM OF PORTAL VEIN THROMBOSIS

Portal vein thrombosis at one time contraindicated liver transplantation; this is no longer the case. Techniques for the replacement of the portal vein or for thrombectomy of a recent thrombus have been described.[19,20] The use of long

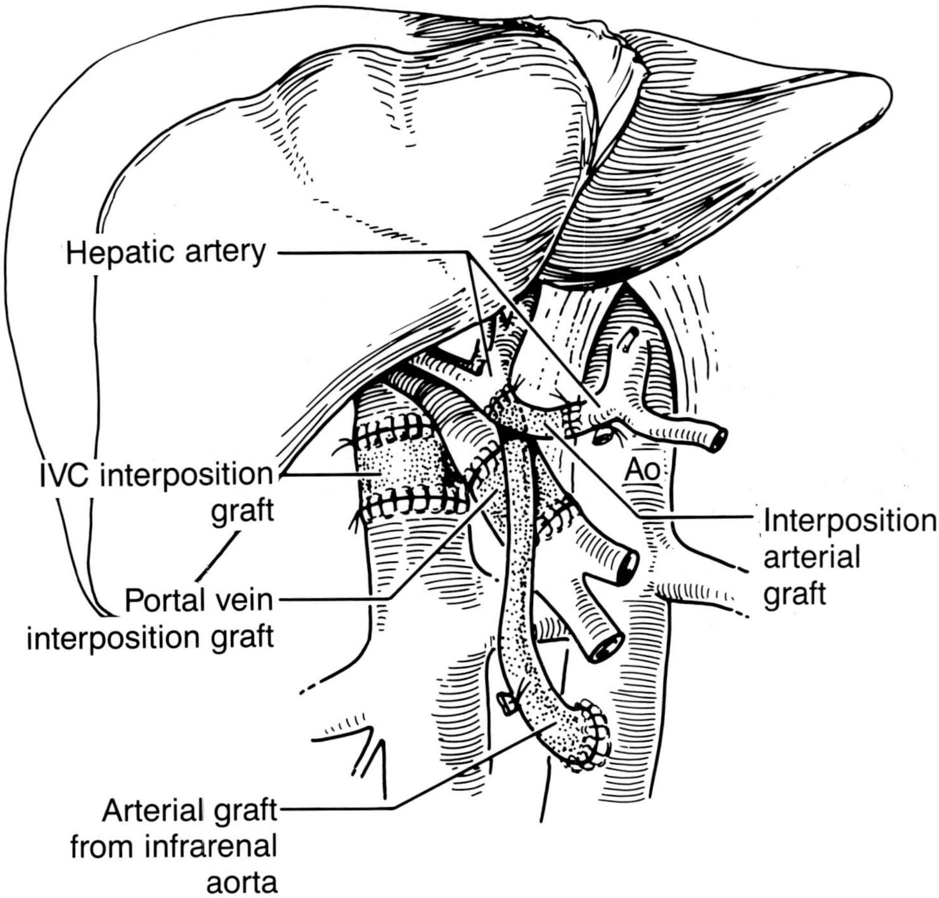

Figure 11-5. Diverse uses of grafts.

iliac vein grafts that can be placed in an extra anatomic position from the superior mesenteric vein and run over the neck of the pancreas have served to decrease the morbidity and mortality attendant with portal vein replacement.[21,22] Portal vein thrombectomy in cases where the thrombosis is less well organized is a simple and effective technique that reserves the proximal portion of the native portal vein for anastomosis. As with the artery, it is important to ensure adequate portal flow; electromagnetic flow measurements are made here as well. Portal flow in the adult should be at least 1 L/min to ensure long- and short-term patency.

The new liver is now in place and completely revascularized. Prior to the reestablishment of biliary continuity, hemostasis must be complete. While in some cases this task may consist of the simple inspection of the anastomoses and suture of a few small bleeding points, in other cases it may require tremendous effort to completely control bleeding. This is dependent on a number of factors, including the preoperative status of the recipient, the degree of preexisting portal hypertension, how well hemostasis was achieved prior to the im-

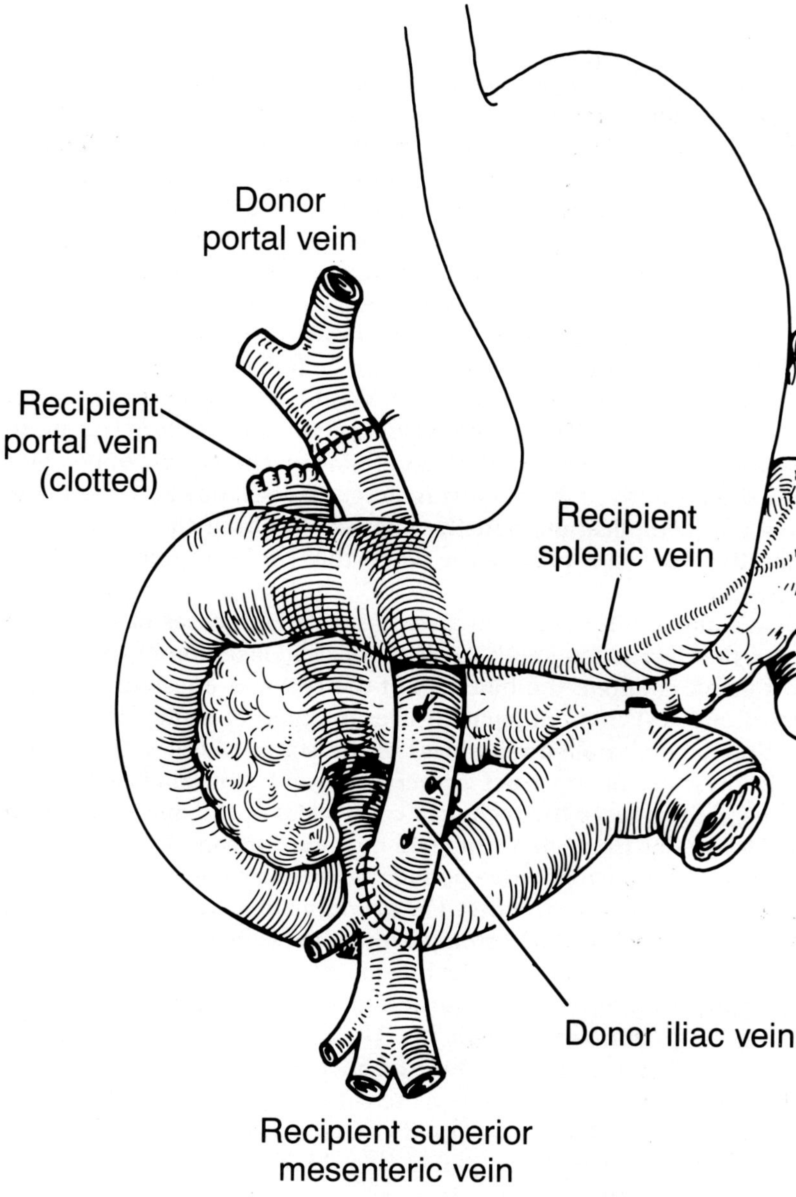

Figure 11-6. Jump graft, portal vein.

plantation of the new liver, how rapidly the new liver begins to function, and whether fibrinolysis develops. If a marginal organ is implanted into a very sick cirrhotic patient with prior surgery, 5–6 hr of work may be needed to achieve hemostasis. Patience on the part of the surgeon, however, is rewarded because when the liver begins to function, the operative field changes dramatically; clots begin to form, small bleeding points previously recalcitrant to surgical measures stop bleeding, and the surgeon knows that the biliary reconstruction can now be completed.

BILIARY RECONSTRUCTION

The reconstruction of the bile duct, once considered the Achilles' heel of liver transplantation,[23,24] is now a routine and simple procedure. If the recipient bile duct is of normal caliber and free of intrinsic disease, a simple donor to recipient duct-to-duct reconstruction can be performed. Most commonly this reconstruction is performed over an indwelling T-tube stent that is exteriorized from the recipient's bile duct through a separate stab wound incision approximately 1 in below the anastomosis. The anastomosis is performed with interrupted absorbable sutures so that "purse-stringing" will not cause an anastomotic stricture. The T-tube acts not only as a stent to prevent possible stricture, but prevents kinking as well. If the two ends of the bile duct can be tailored to meet perfectly without redundancy and are of similar caliber, this end-to-end reconstruction can be performed without a T-tube. This makes visualization of the biliary tree more difficult in the early postoperative period, necessitating an endoscopic or percutaneous approach should study of the duct be required. It does, however, eliminate a potential source of complication, namely, bile leakage from the point where the T-tube exits the duct that may occur when the T-tube is removed three months posttransplant.

If the patient's native bile duct is diseased (especially in cases of sclerosing cholangitis), or if the duct is too small to allow for easy insertion of the T-tube such as in most small children, the bile duct of the donor is anastomosed to a defunctionalized Roux-en-Y loop of jejunum over an internal stent. Liver transplantation can thus be undertaken regardless of the status of the native biliary system; multiple previous biliary tract surgeries do not contraindicate transplantation but merely increases the technical complexity of the operation. With a choledochojejunostomy Roux-en-Y there is no direct means for cholangiographic procedures in the postoperative period; percutaneous methods must be used to visualize the bile duct. In the first 179 primary adult transplantations at our institution, choledochocholedochostomy with an indwelling T-tube was used in 131, without a T-tube in 7, and choledochojejunostomy Roux-en-Y in 41.

Cholangiography is performed to confirm a technically sound biliary reconstruction and may be performed through the T-tube or via the cystic duct in cases with choledochojejunostomy or choledochocholedochostomy without a T-tube. There should be clear visualization of the entire intrahepatic and extrahepatic ductal system with free flow of dye into the duodenum or the jejunum loop. The anastomosis should appear widely patent (Fig. 11-7).

With this completed, the operation is concluded by closing the abdomen after leaving three closed suction drains above and below the liver. The closure should be done with as much attention to detail as the rest of the operation to reduce the risk of postoperative wound infection and sepsis.

SPECIAL CONSIDERATIONS IN PEDIATRIC LIVER TRANSPLANTATION

Although the same in basic concept, liver transplantation in the pediatric population, especially in children weighing $\leq$ 10 kg, presents numerous challenges to

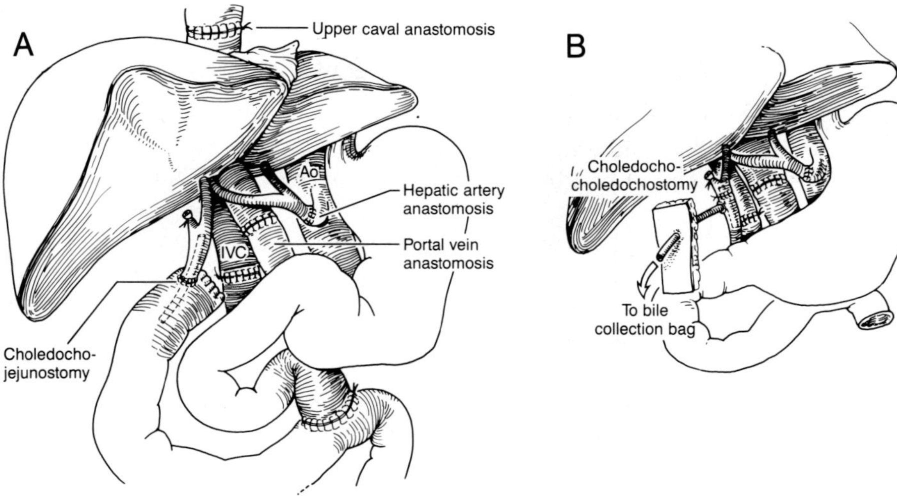

Figure 11-7. The final result.

the transplant team. The prevalence of biliary atresia has created a pool of small children in desperate need of liver transplantation. The relative shortage of small organ donors that allow for whole-organ transplantation has led most pediatric transplant programs to resort to using lobes and segments of adolescent and adult size livers for these patients.[26,27] The most common type of graft used is a left lateral segment graft that can be prepared from a donor weighing 8–10 times as much as the recipient. When the size discrepancy between donor and recipient is not as great, the entire left lobe graft can be used and in a very small number of cases where the discrepancy between donor and recipient is less than 2 to 1, a right lobe graft may be implanted safely. Of special note with the left lateral segment graft is that this segment is used without the vena cava, only the left hepatic vein being used for venous outflow.[28] Is it therefore necessary in performing the recipient hepatectomy to remove the liver from the patient while leaving the entire vena cava intact. This necessitates dissecting out each major and minor hepatic vein with ligation or suture transfixion. The left hepatic vein of the donor segment is then anastomosed to the side of the intact vena cava, allowing for free outflow of blood from the implanted segment. The routine use of segmental reduced-size livers has drastically reduced the number of small babies who died while on the waiting list and, in experienced hands, has yielded short- and long-term survival rates as good as or better than whole-organ transplants.

A few experienced centers have taken the concept of reduced-size liver grafting further to include splitting a single adult organ into two lobes (Fig. 11-8), most commonly the right lobe and the left lateral segment, and implanting these segments into two different recipients. This has never been done on a routine basis as this concept necessitates the mandatory use of venous and arterial grafts on one or the other lobe and there has been reported a high incidence of graft loss.[28] It should be stated, however, that the trials studying the splitting of livers are still in an early stage. As the technical complexities of liver grafting are

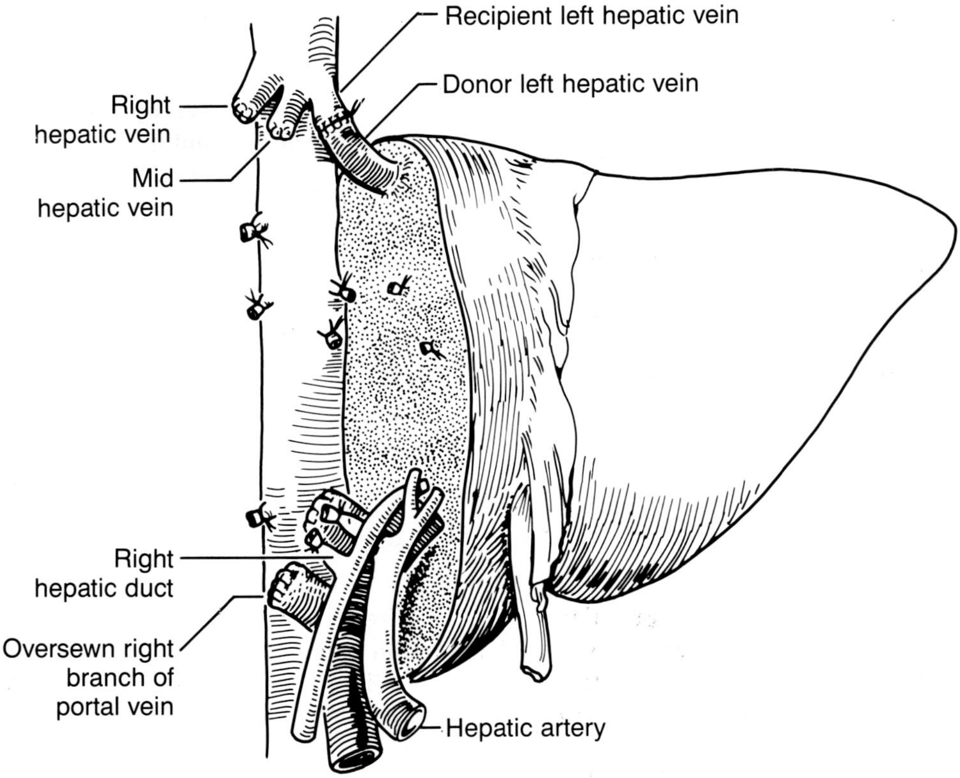

Figure 11-8. Segmental transplantation.

solved, this approach has the great potential of doubling the organ supply if used routinely. A logistical problem associated with this is the need to be able to perform two simultaneous liver transplantations and the physicians, nurses, and other health care workers required to support that effort.

Another major problem in small baby liver transplantation is that of vascular thrombosis due to the diminutive size of the vessels. Historically, the rate of hepatic artery thrombosis was as high as 20 or 30% in babies < 10 kg.[29] With the use of the UW preservation solution and the better endothelial cell preservation it provides, the rate of hepatic artery thrombosis has dropped dramatically,[30] but still remains a significant problem. One of the hidden advantages in using the reduced-size segmental grafts in babies is that their arteries are long and large and can be anastomosed directly to the supraceliac or infrarenal aorta. This type of revascularization has been found to have a low rate of arterial thrombosis presumably because of the better inflow and larger anastomosis possible due to the size of the vessels.

Many children with biliary atresia are found to have very small, atretic portal veins and large venous collaterals. The use of this small native portal vein for inflow is problematic, and liberal use of venous grafts arising from the confluence of the splenic and superior mesenteric veins is wise in this group. In this way, a large, spatulated anastomosis can be constructed, providing the liver graft with vigorous portal inflow.

The final major hurdle in pediatric liver transplantation is mainly in babies with biliary atresia. Because almost all of these children have had previous portoenterostomy (Kasai) procedures that may have required multiple revisions, the recipient hepatectomy can be extraordinarily difficult, and occasionally enterotomies are inadvertently made because of the extensive nature of the adhesions and their vascularity. Most often damaged areas are recognized and repaired at the time of surgery, but occasionally small-bowel segments become devascularized, leading to the syndrome of multiple bowel fistulae in the post operative period, a most difficult clinical problem. It is, therefore, the preference of all pediatric liver transplant surgeons that Kasai-type procedures be performed only once so as to avoid these very difficult problems when it is clear that ultimately liver transplantation will be necessary.

REFERENCES

1. Starzl TE, Demetris AJ: Liver transplantation: a 31 year perspective, part I. *Curr Prob Surg* 3:51–116, 1990.
2. Krom RAF, Gips, CH: Skills and resources needed for liver transplantation. *Hepatology* 4:72–75, 1984.
3. Popper H: Coming of age. *Hepatology* 5:1224–1226, 1985.
4. Darby JM, Stein K, Grenvik A, et al: Approach to management of the heartbeating "brain dead" organ donor. *JAMA* 261:2222–2228, 1989.
5. Soifer BE, Gelf AW: The multiple organ donor: Identification and management. *Ann Intern Med* 110:814–823, 1989.
6. Starzl TE, Miller, CM, Rapaport FT: Algorithm and explantation: approach to the potential organ donor. In American College of Surgeons: *Care of the Surgical Patient, Elective Care;* Chapter XI, Miscellaneous care problems. Reprinted in *Scientific American,* 1990.
7. Starzl TE, Miller CM, Broznick B, et al: An improved technique for multiple organ harvesting. *Surg Gynecol Obstet* 165:343, 1987.
8. Miller CM, Mazzaferro V, Makowka L, et al: Rapid flush technique for donor hepatectomy: safety and efficacy of an improved method of liver recovery for transplantation. *Transplant Proc* 20:948–950, 1988.
9. Lippert H, Pabst R: Arterial Variations in Man: Classification and Frequency, pp. 32–33, Munich, JF Bergmann Verlag, 1985.
10. Todo S, Makowka L, Tzakis AG, et al: Hepatic artery in liver transplantation. *Transplant Proc* 19:2406–2411, 1987.
11. Shaw BW, Iwatsuki S, Starzl TE: Alternative methods of arterialization of the hepatic graft. *Surg Gynecol Obstet* 159:490–494, 1984.
12. Gordon RD, Shaw BW, Iwatsuki S, et al: A simplified technique for revascularization of homografts of the liver with a variant right hepatic artery from the superior mesenteric artery. *Surg Gynecol Obstet* 160:474–476, 1985.
13. Kalayoglu M, Sollinger HW, Stratta RJ, et al: Extended preservation of the liver for clinical transplantation. *Lancet* 1:617–619, 1988.

14. Starzl TE, Iwatsuki S, Van Thiel DH, et al: Evolution of liver transplantation. *Hepatology* 2:614–636, 1982.
15. Griffith BP, Shaw BW, Hardesty RL, et al: Veno-venous bypass without systemic anticoagulation for transplantation of the human liver. *Surg Gynecol Obstet* 160:271, 1985.
16. Klintmalm GB, Olson LM, Paulsen AW, et al: Hepatic arterial thrombosis after liver transplantation: intraoperative electromagnetic blood flow evaluation. *Transplant Proc* 10:616–618, 1988.
17. Yanaga K, Makowka L, Shimada M, et al: Hepatic artery thrombosis following pediatric liver transplantation: assessment of blood flow measurement in allografts. *Hepatology* 3:184–189, 1989.
18. Goldstein RM, Secrest CL, Klintmalm GB, et al: Problematic vascular reconstruction in liver transplantation. Part I. *Arterial Surg* 107:540–543, 1990.
19. Lerut J, Tzakis AG, Bron K, et al: Complications of venous reconstruction in human orthotopic liver transplantation. *Ann Surg* 205:404–414, 1987.
20. Shaw BW, Iwatsuki S, Bron K, et al: Portal vein grafts in hepatic transplantation. *Surg Gynecol Obstet* 161:67–69, 1985.
21. Tzakis A, Todo S, Stieber A, et al: Venous jump grafts for liver transplantation in patients with portal vein thrombosis. *Transplantation* 48:530–531, 1989.
22. Kirsch JP, Howard TK, Klintmalm GB, et al: Problematic vascular reconstruction in liver transplantation. Part II. Portovenous conduits. *Surgery* 107:544–548, 1990.
23. Calne RY: A new technique for biliary drainage in orthotopic liver transplantation utilizing the gallbladder as a pedicle graft conduit between the donor and recipient common bile ducts. *Ann Surg* 184:605–609, 1926.
24. Stratta RJ, Wood RP, Langnas AN, et al: Diagnosis and treatment of biliary tract complications after orthotopic liver transplantation. *Clin Pharmacol Ther* 106:675–684, 1989.
25. Bismuth H, Houssin D. Reduced-sized orthotopic liver grafts in hepatic transplantation in children. *Surgery* 95:367–370, 1984.
26. Broelsch CE, Edmond JC, Thistlethwaite JR: Liver transplantation including the concept of reduced-sized liver transplants in children. *Ann Surg* 208:410–420, 1988
27. Otte JB, DeVille De Goyet J, et al: Size reduction of the donor liver is a safe way to alleviate the shortage of size-matched organs in pediatric liver transplantation. *Ann Surg* 211:146–157, 1990.
28. Edmond JC, Whittington PF, Thistlethwaite JR, et al: Transplantation of two patients with one liver. *Ann Surg* 212:14–22, 1990.
29. Esquivel CO, Koneru B, Karrer F, et al: Liver transplantation before 1 year of age. *J Ped* 110:545–548, 1987.
30. Mazzaferro V, Esquivel CO, Makowka L, et al: Hepatic artery thrombosis after pediatric liver transplantation—a medical or surgical event. *Transplantation* 47:971–977, 1989.

—12—

EVALUATION, COMPLICATIONS, AND THERAPY IN THE IMMEDIATE POSTOPERATIVE PERIOD

Myron E. Schwartz, Cosme Manzarbeitia, and Charles M. Miller

Immediately following transplantation the patient is transferred to the surgical intensive care unit (SICU), where care is supervised jointly by the SICU staff and the transplant team. Arterial and Swan-Ganz catheters are employed routinely, and the urine output is recorded hourly. The patient is maintained on mechanical ventilation until wide awake and showing evidence of good graft function. Intravenous fluids are kept to a minimum compatible with hemodynamic stability; most patients have gross total body fluid overload immediately following surgery. Wound care is performed using sterile technique with gowns, masks, and gloves. The volume and characteristics of wound drainage are monitored daily.

Serum chemistries are analyzed every 8 hr for the first 24–48 hr and then once daily, depending on the condition of the patient. While in the SICU, a daily chest x-ray is performed. Laboratory results and other pertinent information are recorded on a bedside wall chart (see Table 12-1).

THE MOUNT SINAI MEDICAL CENTER
TRANSPLANTATION FLOW SHEET

RECIPIENT NAME ______________________ HOSPITAL NUMBER ______________________

Recipient: Age: ___ Sex: ___ ABO ___ CMV ___

Donor: Age: ___ Sex: ___ ABO ___ CMV ___ PRA ___ Crossmatch _____ # HLA Match ____

ORIGINAL CAUSE OF ORGAN FAILURE ______________________

DATE				TEMP	WEIGHT	Blood Pressure			BLOOD GASES			HEMATOLOGY												BLOOD CHEMISTRIES																	
			Post-op day	High in 24 hr.			24 Hour Volume								Differential																										
YEAR	MONTH	DAY		F°	Lbs	BP	Urine	Bile	PO_2	PCO_2	PH	Hgb / Hct	WBC	Platelets	Seg	Bands	Lymph	Atyp Lymph	Mono	Eos	PT	PTT	Fi-brin-ogen	Na	K	Cl	CO_2	BUN	Creat	Uric Acid	T.P.	Alb	Mg	P / Ca	Amy	Glu	LDH	AP / GGTP	Bili T/D	(ALT) SGPT	(AST) SGOT

TRANSPLANT NUMBER
1st 2nd 3rd

BILIARY/URETERIC ANASTAMOSIS

DATE OF TRANSPLANT

STARTING DATE OF THIS FLOWSHEET

Vascular Technique ______________ ______________

______ month ______ day ______ year ______ month ______ day ______ year

		IMMUNOSUPPRESSIVE THERAPY											MEDICATIONS							PROCEDURES						INVASIVE PROCEDURES		NUTRITION		COMMENTS
		CY-A																												
) T	(AST) SGOT	IV	PO	PRED	Solu Medrol	AZA	FK-506	OKT_3	MALG	C_sA Level	FK Level	T-3 Subsets	Cultures Sent	Results	Antibiotics					Chest X-ray	Cholan-giogram	Sono	Biopsy	Dialysis	Scan	Procedure	Findings	Diet	Calorie Count	

ASSESSMENT OF LIVER FUNCTION IN THE EARLY POSTOPERATIVE PERIOD

The liver plays a central role in the body's metabolism and homeostasis; the manifestations of hepatic dysfunction are, therefore, protean. In the early postoperative period, liver function is clearly reflected in the clinical status of the patient as well as in laboratory tests. The following parameters should be considered:

Acid–Base Status

Poor early graft function is associated with persistent acidosis with elevated lactate levels. A more common finding in the early postoperative period is metabolic alkalosis, most likely due to sodium bicarbonate administered in the operating room after reperfusion of the allograft. With good liver function, these metabolic derangements are corrected over the first 24–48 hr.

Bile Production

Bile production in the early postoperative period is a good barometer of liver function. Since 80–85% of patients will have a T-tube placed within the common duct, bile output and character are readily measured postoperatively. Bile production in a liver with good early function will be ≥ 100 mL/24 hr. Normal bile is somewhat viscous and golden-brown, not unlike motor oil. Scant, green, watery bile is evidence of allograft injury, whether ischemic or immune-mediated. In cases where the biliary reconstruction is via choledochojejunostomy, a transjejunal catheter can be placed across the biliary anastomosis to allow for monitoring of the bile, although this has not been our practice.

Mental Status

Patients with normal mental status before transplant should awaken promptly and fully after surgery. Failure to do so suggests poor early graft function. Patients with advanced hepatic coma preoperatively may take a few days to awaken after surgery, and in such cases mental status is not a reliable indicator of graft function. Ammonia levels are elevated in cases with poor early function, but do not correlate particularly well with mental status.

Correction of Coagulopathy

Regardless of the degree of coagulopathy pretransplant as the result of native liver dysfunction, clotting should normalize rapidly after the new liver is in place. This is evident even on the operating table, and in patients with properly functioning allografts tests of coagulation are near normal by the second postoperative day. The platelet count regularly drops over the first 5–7 days posttransplant, with the degree of thrombocytopenia proportional to the extent of hypersplenism before surgery.

Renal Function

Renal function is intimately linked with liver function, and in patients with poor early graft function renal failure rapidly ensues. The renal dysfunction in patients with the hepatorenal syndrome can in some cases reverse immediately on revascularization of the new liver; more commonly, however, a slower resolution of renal failure occurs. This may be due to renal injury other than the purely physiologic hepatorenal derangement, which was not appreciated preoperatively, and to the nephrotoxic effects of immunosuppressive drugs.

Serum Chemistry

Transaminases (AST and ALT) are released into the circulation from injured or dying hepatocytes. Their levels thus reflect the degree of ischemic injury incurred during the process of transplantation. They generally peak on the second or third postoperative day (POD) and fall rapidly thereafter. Patients in whom allografts suffered no significant injury may exhibit transaminases in the range of 200–300 IU; with severe injury, levels may rise to 5000 IU or more. Bilirubin correlates less well with graft function; its level early after surgery is influenced by the preoperative level and by the amount of transfusion required intraoperatively. By the fourth or fifth day, the bilirubin will generally begin to fall; a climbing bilirubin beyond this point suggests allograft dysfunction or a technical problem with the biliary reconstruction. There is no consistent pattern of elevation for the biliary tract enzymes, alkaline phosphatase and gamma glutamyl transpeptidase, in the perioperative period.

Imaging Techniques

On postoperative day 3, a color-flow duplex ultrasound study is performed to confirm patency of the hepatic artery and portal vein. The absence of an arterial signal should be confirmed by celiac arteriography. It is essential that the surgeon review the films with the radiologist to accurately inform him about anatomic variations or vascular reconstructions which may be present.

On the same day, a T-tube cholangiogram is performed in patients with a T-tube to assess the biliary reconstruction. In patients with Roux-en-Y hepaticojejunostomy, HIDA scan, while not providing precise anatomical information, can be useful in ruling out obstruction or leak.

MANAGEMENT OF THE UNCOMPLICATED POSTOPERATIVE COURSE

Respiratory Care

In uncomplicated cases, the patient is extubated within 24 hr. An arterial line is maintained for 2–3 days for continual blood pressure monitoring and frequent blood gas determinations. Patients with advanced debility before transplant are likely to require prolonged ventilatory support; despite meeting standard criteria for weaning from ventilation, the very wasted patient will predictably fail early efforts at extubation. Atelectasis is seen frequently, and vigorous chest physiotherapy is routine. Patients begun on OKT3 must be observed for the development of noncardiogenic pulmonary edema following the first dose; this complication is much more likely to occur in the setting of fluid overload. A daily chest x-ray is performed while the patient is in the SICU. In patients with poor early graft function, it is prudent to delay extubation, since encephalopathy and resultant aspiration may ensue.

After extubation, a program of respiratory therapy must be instituted to prevent mucous plugging of the airways, especially in debilitated patients. This includes incentive spirometry, chest physiotherapy, and early ambulation. If extubation is not possible within about two weeks, consideration is given to the performance of a tracheostomy.

Renal

Patients with end-stage liver disease commonly exhibit renal dysfunction. While the abnormal physiology responsible for the so-called hepatorenal syndrome reverses rapidly after transplantation, the immunosuppressive agents begun immediately postoperatively may cause significant oliguria. Most patients leave the operating room well, if not overhydrated. Fluid therapy should be guided by the hemodynamic parameters, maintaining an adequate pulmonary capillary wedge pressure. Once hemodynamics are optimized, efforts to further increase the urine output by repeated fluid challenges may result in fluid overload, to the detriment of the patient. "Renal-dose" dopamine is useful, increasing renal perfusion. If massive fluid overload is present, such as may be seen following a long transplant procedure requiring large amounts of transfusion, continuous arteriovenous hemofiltration (CAVH) is a helpful adjunct. Hemodialysis should be instituted early in patients with evidence of oliguric renal failure following transplantation.

Renal failure also develops in the setting of poor graft function. Prostaglandin E_1, when administered in this setting, induces diuresis and improves renal function.[1] This benefit is probably due both to improved liver function and to direct vasodilatory effect of the drug on the kidney.

Moderate to severe intrinsic renal disease (not due to functional causes, i.e., hepatorenal syndrome), can be managed with simultaneous liver-kidney transplantation if the patient meets criteria for both.

Nutrition

Liver transplant candidates are frequently malnourished, with muscle wasting and anergy. After a successful transplant, a return to normal nutritional status is expected; in the severely depleted patients, however, this is a long and sometimes difficult process.[2]

In the uncomplicated case, oral feeding is begun on the first or second postoperative day, starting with fluids and progressing as tolerated to a regular diet. For patients requiring prolonged respiratory support or who are otherwise unable to resume oral intake, alternative routes for the provision of nutrition are needed. Options available include enteral tube feedings and parenteral nutrition; whenever possible use of enteral feeding is preferred. We have avoided gastrostomy and jejunostomy tubes in transplant patients because of concerns about healing in the face of corticosteroids. Early and continual attention to the nutritional requirements of these patients is an important aspect of their care.

Preexisting Diseases

Cardiac

Since liver transplantation is taxing on the cardiovascular system, patients over age 50 and those with a history of cardiac disease are seen preoperatively by a cardiologist. All alcoholic patients also undergo cardiologic evaluation, since cardiomyopathy is prevalent in this group. Because of this careful screening process, cardiac complications are relatively uncommon after transplant.

Myocardial infarction may occur during surgery due to hypotension because of bleeding or on reperfusion. Decreased cardiac output and EKG changes intraoperatively or early in the postoperative period are clues to diagnosis. Transmural infarction is rare; since the patients are prescreened for coronary artery disease, the prognosis is usually good. Diffuse myocardial dysfunction occasionally complicates the postoperative course, most commonly in patients with alcoholic cardiomyopathy which was unrecognized prior to transplantation. Typically, the posttransplant patient demonstrates low peripheral resistance and a high cardiac output; a low output associated with mild hypotension suggests significant cardiac disease.

Diabetes

Diabetes may pose a difficult management problem due to the frequent fluctuations in glucose levels. Corticosteroids, cyclosporine, and FK506 are all diebetogenic. Most patients on an oral hypoglycemic preoperatively will require insulin postoperatively, and many with no previous history develop overt diabetes after transplantation. The treatment of rejection with high-dose steroids predictably throws diabetes out of control. Optimal control of blood glucose levels is as important in these patients as in the general diabetic population.

Respiratory

Patients with severe respiratory dysfunction are not candidates for liver transplantation. Those with less severe impairment benefit from bronchodilators and aggressive chest physiotherapy in the postoperative period. In addition, nutritional support and bronchodilators improve the ease of weaning from the ventilator. Specific treatment for preexisting pulmonary disease, e.g., asthma, should be continued postoperatively. Respiratory dysfunction caused by functional shunting due to liver disease (hepatopulmonary syndrome) resolves postoperatively, but this may take weeks; oxygen therapy may be required and extubation delayed.

Osteoporosis

Osteoporosis can be debilitating in the transplant patient, since the preexisting bone loss characteristic of patients with advanced liver disease is aggravated by the administration of steroids. All patients should receive calcium and vitamin D supplementation. Some transplant recipients demonstrate malabsorption of calcium due to low levels of 1,25-dihydroxyvitamin D and may benefit from exogenous administration of this vitamin. In symptomatic patients, etidronate[3] or calcitonin therapy may be beneficial in halting bone loss.

Liver Biopsy

Liver biopsy provides a quick and precise way of diagnosing the etiology of allograft dysfunction.[4] Specifically, it is of greatest use in the differentiation of acute rejection from infection, as management is totally different. It can also show evidence of ischemic damage, sepsis or biliary tract dysfunction.

Biopsies should be performed by an experienced operator. Technically, they can be performed either percutaneously or laparoscopically. Biopsy should be performed whenever a doubt arises as to the etiology of malfunction of the allograft. Many groups perform protocol biopsies at one week after transplantation to guide in the evaluation and management of patients, and as needed thereafter.

EARLY POSTOPERATIVE COMPLICATIONS

Poor Early Graft Function

Poor early graft function (PEGF) has a clinical spectrum characterized by varying degrees of coma and renal failure associated with lactic acidosis, persistent coagulopathy, poor bile production and marked elevations of AST and ALT. The occurrence of PEGF is unpredictable; its most severe form, requiring retransplantation and termed primary nonfunction (PNF), is seen following approximately 5% of transplant procedures. Possible etiologic factors include liver disease in the donor, technical errors, ischemic injury, and immunologic damage.

Since donors are carefully screened and those with marked abnormalities are rejected, it is not surprising that studies have failed to correlate PEGF with any donor variables.[5] Steatosis, particularly when macrovesicular, is associated with PEGF.[6] In cases where fat is suspected, a biopsy of the donor liver is examined before proceeding with the transplant.

Technical failure is fortunately uncommon, accounting for less than 10% of PEGF in adults. In children, where hepatic artery thrombosis is more common, technical factors are more often the cause of PEGF. Early portal vein thrombosis, although uncommon, can result in a dramatic picture of acute hepatic failure.

Immunologic damage to the graft due to preformed antibodies, so-called hyperacute rejection, was once thought not to occur in liver transplants. While we now recognize this entity, it is unclear to what extent it plays a role in the spectrum of PEGF. Ischemic injury is probably the major cause of PEGF. Ischemia is inherent in the process of organ retrieval, storage, and implantation.

Excessive manipulation of the viscera during the donor operation can compound the problem; careful handling of the tissue and meticulous technique will minimize this factor. Injury may also occur during the cold-ischemic phase.

In its most dramatic form, PEGF is evident in the operating room, manifested by acidosis and coagulopathy. When, over the first two postoperative days, the patient does not awaken and develops renal shutdown, the need for urgent retransplantation is clear. Plasmapheresis with replacement of clotting factors using fresh frozen plasma may improve the clinical picture and provide a larger window within which retransplantation may be performed.

Patients with less severe degrees of PEGF present a much more difficult therapeutic dilemma. They may look reasonably well initially, awakening promptly and displaying mild if any renal dysfunction. Nevertheless, bile production is scant and AST and ALT levels rise above 2500. In our experience, approximately half of this group will eventually recover normal liver function and half will go on to require retransplantation. The development of a second insult to the liver in the form of rejection portends a poor outlook for graft survival for this reason, as well as to protect the kidneys in these patients who are vulnerable to renal failure, conversion to OKT3 immunoprophylaxis is advisable. The administration of prostaglandin E1 has recently been advocated in this setting; it clearly improves renal function, and may be beneficial to the liver as well. In our experience, survival for patients with PEGF requiring retransplantation has been significantly better in those retransplanted within one week than in those redone later. We have reviewed our data in an attempt to define early predictors of the need for ultimate graft replacement. Significant centrilobular necrosis on the postreperfusion liver biopsy that is routinely performed during the transplant procedure, and failure of the prothrombin time to normalize within the first 5 days after transplant, appear to be such predictors. In addition, the development of rejection in a liver with PEGF should lead to serious consideration of retransplantation.

Bleeding

Intraabdominal Bleeding

Since great care is taken to ensure hemostasis before completing the transplant procedure, bleeding is uncommon in the early postoperative period. Nevertheless, despite all precautions, hemoperitoneum occasionally develops shortly after surgery. This most commonly is related to PEGF and the resultant coagulopathy. Diagnosis of this condition is based on the careful and continued monitoring of vital signs, hemodynamic status, serial hematocrit, and drain output. If hemoperitoneum occurs, it is best to reexplore the patient. The presence of blood in the peritoneal cavity perpetuates coagulopathy as well as serves as a nidus for infection. Although a discrete source of bleeding may not be found, evacuation of blood and clots has a salutary effect, and rebleeding is uncommon.

Gastrointestinal

We have seen significant gastrointestinal bleeding in just over 20% of recipients, despite routine prophylaxis with H_2 blockers. While this complication may occur late after transplant (due primarily to opportunistic infections), it is most commonly encountered in the early postoperative period. The most frequent causes have been peptic ulcer, postsclerotherapy ulcer, and bleeding from the intestinal anastomosis of a Roux-en Y loop used for choledochojejunostomy. Aggressive endoscopic diagnosis and therapy should be pursued. Bleeding from a Roux-en-Y loop has required surgical correction in 50% of cases; other causes of bleeding have seldom required surgery.

Vascular Thrombosis

Hepatic Artery

Hepatic artery thrombosis (HAT) is a significant clinical problem, occurring in approximately 5% of liver transplants.[7,8] It is most commonly encountered during the early postoperative period. Technical factors certainly play a role in some cases, particularly in pediatric patients; nothing short of a perfect arterial anastomosis with excellent inflow should be accepted. In our experience, however, most episodes of HAT have been seen in the setting of PEGF or acute rejection, where hepatic arterial flow is reduced and endothelial injury may be present.

HAT rarely presents with a picture of sudden, dramatic liver failure. More commonly the presentation is insidious, with the development of fever and gradually increasing liver enzymes. While the hepatic parenchyma can often survive on portal flow alone, the bile ducts are devoid of portal supply and thus entirely dependent on the hepatic artery. For this reason, the manifestations of HAT are frequently related to the biliary tract, in the form of anastomotic leak, stricture, or intrahepatic duct necrosis with resultant liver abscess. An occasional patient will tolerate HAT with no clinical sequelae, although such cases must be observed for the late development of strictures resembling the picture of sclerosing cholangitis.

Duplex Doppler ultrasound is an effective noninvasive method for evaluating hepatic artery patency, and is performed routinely on POD 1 and POD 7. If a pulsatile arterial flow is seen, the test is reliable. In about 10% of all studies, the artery is not well visualized. If, upon review of the operation, good flow was noted and the surgeon was entirely satisfied with the technical result, nifedipine is administered and the study repeated within 24 hr; the great majority of such cases will have normal findings on the repeat study. If the surgeon has any question about the technical excellence of the arterial reconstruction or if the duplex study repeatedly fails to show the artery, arteriography is indicated.

If diagnosed shortly after thromobosis occurs, emergent revascularization may be successful in salvaging the liver graft.[9] Extreme care must be used in attempting catheter thrombectomy of the delicate hepatic artery, and unless a clear and correctable technical cause for thrombosis is identified an alternative source of inflow using an aortohepatic graft should be considered.

More commonly, retransplantation is required, and should be performed at the merest evidence of HAT-related complication, thus avoiding sepsis and maximizing survival. Retransplantation for HAT should almost always include provision of alternative arterial inflow, usually an aortohepatic graft.

Portal Vein

Portal vein thrombosis is rare. Technical factors may play a role; proper tailoring of the length and lie of the portal vein in preparation for its anastomosis is an art, and if improperly done can lead to kinking. The clinical presentation can range from fulminant hepatic failure to the gradual late development of portal hypertension and its complications with normal liver function. Late stricturing of the portal anastomosis can also occur, leading to portal hypertension. Retransplantation is required for patients with hepatic failure; in those with portal hypertension the liver graft may be preserved, treating complications as required with sclerotherapy or portasystemic shunting.

Biliary System

Bile Leak

This complication has been encountered in 5% of patients in our series. The development of a bile leak for purely technical reasons is unusual, since the anastomosis is doubly checked in the operating room and a cholangiogram is performed. Anastomotic leak is usually associated with either HAT or allograft rejection.[10] Diagnosis is simple in patients with indwelling T-tubes; in those without T-tubes, HIDA scan and percutaneous cholangiography may help in the diagnosis. In addition, duplex ultrasonography should be performed to confirm that the heaptic artery is patent. Conservative management frequently may suffice, but surgical exploration may become necessary if symptoms do not subside on antibiotic treatment. When HAT is present, exteriorization of the bile drainage via tube while awaiting a liver for retransplantation will minimize the development of sepsis. In other cases, conversion to or revision of Roux-en-Y choledochojejunostomy is the correct therapy.

Leakage from the site of entry of the T-tube into the bile duct with resultant peritonitis can develop either as a result of accidental dislodgement of the tube or on its intentional removal 3 months after the transplant procedure. Most such cases are treated successfully with a short course of antibiotic therapy and the endoscopic placement of a temporary nasobiliary stent.

Obstruction

Biliary obstruction is rare; we have seen it in 3% of patients. It is reportedly more common following duct-to-duct reconstruction that after choledochojejunostomy. In some cases, sludge formation and biliary "casts" forming around the T-tube can be complicated.[11] More often, anastomotic strictures are the cause; these usually develop in patients who have experienced significant rejection. HAT should be excluded by Doppler duplex ultrasound. It is important to point out that, radiologically, the donor biliary tree often dilates with time, falsely suggesting obstruction. These patients are asymptomatic, and no therapy is required.

In true obstruction, cholangitis is often the presenting event, and should be treated with antibiotics. Percutaneous and endoscopic methods may be useful in the retrieval of biliary concretions. The role of balloon dilatation and stenting in the long-term management of biliary stricture is not clear; conversion to or revision of Roux-en-Y choledochojejunostomy remains the standard approach.

Neuropsychiatric Dysfunction

Neurologic problems are frequent in the postoperative period. While probably multifactorial in most cases, toxicity of cyclosporine and steroids plays a significant role. The majority of patients experience neurologic symptoms, most commonly tremor, headache, paresthesia, or insomnia. Approximately 10% of patients have experienced seizures; particularly at risk are those with a history of seizure disorders. For new-onset seizures and focal deficits, a full evaluation including CT of the brain and lumbar puncture is indicated. Anticonvulsant therapy is continued for one month and then tapered in patients with no prior history of seizures; recurrence is rare. Fortunately, the various manifestations of neurotoxicity improve over time even with the continued administration of immunosuppressive drugs.

Patients often develop changes in mental status in the early posttransplant period. On occasion, overtly psychotic behavior is seen, with paranoia often a prominent feature. While almost certainly multifactorial, steroids are likely a primary culprit. On rare occasions patients will awaken normally and then over a period of days enter a period of decreased mental status, which may progress to coma and is associated with dramatic and long-lasting weakness and difficulty with speech. This picture in our experience has only been seen in patients who were severely debilitated prior to surgery, and likely represents a manifestation of cyclosporine toxicity.[12]

Infection

Infections in patients following transplantation can be broadly divided into those to which all patients undergoing major surgery are susceptible and those opportunistic infections more or less unique to the immunosuppressed transplant population.

Liver transplant patients are subject to the development of the typical postoperative bacterial infections to which all surgical patients are susceptible—wound infection, pneumonia, urinary tract infection, intraabdominal abscess, and catheter sepsis. Therapy for these infections follows the traditional guidelines of adequate drainage (where applicable) and appropriate antibiotic therapy guided by culture results.

Opportunistic organisms of concern include viruses, fungi, and protozoans. Cytomegalovirus (CMV) has traditionally been a major cause of morbidity and mortality in transplant patients. Serologic evidence of exposure to this virus is evident in a large segment of the population; in our experience, 69% of transplant candidates and 52% of liver donors have antibodies to CMV. Whether by reactivation or following introduction of the virus via blood products or the donor organ, immunosuppression may induce the development of clinical infection. Manifestations may include hepatitis, pneumonitis, gastroenteritis, and colitis, as well as a picture of generalized sepsis. CMV disease most commonly occurs in patients who have received large amounts of immunosuppressive medication, often including OKT3, for the treatment of rejection. While reports have demonstrated shedding of CMV virus as detected on routine surveillance cultures in over 50% of recipients, clinical disease is less common; we have documented CMV disease in 20% of our liver transplant patients. The mean interval for the development of CMV disease following transplantation has been about 50 days. The introduction of the effective anti-CMV agent ganciclovir has markedly changed the outlook for patients with CMV disease;[13] mortality due to CMV is now extremely rare. Effective prophylactic regimens have also had significant impact in reducing the incidence of CMV disease. High-dose acyclovir (800 mg q6h) is now widely used for this purpose;[14] in addition, we add human immune globulin for CMV-negative recipients. Trials are currently underway evaluating ganciclovir for CMV prophylaxis. In some centers 2 weeks of intravenous ganciclovir is given immediately posttransplant.

Herpes simplex virus can cause a devastating hepatitis in the early posttransplant period, usually within the first 2 weeks.[15] The incidence of herpes hepatitis is approximately 1%. If diagnosed early, therapy with high-dose acyclovir and, if necessary, retransplantation, may yield success, but this infection is often rapidly fatal.

Epstein-Barr (EBV) virus can produce a hepatitis which is generally not clinically severe and has been reported to occur at a mean of 264 days posttransplant. Of far greater significance is EBV-induced proliferation of lymphocytes in the immunosuppressed patient.[16] This can range from a reversible, polyclonal state to full-blown lymphoma. Although it can be seen as early as 6 weeks posttransplant, the mean time to the occurrence of lymphoma is 15 months following transplant. The presentation is frequently related to involvement of the gastrointestinal tract, although lymph node involvement is common; in unchecked cases, all organ systems may be infiltrated. The key to therapy is early recognition of the problem and reduction of immunosuppression; tumor regression or disappearance may result from this alone. Excision of large tumors is beneficial; the role of chemotherapy is not clearly defined. Therapy with the antiviral agents acyclovir and ganciclovir is generally added, although these agents are not dramatically effective against EBV.

Fungal infections occur primarily in sick recipients, either those who require prolonged hospitalization prior to transplantation or those who have developed poor early graft function and/or bacterial infection early after transplant.[17] *Candida* is by far the most common organism, and can be identified in the respiratory tract, wounds, peritoneal cavity, and urine, as well as in blood cultures. All patients receive nystatin orally as prophylaxis; high-risk patients may deserve systemic antifungal prophylaxis. Amphotericin-B is the standard therapy for systemic candidiasis; although this agent has known toxicity and must be respected, its liberal use on the transplant service has been associated with remarkably few complications. The new agent fluconazole is active against *Candida* and has little in the way of toxicity.[18] Randomized trials of this drug for prevention of fungal infections after transplantation are underway. Infections with other fungi are less commonly noted. Aspergillus is a particularly troublesome organism; frequent sites of involvement include the lungs and the central nervous system.

Diagnosis is difficult, often requiring biopsy, and therapy with amphotericin is less than satisfactory in many cases.

Pneumocystis carinii is a protozoan that frequently causes pneumonia in immunosuppressed patients. Involvement is bilateral; while chest x-ray may be unremarkable initially, gallium scans are reliably abnormal. The diagnosis is confirmed by finding the organism in bronchial washing or on transbronchial biopsy. Therapy is with intravenous sulfamethoxazole/trimemethoprim, with pentamidine added in resistant cases. All transplant patients should receive lifelong prophylaxis against pneumocystis with either sulfamethoxazole/trimemethoprim, inhaled pentamidine, or dapsone, since the period of risk for this infection is indefinite.

REFERENCES

1. Grieg PD, Woolf GM, Sinclair T, et al: Treatment of primary liver graft nonfunction with prostaglandin E1. *Transplantation* 48:447–453, 1989.
2. Reilly J, Mehta R, Teperman L, et al: Nutritional support after liver transplantation: a randomized, prospective trial. *J Parenter Enteral Nutrition* 14:386–391, 1990.
3. Storm T, Thamsborg G, Steiniche T, et al: Effect of intermittent cyclical etidronate therapy on bone mass and fracture rate in women with postmenopausal osteoporosis. *New Engl J Med* 322:1265–1271, 1990.
4. Sankary HN, Foster P, Ashmann M, et al: Can criteria present on hepatic allograft biopsy determine the presence or absence of rejection?*Ann Surg* 21:2284–2285, 1989.
5. Makowka L, Gordon RD, Todo S, et al: Analysis of donor criteria for the prediction of outcome in clinical liver transplantation. *Transplant Proc* 19:2378–2382, 1987.
6. D'Alessandro AM, Kalayoglu M, Sollinger HW, et al: The predictive value of donor liver biopsies on the development of primary nonfunction after liver transplantation. *Transplant Proc* 23:1536–1537, 1991.
7. Tzakis AG, Gordon RD, Shaw BW, et al: Clinical presentation of hepatic artery thromobosis after liver transplantation in the cyclosporine era. *Transplantation* 40:667–671, 1985.
8. Hesselnik EJ, Klompmaker IJ, Grond J, et al: Hepatic artery thromobosis after orthotopic liver transplantation: a fatal complication or symptomless event? *Transplant Proc* 21:2462, 1989.
9. Marujo WC, Langnas AN, Wood RP, et al: Vascular complications following orthotopic liver transplantation: outcome and the role of urgent revascularization. *Transplant Proc* 23:1484–1486, 1991.
10. Vicente E, Perkins JD, Sterioff S, et al: Biliary tract complications following orthotopic liver transplantation. *Clin Transplant* 1:138–142, 1987.
11. Chen Ch-L, Wang K-L, Chuang J-N, et al: Biliary sludge-cast formation following liver transplantation. *Hepatogastroenterol* 35:22–24, 1988.
12. Boon AP, Adams DH, Buckels JAC, et al: Neuropathological findings in autopsies after liver transplantation. *Transplant Proc* 23:1471–1472, 1991.
13. Harbison MA, De Girolami P, Jenkins RL, et al: Ganciclovir therapy of severe cytomegalovirus infections in solid organ transplant recipients. *Transplantation* 46:82–88, 1988.
14. Balfour HH, Chace BA, Stapleton JT, et al: A randomized, placebo-controlled trial

of oral acyclovir for the prevention of cytomegalovirus disease in recipients of renal allografts. *New Engl J Med* 320:1381–1387, 1989.

15. Markin RS, Langnas AN, Donovan JP, et al: Opportunistic viral hepatitis in liver transplant recipients. *Transplant Proc* 23:1520–1521, 1991.
16. Langnas AN, Castaldo P, Markin RS, et al: The spectrum of Epstein-Barr virus infection with hepatitis following liver transplantation. *Transplant Proc* 23:1513–1514, 1991.
17. Castaldo P, Stratta RJ, Wood RP, et al: Fungal disease in liver transplant recipients: a multivariate analysis of risk factors. *Transplant Proc* 23:1517–1519, 1991.
18. Conti DJ, Tolkoff-Rubin NE, Baker GP, et al: Successful treatment of invasive fungal infection with fluconazole in organ transplant recipients. *Transplantation;* 48:692–695, 1989.

—13—

IMMUNOSUPPRESSION AND REJECTION

Myron E. Schwartz,
Cosme Manzarbeitia,
and Charles M. Miller

It is the goal of this chapter to outline the clinical practice of immunosuppression following liver transplantation. At the current state of the art, immunosuppression requires the balanced administration of multiple agents to prevent and treat rejection. A brief description of the major agents currently used is warranted before detailing their clinical application.

IMMUNOSUPPRESSIVE AGENTS

Corticosteroids

Adrenal corticosteroids (steroids) are hormones that exert profound effects on virtually every organ system of the human body. Hydrocortisone and its synthetic analogues prednisone and methylprednisolone *interfere with the normal immune response* in a number of ways. Steroids prevent the proliferation of T-cells in response to foreign antigens by interfering with both the release of and the response to the lymphokine interleukin-2. They also have *powerful nonspecific antiinflammatory activity* that lessens the rejection response. Major side effects include edema, hyperglycemia, muscle weakness, behavioral disturbances, cataract formation, and osteoporosis. These agents are well absorbed orally and may be administered parenterally or by mouth in equivalent dosages.

Azathioprine

Azathioprine is a purine analog that acts as an antimetabolite, interfering with nucleic acid synthesis. As such, it interferes with the rapid proliferation of lymphocytes that follows exposure to foreign antigen. Azathioprine is *useful only in the prevention* of rejection; it is ineffective in the reversal of the acute rejection process. The major toxicity of azathioprine is bone marrow suppression, particularly leukopenia. Other side effects include drug-induced hepatitis and alopecia. This drug is well-absorbed orally and is given either by mouth or by vein in equivalent dosages.

Cyclosporine

Cyclosporine (CyA) is a peptide fungal derivative that was discovered in 1972.[1] As compared to steroids and azathioprine, CyA is considerably more *selective in its inhibition of immune responses.* Interleukin-2 synthesis is impaired, preventing or curtailing the response to foreign antigens. Suppressor T-cells, however, are not inhibited. Defenses against bacterial infection are also left relatively intact. The most significant toxicity is to the kidneys, and is a major factor limiting use of the drug. Other common side effects include headache, tremor, hypertension, hypercholesterolemia, hyperglycemia, excessive hair growth, and gingival hyperplasia. CyA is variably absorbed after oral administration; its absorption is dependent on the presence of bile.[2] The oral to parenteral bioequivalence ratio is approximately 3:1. The absorption and metabolism of CyA may be influenced by a number of commonly used drugs. Cholestyramine is a resin which binds bile salts and is used to lower the serum cholesterol or to reduce the itching associated with cholestasis. It may bind CyA and thus lower its level. Attempts to increase CyA absorption by the concomitant administration of bile salts (ursodeoxycholic acid) have met with limited success and is used infrequently. Since CyA is metabolized by the cytochrome p-450 system in the liver, the administration of agents such as phenobarbital or dilantin, which induce this system, will lower CyA levels. Drugs like the antifungal ketoconazole and the calcium channel blocker verapamil, on the other hand, will result in higher CyA levels.

Cyclophosphamide

This alkylating agent causes structural damage to DNA and is thus cytotoxic to rapidly proliferating tissues. As compared to other agents, it is relatively more suppressive of the humoral immune response. Cyclophosphamide is quite toxic. Marrow suppression is routinely seen. Nausea and vomiting, hemorrhagic cystitis, and alopecia are also common.

Muromonab-CD3 (OKT3)

OKT3 is a monoclonal antibody produced in mice and directed against the CD3 complex, an integral part of the antigen recognition structure found on the surface of T-cells. Administration of this agent results in *rapid depletion of T-cells* from the circulation. The first dose is typically followed by fever and tachycardia; pulmonary edema may occur in the setting of volume overload. Premedication with high-dose steroids ameliorates these symptoms. Treatment is for a limited period, generally 10–14 days. During therapy with OKT3 T-cells may repopulate, but without the CD3 complex necessary for normal function. Monitoring T-cell subsets is useful in documenting the desired therapeutic effect in cases of suboptimal response.[3] Other side effects include headache and seizures. The development of anti-mouse determinant antibodies in response to OKT3 may limit the ability to reuse this drug;[4] continuation of CyA and steroids during OKT3 administration may decrease the likelihood of antibody production. Available only for IV administration, the usual dose is 5 mg/day.

Antithymocyte Globulin, Antilymphocyte Globulin

These agents are prepared by administering human lymphocytes to horses or rabbits and purifying the resultant immune globulins. *A heterogeneous group of antibodies to multiple determinants* is produced. Treatment is limited to 10–14 days. While allergic reactions are common, a first-dose effect such as is seen with OKT3 is not encountered. These agents are administered intravenously and are dosed according to weight.

FK506

This investigational drug is a fungal derivative, a macrolide, related structurally to erythromycin. FK506 can *both prevent and reverse acute rejection*. Its immunosuppressive activity is mediated, like CyA, through *inhibition of the action of interleukin-2*. Renal and neurotoxicity are significant with FK506 and it is apparently diabetogenic, similar to CyA. Unlike CyA, FK506 does not seem to cause hypertension or to raise serum cholesterol levels. FK506 is about 100 times as potent as CyA and is not dependent on bile for its oral absorption. Although quite variable, the oral to parenteral dosage ratio is roughly 3:1. While not yet approved for clinical use in the United States, a significant body of literature already exists on the use of this agent based primarily on studies performed at the University of Pittsburgh.[5,6] A multicenter trial in the United States and in Europe is currently underway studying this drug both as rescue therapy and as primary immunosuppression.

MULTIDRUG THERAPY

Currently CyA is the backbone of modern immunosuppressive therapy. The introduction of this drug marked the beginning of the contemporary era of liver transplantation, yielding results an order of magnitude greater than had ever been achieved with azathioprine and steroids. Nevertheless, the toxicity of CyA limits its use as a single agent.[7] Early on, it was determined that the addition of corticosteroids allowed reduction of CyA dosage, thus limiting toxicity. A number of centers use a regimen of CyA and steroids for routine immunosuppression.[8] Increasingly, transplant centers add azathioprine to CyA and steroids in a so-called triple drug regimen in an attempt to further reduce the incidence of rejection while limiting adverse drug effects.[9] Triple therapy allows a bit more latitude in the adjustment of CyA levels and permits a more rapid reduction in steroid dosage. The early experience with FK506 suggests that this drug may provide adequate immunosuppression (with tolerable side effects) without the addition of azathioprine and with markedly reduced steroid dosages. If so, this would represent a significant advance.

IMMUNOSUPPRESSION PROTOCOLS

Each transplant center has its own way of handling immunosuppression, and each feels that its own approach is by far the best. While it is doubtful that any modern CyA-based regimen is markedly superior to any others, there is a clear value in the adoption of and the conformity to protocols for immunosuppression within each transplant program. Such a policy simplifies patient management while facilitating meaningful evaluation of results.

IMMUNOSUPPRESSION IN THE PERITRANSPLANT PERIOD

A triple drug regimen is routinely employed to initiate immunosuppression. Drug administration ideally begins before exposure to foreign antigens, i.e., preoperatively. In our institution methylprednisolone 50 mg and azathioprine 2 mg/kg are given intravenously, and CyA 10 mg/kg is administered orally prior to surgery. Methylprednisolone 500 mg is given immediately following reperfusion of the liver graft; CyA is withheld until adequate urine output is noted and the new liver has begun to function as evidenced by bile production and the normalization of clotting.

A high level of CyA is desirable in the early posttransplant period; a dose of 2.5 mg/kg IV q12h is begun and is adjusted to maintain levels of 800–1000 by a nonselective assay (TDX). Methylprednisolone dosage is tapered over 6 days to 20 mg/day, either PO (prednisone) or IV (methylprednisolone) as outlined in Table 13-1. Azathioprine is continued at 2 mg/kg IV or PO, with downward adjustment for leukopenia. Oral CyA, which is less nephrotoxic than the IV preparation, is begun by the second or third postoperative day. The absorption of CyA is variable; under ideal conditions the bio-availability of a PO dose averages about 30%, so an initial dose of 7 mg/kg PO q12h is employed. CyA absorption is heavily bile-dependent; it is difficult to achieve therapeutic levels via PO administration alone when the bile is diverted externally, as with an open T-tube following transplantation with a duct-to-duct anastomosis. IV administration should be continued until the T-tube is clamped and adequate absorption is demonstrated.

As an alternative, immunosuppression may begin with the use of OKT3 monoclonal antibody instead of CyA.[10,11] The use of OKT3 allows for a more rapid taper of steroids, as outlined in Table 13-2; azathioprine is omitted during the first week. OKT3 is initiated intraoperatively following the administration of

TABLE 13-1. Tapering Steroid Regimen for Induction of Immunosuppression (Prednisone or Methylprednisolone)

Initial dose 1 g (pediatric: 20 mg/kg), then:		
Postop day	*Dose: adults*	*Dose: pediatric (<20 kg)*
1	50 mg q6h	10 mg/kg q6h
2	40 mg q6h	8 mg/kg q6h
3	30 mg q6h	6 mg/kg q6h
4	20 mg q6h	4 mg/kg q6h
5	10 mg q6h	2 mg/kg q6h
Thereafter	20 mg qd	0.3 mg/kg qd

methylprednisolone 200 mg; the typical first-dose reaction is not observed. Patients treated with this regimen probably experience less early rejection. With current prophylaxis against CMV, there is little if any increased risk of infection. The risk of later development of malignancy is unclear, but may be increased. OKT3 is the primary agent used to treat steroid-resistant rejection, and its reuse, while often clinically effective, can be hampered by the development of antimurine antibodies in the transplant recipient after the first exposure. For this reason, the OKT3 regimen is reserved for the following special circumstances:

1. The patient with compromised renal function. Functional renal impairment (hepatorenal syndrome) is not uncommon in patients with advanced liver disease. In patients in whom this condition has progressed to oligo- or anuria with significantly elevated creatinine, the OKT3 regimen allows for a period of recovery for the kidneys prior to the institution of CyA and may prevent the need for dialysis in the early postoperative period.
2. The patient with poor early graft function. Renal failure rapidly ensues when an hepatic allograft fails to function immediately, and OKT3 in this situation spares an additional insult to the kidneys. Additionally, should the liver begin to recover, maximal protection against early rejection is essential since early rejection in a liver that has suffered significant ischemic injury can result in severely compromised graft function with a poor outcome.

TABLE 13-2. Alternative Steroid Regimen for Use with OKT3 Induction (Methylprednisolone)

Administer first dose of OKT3 5 mg in OR with 200 mg methylprednisolone (10 mg/kg for children <20 kg) as premedication, then begin daily OKT3 for 10–14 days with the following steroid dosages used as premedication:		
Postop day	*Dose: adults*	*Dose: pediatric (<20 kg)*
1	200 mg	10 mg/kg
2	50 mg	2 mg/kg
3–14	20 mg	0.3 mg/kg

IMMUNOSUPPRESSION IN THE EARLY POSTOPERATIVE PERIOD

After the tapering of steroids over the first six days, a dose of prednisone 20 mg/day is maintained. Azathioprine is continued at 2 mg/kg, with downward adjustment if the leukocyte count drops below 4000 mm^{-3}. CyA levels are maintained between 800 and 1000; side effects may warrant lower cyclosporine levels. In patients receiving initial therapy with OKT3, CyA is begun orally on the third or fourth day postoperatively; azathioprine 2 mg/kg is begun 2 days prior to discontinuing OKT3.

ACUTE REJECTION

Diagnosis

Clinically evident rejection is observed in over half of all recipients.[12] It is probably a reasonable goal to aim for a 50% rejection rate; using currently available immunosuppressive agents, attempts to further reduce the incidence of rejection would likely be paid for in increased infection and cancer rates. The typical acute cellular rejection, which requires recognition and processing of foreign antigens and the proliferation of T-lymphocytes directed against them, is rarely observed before the fifth postoperative day. Rejection is typically manifested by fever, with decreased bile output (if observable), and elevation of transaminases, alkaline phosphatase activity, and bilirubin. Although the diagnosis of rejection may seem evident based on the clinical picture, each transplant physician learns early the need for corroborative histologic evidence.[13] A number of conditions can mimic rejection and should be considered when liver function[14] becomes abnormal.

In the early posttransplant period, vascular thrombosis, most commonly of the hepatic artery, should be sought. Duplex Doppler ultrasound study is generally satisfactory for this purpose, but angiography should be performed if the duplex study is inconclusive. Biliary complications are also notorious masqueraders of rejection, and visualization of the bile duct by T-tube cholangiography, endoscopic retrograde cholangiopancreatography, or percutaneous transhepatic cholangiography should be performed. Hepatitis must be distinguished from rejection on biopsy; this differentiation can tax even the most experienced hepatopathologist. Herpes simplex, EBV, and adenovirus can produce early, severe liver dysfunction; hepatitis B and C, either recurrent or de novo acquired during the transplant process, generally develop between 3 and 6 months postoperatively. Distinguishing these conditions from rejection is crucial since therapy differs greatly.

Treatment

The first-line therapy against acute rejection is high-dose corticosteroids. One gram of methylprednisolone is administered initially and may be repeated the following day, after which a tapering regimen like that used immediately after transplantation is employed (Table 13-1).

If the response is unsatisfactory, or if the rejection flares again soon after completion of the steroid taper, antilymphocyte antibodies (OKT3, ALG, or ATG) are employed.[15] OKT3 therapy is successful in reversing 90% of rejections that have not responded adequately to steroids. In patients who do not respond to OKT3 the diagnosis of rejection should be reconfirmed, and the adequacy of OKT3 effect should be confirmed by studying T-cell subsets. The presence of antimurine antibodies does not preclude the use of OKT3 but may necessitate higher than usual dosage.

In the patient who continues to manifest rejection after completion of a course of OKT3, the physican begins to sail in less well-charted waters. Another steroid recycle may finally overcome the problem; time is on our side, since the tendency to reject decreases with the passage of time. A number of centers have begun to gain experience using FK506 in the treatment of refractory rejection, and this agent appears promising. One of the more difficult judgments that must be made by the transplant surgeon is when to abandon efforts to salvage an organ and proceed with retransplantation.

ANTIBODY-MEDIATED REJECTION

While acute rejection is typically mediated by T-lymphocytes, antibodies play a role in the rejection process in a number of different settings.

Hyperacute Rejection

A major problem in renal transplantation, hyperacute rejection results when preformed antibodies to donor antigens cause diffuse small vessel thrombosis and immediate graft failure. This entity was long believed not to occur in liver transplantation, but has been increasingly recognized recently.[16] The likelihood of hyperacute rejection is significantly increased in transplants performed across ABO blood group barriers.[17] It is difficult to distinguish between hyperacute rejection and the poor early graft function due to ischemic graft injury. The presence of a positive crossmatch between the donor and recipient lends support to the diagnosis of hyperacute rejection; immunoglobulin may be observed lining the hepatic sinusoids using immunofluorescence studies on liver biopsy. Plasmapheresis, by clearing antibodies from the circulation, may be beneficial.

Antibody-Mediated Acute Rejection

Occasionally, antibodies play a significant or even a dominant role in the picture of acute rejection. Typical cellular rejection is present concomitantly, but immunofluorescence studies reveal the presence of immunoglobulin lining the hepatic sinusoids. This type of rejection may not respond adequately to the usual therapeutic measures. We have found the short-term use of cyclophosphamide, which has known anti-B-cell activity, is a useful adjunct in these cases. Plasmapheresis, by clearing circulating antibodies, may also have a role.

Chronic Rejection

Chronic rejection is a clinical entity characterized by progressive destruction of the vasculature and, secondarily, of the bile ducts without the intense cellular infiltration of the portal tracts seen in typical acute rejection. The term "chronic" is misleading in that this phenomenon may occur relatively early after transplant (within the first few months) and may progress rapidly, while acute rejection can present in the later posttransplant period. The pathophysiology of chronic rejection is poorly understood, although it is believed to be mediated primarily through antibodies.[18] In the advanced stages of chronic rejection the bile ducts virtually disappear, hence the terminology "vanishing bile duct syndrome" (VBDS). Although there are reports of spontaneous resolution of VBDS, progressive chronic rejection has classically been considered an indication for retransplantation. Even with retransplantation, the outlook has been marred by the frequent recurrence of VBDS. Hopeful reports have begun to appear in the literature that FK506, particularly when initiated relatively early in the course of VBDS (with the bilirubin ≤10 mg/dL), may be successful in reversing the rejection in a significant proportion of patients.

IMMUNOSUPPRESSION IN THE FACE OF INFECTION

Infection is, unfortunately, all too common in transplant recipients;[19] when infection develops, the question inevitably arises: "What should we do with the immunosuppression?" The answer is by no means always clear, but some general guidelines can safely be laid down for the reader's consideration.

Bacterial Infection

In the face of localized bacterial or fungal infection without evidence of systemic illness, appropriate local therapy and antibiotics are given without any reduction in immunosuppression. If significant generalized infection develops, immunosuppression should be reduced. CyA, which is relatively sparing of the defenses against bacterial infection, should be maintained while azathioprine and steroids are reduced. In overwhelming sepsis, all immunosuppression must be withheld except for perhaps a minimal dose of steroids to avoid Addisonian crisis. Rejection is rarely seen to develop in this setting.

Cytomegalovirus

Cytomegalovirus (CMV) infection was long considered a major problem in transplantation.[20] Recently, with the development of effective regimens for prophylaxis and treatment, CMV has become less of a threat;[21] it nevertheless remains a significant source of posttransplant morbidity. Predominant manifestations include pneumonia, hepatitis, and gastrointestinal tract involvement. Reports have linked the occurrence of CMV infection with an increased incidence of rejection;

this association is likely in part due to the lowering of immunosuppression that has in the past been routine in the treatment of CMV. Ganciclovir, the anti-CMV agent of choice, frequently causes a reduction in the granulocyte count, as does CMV infection itself. For this reason, azathioprine is reduced or withheld during treatment of CMV infection. Unless the patient is gravely ill, the immunosuppression should otherwise be maintained at preinfection levels throughout the course of therapy.

Hepatitis

Hepatitis B in a transplant recipient, whether recurrent in a patient transplanted for hepatitis B cirrhosis or acquired de novo, runs a variable course. While it is rational to imagine that immunosuppression might be beneficial, since liver damage in hepatitis B is to some extent immune-mediated, this is not in fact the case. Patients with hepatitis B show evidence of immunosuppression as a result of their infection and have been reported to manifest rejection less often than other patients. Nevertheless, they are not free of the risk of rejection, and immunosuppression should be maintained according to standard protocol.

There is considerable confusion surrounding the diagnosis and treatment of hepatitis C in transplant recipients. Only within the past year, with the advent of tests to detect antibodies to the hepatitis C virus in the serum and viral RNA within infected hepatocytes [by polymerase chain reaction (PCR) methodology] have we begun to make some sense out of the patient found to have "hepatitis" on liver biopsy. There are clearly cases of hepatitis C, both recurrent and newly acquired, in transplant recipients. In such cases, where infection is documented by finding viral RNA in the liver, immunosuppression is maintained according to standard protocol; there may be a role for interferon in cases of persistent and active infection.[22] We have found many cases, however, in which the biopsy diagnosis of hepatitis was not confirmed by the PCR viral RNA assay. While there may be other viruses not as yet detectable, the fact that many of these patients respond to increased immunosuppression with lasting normalization of liver function has led us to conclude that some of the histologic findings classically associated with hepatitis may in fact be manifestations of rejection. Increasing the immunosuppression may in fact serve as a therapeutic trial in such cases.

EBV-Related Lymphoproliferative Disorder (LPD) and Lymphoma

Epstein-Barr virus (EBV) can cause hepatitis in the transplant recipient that is usually self-limited.[23] Much more problematic is EBV-induced proliferation of lymphocytes, a spectrum that ranges from a reversible polyclonal proliferation to a full-blown monoclonal lymphoma.[24] LPD is de facto evidence of overimmunosuppression, and is most commonly seen in patients who have undergone treatment of repeated rejection episodes, which have included OKT3 therapy.[25] This is one instance where a reduction in immunosuppression is clearly in order; lowering the immunosuppression alone, with no further treatment, will in many cases result in regression of LPD.[26]

TABLE 13-3. Dosage Reduction Schedule Following Transplantation

			Prednisone	
Postop day	*CyA level*[a]	*AZA (mg/kg)*	*Adult mg*	*Pediatric mg/kg*
7–60	800–1200	1–2	20	0.2
61–120	600–900	1–2	15	0.2
121–180	500–800	1–2	15	0.2
181–360	300–600	1–2	12.5	0.2
360+	200–400	1–2	10	0.2

[a]TDX method; absolute levels will vary among centers.
All are given as a single daily dose.

IMMUNOSUPPRESSION IN THE LATE POSTTRANSPLANT PERIOD

The goal of inducing specific tolerance to transplanted organs remains elusive. Nevertheless, a relationship develops between host and allograft such that, with the passage of time, less immunosuppression is required to maintain normal graft function. Patients treated with standard triple therapy (i.e., CyA–prednisone–azathioprine) are maintained on this regimen indefinitely. By using low doses of all three drugs rather than attempting to eliminate any one of them, we believe that the risks of both rejection and toxicity are reduced. General guidelines for dosage reduction are outlined in Table 13-3. Considering the early experience with FK506, the hope has been raised that this drug may prove satisfactory as monotherapy;[27] currently, however, most patients treated with FK506 have also been maintained on low-dose steroids.

Although it may be preferable to continue triple therapy, an occasional patient develops intolerable side effects due to a component of the immunosuppressive regimen. CyA is most commonly at issue in this regard. In patients with creatinine levels >2.0, reduced CyA levels may be accepted in conjunction with a higher dose of azathioprine. In the rare circumstance where CyA is not tolerated at all, usually due to severe neurotoxicity, patients may be carried on steroids and azathioprine alone, with an admittedly increased risk of rejection. While reduction of prednisone dosage to 5 mg/day is usually possible, the elimination of steroids significantly increases the likelihood of rejection. Azathioprine dosage may need to be lowered because of marrow suppression, but it is rarely necessary to discontinue this drug due to side effects.

IMMUNOSUPPRESSION IN PEDIATRIC PATIENTS

The principles of immunosuppression in children are no different from those in adults. Although the fetus and perhaps even the newborn presents an immunologically privileged milieu, by the age at which we begin to contemplate transplantation (about 6 months), the infant has the capability to mount a vigorous rejection response. Higher corticosteroid doses on a per kilogram basis are required in young children than in adults for the induction of immunosuppression and for the treatment of rejection. In the later posttransplant period, an effort is made to carry children on alternate-day steroids to optimize growth. CyA levels and azathioprine doses are maintained similar to the adult range. Large oral doses of CyA may be required to attain therapeutic levels, since its absorption is often poor in infants. CyA absorption has been related to small intestinal length,[28] and since the most common indication for transplantation in these patients is biliary atresia, requiring Roux-en-Y choledochojejunostomy, most babies transplanted have a shortened small bowel. In addition to difficulty with absorption, infants frequently metabolize CyA rapidly; administering the drug in three daily doses alleviates this problem. Table 13-3 details our pediatric immunosuppression protocol.

MAJOR SIDE EFFECTS OF IMMUNOSUPPRESSION

Hypertension

Close to half of all patients treated with CyA will develop clinically significant hypertension (BP $>$ 140/90).[29] The implications for treatment of this hypertension are no different from those of the general population; considering the concomitant renal dysfunction usually present, control of blood pressure is especially important in transplant patient. In patients who were normotensive prior to transplantation, there is little doubt as to the etiology, and extensive workup is not required. Patients with blood pressure consistently above 140/90 are begun on a low daily dose of a diuretic (we prefer furosemide 20 mg). If after one week the blood pressure remains elevated, nifedipine 30 mg in an extended-release capsule is begun and the dose increased weekly to a maximum of 90 mg/day or until the blood pressure is controlled. If hypertension persists, an angiotensin-converting enzyme inhibitor is added; our choice is lisinopril at a dose of 10 mg/day, which may be increased up to 40 mg/day until control is achieved. In diabetics and in patients with evidence of congestive heart failure, lisinopril is used initially in preference to nifedipine.

Unwanted Hair Growth

This side effect of CyA is troublesome primarily in children and female recipients. Depilatory creams are the best remedy. FK506 apparently does not cause hypertrichosis.

Renal Dysfunction

Most patients treated with CyA demonstrate a measurable decrease in renal function,[30,31] with a mean decrement in the glomerular filtration rate of about 20%. The major insult to the kidneys by CyA takes place within the first 3 months after transplantation; beyond this point, renal function usually stabilizes despite continuation of CyA. Apart from lowering the CyA levels, a number of pharmacologic interventions have been proposed to counteract this nephrotoxicity. Prostaglandins E1 and E2 have been used in the early postoperative period to reverse the renal vasoconstriction, which is the basis for acute CyA nephrotoxicity,[32] often with gratifying results. Nifedipine has a similar action, but its use on a more long-term basis in an attempt to limit chronic nephrotoxicity has been less successful.

REFERENCES

1. Oates JA, Wood AJJ, Kahan BD: Drug therapy; cyclosporine. *New Engl J Med* 321:1725–1738, 1989.
2. Mehta MU, Venkataramanan R, Burckart GJ, et al: Effect of bile on cyclosporine in liver transplant patients. *Br J Clin Pharmacol* 25:579–584, 1988.
3. Colonna JO, Millis JM, Martello J, et al: The successful use of repeated courses of OKT3 using T3 cells to adjust dose. *Ann Surg* 21:2247–2248, 1989.
4. Schroeder TJ, First MR, Mansour ME, et al: Antimurine antibody formation following OKT3 therapy. *Transplantation* 49:48–51, 1990.
5. Todo S, Fung JJ, Demetris AJ, et al: Early trials with FK506 as primary treatment in liver transplantation. *Transplant Proc* 22:13–16, 1990.
6. Starzl TE, Fung, J, Vankataramanan R, et al: FK506 for liver, kidney and pancreas transplantation. *Lancet* 1000–1004, 1989.
7. Calne RY, Rolles K, Thiru S, et al: Cyclosporine A initially as the only immunosuppressant in 34 recipients of cadaveric organs: 32 kidneys, 2 pancreases, and 2 livers. *Lancet* 2:1033–1036, 1979.
8. Klompmaker IJ, Haagsma EB, Gouw ASH, et al: Azathioprine and prednisone immunosuppression versus maintenance triple therapy including cyclosporine for orthotopic liver transplantation. *Transplant Proc* 48:814–818, 1989.
9. Guggenheim J, Samuel D, Saliba F, et al: Use of cyclosporine A in combination with low-dose corticosteroids and azathioprine in liver transplantation. *Transplant Proc* 3:366–368, 1988.
10. Cosimi AB, Jenkins RL, Rohrer RJ, et al: A randomized clinical trial of prophylactic OKT3 monoclonal antibody in liver allograft recipients. *Arch Surg* 125:781–785, 1990.
11. Millis JM, McDiarmid SV, Hiatt JR, et al: Randomized prospective trial of OKT3 for early prophylaxis of rejection after liver transplantation. *Transplantation* 4:82–88, 1989.
12. Grant D, Ghent C, Duff J, et al: Liver transplantation: the problem of rejection. *Transplant Proc* 18:163–166, 1986.
13. Sankary HN, Foster P, Ashmann M, et al: Can criteria present on hepatic allograft biopsy determine the presence or absence of rejection? *Ann Surg* 21:2284–2285, 1989.
14. Esquivel CO, Jaffe R, Gordon RD, et al: Liver rejection and its differentiation from other causes of graft dysfunction. *Semin Liver Dis* 5:369–374, 1985.
15. Cosimi AB, Cho SI, Delmonico FL, et al: A randomized clinical trial comparing OKT3

and steroids for treatment of hepatic allograft rejection. *Transplantation* 43:91–95, 1987.

16. Demetris AJ, Jaffe R, Tzakis A, et al: Antibody-mediated rejection of human orthotopic liver grafts. *Am J Pathol* 132:400–502, 1988.
17. Rego J, Prevost F, Rumeau JL, et al: Hyperacute rejection after ABO-incompatible orthotopic liver transplantation. *Transplant Proc* 19:4589–4590, 1987.
18. Oguma S, Zerbe T, Banner B, et al: Chronic liver allograft rejection and obliterative arteriopathy: possible pathogenic mechanisms. *Transplant Proc* 21:2203–2207, 1989.
19. Colonna JO, Winston DJ, Brill JE, et al: Infectious complications in liver transplantation. *Arch Surg* 123:360–364, 1988.
20. Bronster O, Makowka L, Jaffe R, et al: Occurrence of cytomegalovirus hepatitis in liver transplant patients. *J Med Virol* 24:423–434, 1988.
21. Harbison MA, DeGirolami P, Jenkins RL, et al: Ganciclovir therapy of severe cytomegalovirus infections solid-organ transplant recipients. *Transplantation* 46:82–88, 1988.
22. Davis GL, Balart LA, Schiff ER, et al. Treatment of chronic hepatitis C with recombinant interferon alfa. *New Engl J Med* 321:1501–1506, 1989.
23. Lamy ME, Favart AM, Cornu C, et al: Epstein-Barr virus infection in 59 orthotopic liver transplant patients. *Med. Microbiol. Immunol.* (Berlin) 179:L137–144, 1990.
24. Hanto DW, Frizzera G, Gajl-Peczalska KJ, et al: Epstein-Barr virus-induced B-cell lymphoma after renal transplantation. *New Engl J Med* 306:913–918, 1989.
25. Swinnen LJ, Constanzo-Nordin MR, Fisher SG, et al: Increased incidence of lymphoproliferative disorder after immunosuppression with the monoclonal antibody OKT3 in cardiac-transplant recipients. *New Engl J Med* 323:1723–1728, 1990.
26. Starzl TE, Porter KA, Iwatsuki S, et al: Reversibility of lymphomas and lymphoproliferative lesions developing under cyclosporine-steroid therapy. *Lancet* 1:583–587, 1984.
27. Shapiro R, Fung JJ, Jain AB, et al: The side effects of FK506 in humans. *Transplant Proc* 22:35–36, 1990.
28. Whittington PF, Emond JC, Whittington SH, et al: Small-bowel length and the dose of cyclosporine in children after liver transplantation. *New Engl J Med* 322:733–738, 1990.
29. Mark AL. Cyclosporine, sympathetic activity, and hypertension. *New Engl J Med* 323:748–750, 1990.
30. Mihatsch MJ, Thiel G, Ryffel B: Cyclosporine nephrotoxicity. *Adv Nephrol* 17:303–320, 1988.
31. Dische FE, Neuberger J, Keating J, et al: Kidney pathology in liver allograft recipients after long-term treatment with cyclosporine A. *Lab Invest* 58:395–402, 1988.
32. Pomer S, Rohl L, Hull W, et al: Reduction of cyclosporine nephrotoxicity by prostaglandin E2 after experimental renal transplantation. *Transplant Proc* 19:4041–4042, 1987.

—14—

LATE POSTOPERATIVE (OUTPATIENT) MANAGEMENT

Franklin M. Klion and Thomas L. Fabry

After discharge from the hospital the transplant center follows the patient closely (usually weekly), and at 3 months, stable patients without evidence of rejection are discharged to the management of their local physician. Close interaction between the local physician and the transplant center is essential to avoid problems with rejection and infection.

WELL-PATIENT MANAGEMENT

DAILY ACTIVITIES

The majority of patients should be able to return to their daily activities by the third month after a single transplantation with some modification of their lifestyle. Patients are independent in their activities of daily living (ADL) and in their mobility. The diminished endurance experienced pretransplant is corrected in most patients and work is limited mostly by impaired limb function and lack of concentration.[1] Professional and blue collar workers as well as homemakers can resume their usual schedule without significant limitations of their activity.[2] Gender has no influence on rehabilitation.

Patients who required more than one transplantation tend to have more disability, with more difficult rehabilitation. Less than half can resume pretransplant activities. Two years after transplantation 85% of the survivors of a single transplant and 43% of multiple transplants were working in or outside their home.[3]

Three years after surgery the quality of life has significantly improved for all liver transplant patients, although on test scores they did not recover to the level of normal individuals. However, the differences were not clinically significant.[4]

Lifestyles have to be modified to accommodate participation in support groups,[5] and regular visits to the physician's office to monitor immunosuppression and liver function. Patients cannot temporize if medical problems develop and even minor illnesses require prompt attention.

Similar results were obtained in the United Kingdom. Mobility was slightly impaired, while emotional satisfaction was better compared to the general population. However, the overall quality of life was equivalent to that of the general population.[6]

The overall result of transplantation on the quality of life is excellent.[7] Surviving patients have a significant improvement in their quality of life and rate their quality of life better than do patients with chronic liver disease. Even in the face of some somatic restrictions, long-term survivors achieve a quality of life as high as healthy controls. A psychotherapeutic support program assists with rehabilitation and return to normal daily activities.

DIET AND EXERCISE

Nutritional regimen is aimed at correcting the pretransplantation malnutrition and coping with the nutrition related problems of immunosuppression: edema, obesity, hypercholesterolemia, diabetes, hypertension, and osteoporosis.

Most patients tolerate a regular diet.[8] Some patients have edema for several months after transplantation. Although prednisone may contribute, other, yet unrecognized factors may be responsible. A reduced salt (usually no added salt) diet is indicated. Intermittent use of loop diuretics can be beneficial. Prednisone may unmask latent diabetes, and a diabetic diet or insulin may be necessary.

The amount and type of activity has to be guided by disabilities other than the transplantation. For instance, patients with osteoporosis are at increased risk of bone fracture. Otherwise activities should be unrestricted and regular physical exercise encouraged. Contact sports are contraindicated.

IMMUNOSUPPRESSION MONITORING

Serum samples for levels of immunosuppression drugs have to be monitored either at the transplant center or at a reliable local commercial laboratory under direct supervision from the center. Even though the local physician may become proficient with selecting and dosing immunosuppressive medication, the patient is best served by having a responsible physician at the transplant center control all drugs and dosage changes.

INTERCURRENT ACUTE ILLNESS

Since fever or new symptoms can signal significant or possible life-threatening problems, such as rejection or hepatitis, they should be promptly investigated. Blood count, chemistries, and chest x-ray are routine initial tests. If these tests

TABLE 14-1. When Should the Transplant Center be Contacted

Fever
Abnormal liver function tests
Diarrhea not responding to simple management
Pregnancy
Elective surgery
Persistant pain
Anemia
Any unexplained signs or symptoms

are normal, and the diagnosis of a viral syndrome is made, symptomatic treatment may be initiated locally. Otherwise the transplant center should be contacted, if only for telephone consultation (Table 14-1).

One frequent symptom in the early convalescent period is mild or recurrent diarrhea. Symptomatic treatment may be started, after the stool is cultured and examined for ova and parasites and C. *difficele* toxin. If any of the stool tests are abnormal or antibiotic treatment is indicated the transplant center should be consulted. Alternatively the patient should be referred to the transplant center for further diagnosis and treatment. These patients are immunosuppressed and opportunistic infections (discussed in "Opportunistic Infections" section, below) are frequent.

DENTAL PROBLEMS[9]

A protocol has been developed for the dental management of liver transplant patients.[10] Regular dental examinations, especially to detect periodontal disease, are required and prompt management of even minor gingival problems is essential. Antibiotic prophylaxis is used on an empirical basis for dental procedures because of concern that multiple vascular anastomosis are prone to infection.

EYE DISEASES

Routine annual eye examinations are recommended since most patients are on steroids which can cause cataracts.

NONHEPATIC SURGERY

Transplantees can undergo anesthesia and nonabdominal surgery without technical difficulties. Abdominal surgery is difficult due to the adhesions resulting from the transplant surgery. Because of problems relating to the management of immunosuppression surgery is best performed at the transplant center.

PROPHYLAXIS AND VACCINATIONS

Patients are maintained on multiple drugs for prophylaxis of frequently encountered infections, unless a drug allergy develops. Single-strength trimethoprim/

sulfasaxole once daily or aerosol pentamidine monthly is given to prevent pneumocystis pneumonia. Acyclovir, 800 mg 4 times daily is used for prophylaxis of cytomegalovirus infections.[11] The dose is reduced to 200 mg after 12 weeks. Mycelex troches are effective for the prevention of oral candidiasis.

Patients should be protected from the annual influenza epidemic with vaccination every autumn. (Hepatitis B vaccine and polyvalent pneumococcal vaccine are administered pretransplantation. Immunity to measles, mumps, rubella, and polio is tested before transplantation, and vaccine is administered to nonimmune patients.)

In addition, aspirin, 81 mg once daily, is given to prevent hepatic artery thrombosis.

PREGNANCY

Menstrual function returns within 10 months[12,13] after liver transplantation in women of child-bearing age, even if they were amenorrheic before the surgery.

Normal pregnancy is therefore possible and has been reported as soon as 5 months after surgery.[14] In most patients immunosuppression with prednisone, cyclosporine, and azathioprine is continued during pregnancy. Major medical problems during pregnancy are hypertension, anemia, and hyperbilirubinemia. Rejections were successfully treated with corticosteroids.[15]

Preterm delivery was more frequent than expected in these patients.[14] Cesarean sections were also more frequent, with toxemia of pregnancy and early rupture of the membranes being the principal indications. Pregnancy had no adverse effect on the postpartum health of the mothers.

All the children were well developed and progressed with normal developmental milestones. Evidence of genetic damage to the children has not been observed;[14] however, the number of pregnancies reviewed was small. None of the children are child bearing age yet, so their reproductive potential is unknown.

Intrapartum orthotopic liver transplantations have been reported (for fulminant hepatic failure) with good outcome of the pregnancy.[16]

Oral birth control medication is contraindicated posttransplantation because of the possibility of thrombotic phenomena, exacerbation of hypertension, and drug interactions.

No data have been published on pregnancy while the patient is on FK506 immunosuppression. Male fertility has not been studied posttransplantation.

TRAVEL

Ability to travel depends on the length of time post transplantation and medical stability. 3-6 months after transplantation the medically stable patient is able to travel, even overseas. Restrictions apply though: the transplant center has to be notified and their approval obtained. In turn the transplant center will provide the patient with contacts to the local transplant center at the destination. In case of emergency the patient may have to cut short the travel.

TABLE 14-2. Complications of Immunosuppression

Hypertension
Renal impairment
Metabolic
obesity
diabetes
bone disease
Neoplastic
Opportunistic infections
bacterial
protozoal
viral
fungal
Neurologic
Skin and mucus membranes
hirsutism
gingival hypertrophy
condyloma

MEDICAL COMPLICATIONS OF LIVER TRANSPLANTATION

MANAGEMENT OF THE SIDE EFFECTS OF IMMUNOSUPPRESSION

Immunosuppression is associated with many adverse effects, including hypertension, nephrotoxicity, neurotoxicity malignancy, opportunistic infections, and bone disease (Table 14-2). Data collected from patients treated with cyclosporine forms much of the basis for the management of these side effects. However, it is likely that the observations noted with cyclosporine will apply to other drugs as well (Table 14-3 and Table 14-4).[17]

Bone Disease

Atraumatic bone fracture and avascular necrosis is frequent after liver transplantation. Bone disease leading to vertebral collapse occurred in 38% of the patients. Some of the collapse developed in previously normal vertebra.[18]

Hepatic osteodystrophy is most prevalent with cholestatic liver disease, especially with primary biliary cirrhosis.[19] Osteoporosis, in a fracture pattern resembling postmenopausal osteoporosis, is frequent. Steroid treatment and bed rest following transplantation accelerate the progress of osteoporosis. In the first 3–6 months after surgery bone mineral density levels decrease further. This trend subsequently reverses and by one year post transplantation bone density levels increase, resulting in a decreased incidence of fractures. Osteomalacia is relatively uncommon.[20]

Adequate dietary intake of calcium and vitamin D helps in the prevention of osteoporosis. Treatment can be instituted with vitamin D (400 units) and

TABLE 14-3. Signs and Symptoms Associated With Cyclosporine Therapy

Neurologic:
tremor
paresthesia or burning of palms or soles
headache
flushing
depression
confusion
somnolence
seizures
visual disturbance
disorientation
coma
paresis
pseudo-psychosis: e.g. inappropriate behaviour
Gastrointestinal:
bloating
nausea
vomiting
Dematologic:
hypertrichosis of face, arm, shoulder and back
coarsening of facial features (mostly in children)
gingival hyperplasia
condyloma
Endocrine:
polyuria
hyperglycemia
Hypersensitivity to the oil base:
crushing chest pain
dyspnea
flushing

calcium (2.5 g of carbonate daily equivalent to 1 g of elemental calcium) after assessment for bone density, and measurement of serum 1,25-dihydroxy vitamin D and its metabolites. Calcitonin and etidronate have been proven effective in reversing postmenopausal osteoporosis, but further studies are required to prove their efficacy in steroid induced osteoporosis and posttransplant patients.

Hypertension and Impaired Renal Function

Hypertension and decreased renal function is a common complication of cyclosporine therapy. It is a consequence of the cyclosporine-induced arterial vasoconstriction. Two-thirds of the patients in one study[2] developed hypertension that was easily controlled medically.

A similar number of patients had nephrotoxicity with elevation of serum creatinine. Reducing the dose of cyclosporine and including azathioprine in the immunosuppression regimen stabilized renal function. Treatment with calcium channel blockers (nifepedine, which has the least interaction with cyclosporine

TABLE 14-4. Signs and Symptoms Associated with FK506 Therapy

Neurologic:
Seizure
Tremor
Hyperesthesia
Muscle weakness
Insomnia
Blurred vision
Photophobia
Paranoid psychosis
Expressive dysphasia
Gastrointestinal:
Bloating
Nausea
Vomiting
Dermatologic:
Hypertrichosis (rare)
Pruritus
Endocrine:
Hyperglycemia

is the drug of choice) is also effective. Prostaglandins have recently been shown to reverse the vasoconstriction effect of cyclosporine.[21]

In early reports FK506 had significant nephrotoxicity. However, with reduced intravenous induction doses and close pharmacologic monitoring, nephrotoxicity can be controlled.[22] When used for primary immunosuppression, the incidence of hypertension is low.[23] However, nephrotoxicity is aggravated when immunosuppression is changed from cyclosporine to FK506.[17]

Neurologic Manifestations

Seizures, coma, confusion, cortical blindness and quadriplegia are among the severe neurologic manifestations of cyclosporine toxicity. Seizures are present in up to one-third of the patients.[24] All these side effect are due to severe, diffuse disorder of the white matter[24a] and reversed by the discontinuation or reduction of cyclosporine therapy.[25] Tremor and dysesthesia are also improved by reduction of the dose of immunosuppressive medication.

Psychosis can occur and may be due to steroids or cyclosporine. Psychiatric consultation should be obtained. Treatment with psychoactive agents such as Haldol (haloperidol) are not very effective and frequently lead to obtundation. Occasionally they are required in the agitated, hyperactive patient. Frequently reduction of the steroid dose controls the psychosis.

Persistent headaches must be carefully evaluated. Central nervous system involvement with fungal,[26] viral,[27] and bacterial[28] infections, lymphoma, and other vascular or neoplastic lesions have to be excluded. A complete neurologic evaluation, including CAT scan and MRI of the brain, is often necessary before symptomatic treatment is initiated. When an organic cause has been excluded, a nonsteroidal antiinflammatory agent (NSAID), a calcium channel blocker, or a beta blocker can be tried as an empiric treatment.[25]

Cortical blindness occurred in a patient and was reversed by discontinuation of cyclosporine. Central nervous system demyelination was a late complication in the same patient.[29]

Cyclosporine circulates in association with lipoprotein; its neurotoxicity is enhanced by hypocholesterolemia, especially when serum levels are < 120 mg/dl.[25,30,31]

Skin and Mucous Membrane Problems

Hirsutism is frequently encountered during steroid and cyclosporine treatment. About half of the patients have hypertrichosis involving the face, arms, shoulders, and back. Cosmetic treatment can adequately resolve the problems, but many patients tolerate mild to moderate hirsutism.

Rhinorrhea is a common side effect of cyclosporin therapy and requires no treatment.

Gingival hypertrophy requiring dental treatment is moderately frequent (see above). It is due to increased production of collagen by the already increased number of fibroblasts. In patients with poor oral hygiene, the inflammatory interaction between fibroblast and lymphocytes exacerbates the problem.[32]

Condylomata is seen with moderate frequency.[32a]

Obesity, Diabetes, and Hypercholesterolemia

Obesity often results in fatty liver, hypertension, or diabetes and may complicate the management of the posttransplant patient. Two-thirds of the 28 transplanted patients in a series[33] were found to be overweight. All patients who were overweight pretransplantation were also overweight posttransplantation. Weight control is an important management problem of the otherwise well liver recipient.

Both cyclosporine and prednisone are diabetogenic and new onset of diabetes, occasionally insulin-dependent, occurs.[2]

Cyclosporine enhances cholesterol biosynthesis,[34] and moderate increases of serum cholesterol are observed in patients taking this drug. Prednisone and obesity may be contributing factors. FK506 immunosuppression significantly decreased cholesterol levels.[35]

Neoplasia

The overall incidence of de novo neoplasm after transplantation is 6%. However, only 1% of the patients die from this cause.[36]

The incidence of lymphoma is increased during chronic immunosuppression, with disproportionate increase in non-Hodgkin's lymphomas. Most of these are of central nervous system or gastrointestinal origin. The cyclosporine/steroid treated group had twice as many (20%) lymphomas as the azathioprine-treated group.[36] Patients who received repeated courses of OKT3 for the treatment of rejection had a particularly high incidence of lymphoma.[37]

Several other groups of cancers, relatively uncommon in the general population (Kaposi's sarcoma; squamous cell carcinoma of lip and skin; carcinoma of vulva, kidney, and the hepatobiliary system) occur more frequently posttransplantation. If hepatitis B recurs, the development of hepatocellular carcinoma may be accelerated by immunosuppression.[38]

Decreased immunosuppression reverses the development of lymphomas. For a discussion of the pathology of these tumors, see the chapter by Thung and Gerber (Chapter 17).

Opportunistic Infections

Bacterial Infections

Bacterial infections are most common in the first 2 months postransplantation and are related to the dose of immunosuppression and duration of the operation.[39] Following discharge, bacterial infections are caused by the organisms usually found in the general population and are not increased in frequency.[40]

Protozoan Infection

Immunosuppressed patients are at high risk for *Pneumocystis carinii* pneumonia. It is relatively rare posttransplantation, since all patients are on a prophylactic regimen. If the prophylaxis is interrupted, while the patient is immunosuppressed, pneumocystis pneumonia is frequent. Multiple techniques are needed for diagnosis: specific culture media, histology, cytology, and serology.[40]

Fungal Infections[41]

There is a strong relationship between the number of severe fungal infections and prolonged course(s) of antibiotic treatment.[42] The most frequent species are *Candida* and *Aspergillus*[43]. Most common sites are skin, lung, and mucous membranes (including the gastrointestinal and urinary tracts). Bronchoalveolar lavage is useful in establishing the diagnosis of pulmonary infections. Hospitalization for diagnosis and treatment is almost always required. A case of disseminated coccidioidomycosis along with rare cases of infections with *Mucor* and *Cryptococcus neoformans* have been reported.[44] The incidence of fungal infections declines with time after surgery.[45]

Cytomegalovirus[46]

Infections with cytomegalovirus (CMV) involve multiple organs, including lung, liver, and the gastrointestinal tract. Most infections occur within the first 3 months after surgery and during rejection episodes.[47]

CMV involvement of the liver is the most common and most life-threatening. The most severe infections occur when the donor's serology is positive for CMV

TABLE 14-5. Late Medical Complications of Liver Transplantation

Complications of immunosuppression
Hepatic artery thrombosis
Recurrent disease
Chronic rejection
Disease acquired from donor liver
Biliary strictures

infection and the recipient is seronegative for CMV. Hepatitis presents with malaise, low-grade fever, leukopenia, and abnormal liver functions test. Liver biopsy is necessary for diagnosis. The mean occurrence of CMV hepatitis is 38 days after surgery.[48]

Diarrhea or bleeding is a common presenting symptom of cytomegalic involvement of the gastrointestinal tract. Ulcerations are frequent,[49] and hepatitis may be coincidental. The colonic mucosa, however, may appear grossly unusual on colonoscopic exam and multiple biopsies are required. Involvement of the colon may be limited to the right side only. CMV may also involve the esophagus, stomach and duodenum. Inclusion bodies in biopsy specimen are diagnostic of active disease.[50] The diagnosis can also be made by immunohistochemical staining or culture of the biopsy specimen. Newer techniques using a DNA probe or the polymerase chain reaction (PCR) are being evaluated to assist in diagnosis.[51]

Gangciclovir is the treatment of choice for active disease.[52]

Herpes Simplex Virus (HSV)

Herpes hepatitis, although rare, occurs soon after transplantation and is fulminant.[53,54] There is no effective treatment available although a few patients who only had local liver injury survived with antiviral therapy.[54a] Retransplantation may be attempted, but the results are poor. HSV pneumonia is fatal in over 60% of cases.[54b] Dysphagia is a sign of HSV esophagitis.[54c]

Epstein-Barr Virus[55,56]

This virus causes a spectrum of illness from the classical mononucleosis like syndrome to B-cell proliferative disease to full blown malignant lymphoma. The mononucleosis like syndrome may have atypical features, including jaw pain, joint effusions, pneumonitis, and encephalitis. Acyclovir is an effective treatment. B-cell proliferative syndromes, polyclonal in nature, require reduction of immunosuppression. The true B-cell lymphoma, monoclonal, responds poorly to chemotherapy.[56a]

HEPATIC ARTERY THROMBOSIS

Hepatic artery thrombosis may mimic hepatitis or allograft dysfunction or may be found on a screening ultrasound study.[57] It is frequently associated with intra-abdominal infections and is more frequent after multiple episodes of rejection.[58] Vascular compromise of the graft is a major etiology of graft failure; therefore, early diagnosis is crucial for graft salvage. Since these changes seldom are medically reversible, prompt surgical intervention is necessary. Revascularization can be attempted, but retransplantation may be required. The overall mortality is 70%.

RECURRENT DISEASE

Primary Biliary Cirrhosis

Mitochondrial antibody disappears after liver transplantation, but recurs with decreased titers in the first postoperative year in 90% of the patients. Contoversy exists about clinical recurrence.[59,60] Within the first year after transplantation differentiation from acute or chronic rejection would be difficult. Neuberger et al.[61] reported clinical and pathologic recurrence. This was questioned by Van Thiel et al.[62] However, primary biliary cirrhosis is a slowly progressing disease with insidious onset; therefore, recurrence may take decades.

Sclerosing Cholangitis and Ulcerative Colitis

Primary sclerosing cholangitis cannot be diagnosed after biliary surgery because any abnormality of the bile duct may be due to the surgery. However, patients who were transplanted for end-stage liver disease secondary to PSC have an increased incidence of biliary complications.

Cholangiocarcinoma, irrespective of its size, has a very poor prognosis and recurs soon after transplantation.[63]

Colitis may recur in the posttransplant patient, even under the influence of immunosuppression. Similarly colon cancer in ulcerative colitis has been reported after transplantation.[64] Therefore surveillance for colon cancer should continue in the transplant patient.

Hepatitis

Patients who are transplanted for hepatitis B cirrhosis, but have antibody for hepatitis B surface antigen will not develop recurrent disease. The recurrence rate in surface antigen–positive patients with evidence of viral replication (i.e., who are positive for hepatitis B e antigen or have significant titers of hepatitis B virus DNA), is 80–90% in one year. This rate is reduced to 40–50% if viral replication is not evident before transplant.[65-69]

Recurrent hepatitis B in the posttransplant patient usually develops into chronic active hepatitis, but occasional cases are fulminant. Less than 10% become chronic carriers and have normal histology on liver biopsy. A variant of recurrent hepatitis B characterized by minimal inflammation and significant fibrosis and cholestatis has been described by the group at Kings College Hospital in London. This suggests a nonimmune mediated, cytopathic mechanism.[70] Progression to cirrhosis occurs at an accelerated rate and requires retransplantation. This cycle is repeated with increasing frequency resulting in multiple transplantation at shorter and shorter intervals.

Pancreatitis can also occur secondary to recurrent hepatitis B infection.[70a] Drug induced pancreatitis may be due to azathioprine. Cyclosporine and FK506 are less likely to produce clinically significant disease.

Therapeutic trials using hyperimmune B globulin, stimulation of antibody production by hepatitis B vaccine, and α-interferon treatment in the pre- and posttransplant period have not as yet shown an improvement in prognosis, but further controlled studies are warranted.[67]

A few cases of recurrent hepatitis C have been reported.[68,71] Other workers suggested that posttransplantation hepatitis C is unrelated to the presense of hepatitis C in the native liver of the recipient.[72] Unlike hepatitis B, recurrent hepatitis C has a clinical course similar to that of nontransplanted hepatitis C cases and retransplantation is less likely to be required.

Theoretically one could consider treatment with interferon to suppress or eliminate the virus if active, biopsy-proven hepatitis C is present. Controlled studies to prove this point are needed.

Incidentally, aplastic anemia has been reported, as a unique complication, after transplantation for fulminant hepatitis C.[73,74]

Recurrent hepatitis in patients transplanted for acute hepatitis D has a more benign course.[66] On the other hand only two out of seven patients who were transplanted for hepatitis D cirrhosis cleared both the hepatitis B and D virus and survived for more than one year. The other five died of recurrent hepatitis D.[75] Recurrence of autoimmune hepatitis appears to be rare.

Malignancy

Hepatocellular carcinoma most frequently recurs as metastatic disease. Overall recurrence rates are up to 50% in some series.[76] Small $<$5 cm) lesions usually are an incidental finding in the resected liver and have a better prognosis.

Epitheliod hemangioendothelioma, which usually has a poor prognosis, may not recur for 2 years or longer.

Fibrolamellar carcinoma is rarely metastatic and because it tends to recur late is thought to be associated with a long survival.

Alcoholism

The rate of recidivism is about 10-20%. Patients who were drinking up to the time of transplantation are more likely to return to drinking.[76a] No information is available as to the consequences, i.e., recurrent alcoholic liver disease, in patients who drink alcohol posttransplant. However, recurrent drinking poses a problem with the management of immunosuppression because it interferes both with compliance and drug therapy. Alcohol also interferes with the absorption and metabolism of cyclosporine.

Budd-Chiari Syndrome

Recurrence rates, which may depend on etiology, are not known. Patients transplanted for complications of Budd-Chiari syndrome need treatment to prevent recurrence. Lifetime anticoagulation with Coumadin is required.[76b] In patients with underlying myeloproliferative disease an alternative therapy with hydroxyurea and aspirin has been advocated to reduce the number and function of platelets.

CHRONIC REJECTION

Chronic rejection should always be suspected in patients with elevated liver enzymes. Persistent jaundice associated with abnormal liver enzymes may herald severe rejection associated with the vanishing bile duct syndrome. It is more frequent in the first 2 years after transplanation. Referral to the transplant center and hospitalization is necessary for diagnosis and treatment. If a liver biopsy confirms rejection, then the treatment will be decided by the transplant center staff. Sometimes only an increase of the dose of FK506 is necessary. Mild rejection may be treated with high-dose steroid intravenously. Moderate or severe rejection require combination of steroids, FK506 or OKT3. For detailed discussion see Chapter 13 by Schwartz, Manzarbeitia and Miller. Enhanced arteriosclerosis is a manifestation of chronic rejection.

DISEASES TRANSMITTED BY LIVER TRANSPLANTATION

It is not unexpected that illness either thought not to involve the liver or clinically not detected in the donor pre-transplant may be transmitted to the recipient. Penn has reported several cases of malignancies transmitted with donor organs.

Factor 11 deficiency,[78] idiopathic thrombocytopenic purpura (ITP),[79] hepatitis C[80], Gilbert's syndrome[81] and cerebral neoplasm[82] all have been transmitted from a donor to the liver transplant recipient. Retransplantation was performed in most of these cases. In addition infectious diseases are more commonly transmitted.

REFERENCES

1. Robinson LR, Switala J, Tarter RE, Nicholas JJ: Functional outcome after liver transplantation: a preliminary report. *Arch Phys Med Rehab* 71:426–427, 1990.
2. Eid AR, Steffen R, Porayko MK, et al: Beyond 1 year after liver transplantation. *Mayo Clin Proc* 64:446–450, 1989.
3. Tarter RE, Erbs S, Biller PA, Switala JA, Van Thiel DH: The quality of life following liver transplantation: a preliminary report. *Gastroenterol Clin Am* 17:207–217, 1988.
4. Tarter RE, Switala J, Arria A, Plail I, Van Thiel D: Quality of life before and after orthotopic hepatic transplantation. *Arch Intern Med* 151:1521–1526, 1991.
5. Kuchler T, Kober B, Brolsch C, Henne Bruns D, Kremer B: Quality of life after liver transplantation: can a psychosocial support program contribute? *Transplant Proc* 23:1541–1544, 1991.

6. Lowe D, O'Grady JG, McEwen J, Williams R: Quality of life following liver transplantation: a preliminary report. *J R Coll Physicians Lond* 24:43–46, 1990.
7. Kober B, Kuchler T, Broelsch C, Kremer B, Henne Bruns D: A psychological support concept and quality of life research in a liver transplantation program: an interdisciplinary multicenter study. *Psychother Psychosom* 54:117–131, 1990.
8. Hasse J: Role of the dietitian in the nutrition management of adults after liver transplantation. *J Am Diet Assoc* 91:473–476, 1991.
9. Gragiulo AV, Schaffner JA, Robinson JA: Gingival and systemic manifestations of chronic liver disease: pre- & post-liver transplant. *Periodont Case Rep* 10:13–18, 1988.
10. Svirsky JA, Saravia ME: Dental management of patients after liver transplantation. *Oral Surg Oral Med Oral Pathol* 67:541–546, 1989.
11. Stratta RJ, Shaefer MS, Cushing KA, et al: Successful prophylaxis of cytomegalovirus disease after primary CMV exposure in liver transplant recipients. *Transplantation* 51:90–97, 1991.
12. Cundy TF, O'Grady JG, Williams R: Recovery of menstruation and pregnancy after liver transplantation. *Gut* 31:337–338, 1990.
13. de Koning ND, Haagsma EB: Normalization of menstrual pattern after liver transplanation: consequences for contraception. *Digestion* 46:239–241, 1990.
14. Scantlebury V, Gordon R, Tzakis A, et al: Childbearing after liver transplantation. *Transplantation* 49:317–321, 1990.
15. Laifer SA, Darby MJ, Scantlebury VP, Harger JH, Caritis SN: Pregnancy and liver transplantation. *Obstet Gynecol* 76:1083–1088, 1990.
16. Fair J, Klein AS, Feng T, Merritt WT, Burdick JF: Intrapartum orthotopic liver transplantation with successful outcome of pregnancy. *Transplantation* 50:534–535, 1990.
17. Todo S, Fung JJ, Starzl TE, et al: Liver, kidney, and thoracic organ transplantation under FK 506. *Ann Surg* 212:295–305, 1990.
18. Haagsma EB, Thijn CJ, Post JG, Slooff MJ, Gips CH: Bone disease after orthotopic liver transplantation. *J Hepatol* 6:94–100, 1988.
19. Maddrey WC: Bone disease in patients with primary biliary cirrhosis. *Prog Liver Dis* 9:537–554, 1990.
20. Porayko MK, Wiesner RH, Hay JE, et al: Bone disease in liver transplant recipients: incidence, timing, and risk factors. *Transplant Proc* 23:1462–1465, 1991.
21. Paller MS: The prostaglandin E1 analogue, misoprostol analogue reverses acute cyclosporin nephrotoxicity. *Transplant Proc* 20(3 suppl 3):634–637, 1988.
22. Abu Elmagd K, Fung JJ, Alessiani M, et al: The effect of graft function on FK506 plasma levels, dosages, and renal function, with particular reference to the liver. *Transplantation* 52:71–77, 1991.
23. McCauley J, Takaya S, Fung J, et al: The question of FK 506 nephrotoxicity after liver transplantation. *Transplant Proc* 23:1444–1447, 1991.
24. Martinez AJ, Estol C, Faris AA: Neurologic complications of liver transplantation. *Neurol Clin* 6:327–348, 1988.
24a. Truwit CL, Denaro CP, Lake JR, DeMarco T: MR imaging of reversible cyclosporin A-induced neurotoxicity. *Am J Neuroradiol* 12:651–659, 1991.
25. de Groen PC, Aksamit AJ, Rakela J, Forbes GS, Krom RA: Central nervous system toxicity after liver transplantation. The role of cyclosporine and cholesterol. *New Engl J Med* 317:861–866, 1987.

26. Boon AP, Adams DH, Buckels J, McMaster P: Cerebral aspergillosis in liver transplantation see comments. *J Clin Pathol* 43:114–118, 1990.

27. Power C, Poland SD, Kassim KH, Kaufmann JC, Rice GP: Encephalopathy in liver transplantation: neuropathology and CMV infection. *Can J Neurol Sci* 17:378–381, 1990.

28. Raby N, Forbes G, Williams R: Nocardia infection in patients with liver transplants or chronic liver disease: radiologic findings. *Radiology* 174:713–714, 1990.

29. Wilson SE, de Groen PC, Aksamit AJ, Wiesner RH, Garrity JA, Krom RA: Cyclosporine A-induced reversible cortical blindness. *J Clin Neuro Ophthalmol* 8:215–220, 1988.

30. Cooper DK, Novitzky D, Davis L, et al: Does central nervous system toxicity occur in transplant patients with hypocholesterolemia receiving cyclosporine? *J Heart Transplant* 8:221–224, 1989.

31. de Groen PC: Cyclosporine, low-density lipoprotein, and cholesterol. *Mayo Clin Proc* 63:1012–1021, 1988.

32. Wysocki GP, Gretzinger HA, Laupacis A, et al: Fibrous hyperplasia of the gingiva; a side effect of cyclosporine A therapy. *Oral Surg Oral Med Oral Pathol* 55:274–278, 1983.

32a. Gentile G, Formelli G, Selva S: Atypical picture of cervico-vaginal condylomatosis in a patient submitted to hepatic transplant. A case report. *Clin Exp Obstet Gynecol* 17:155–157, 1990.

33. Palmer M, Schaffner F, Thung TN: Excessive weight gain after liver transplantation. *Transplantation* 51:797–800, 1991.

34. Ballantyne CM, Podet EJ, Patsch WP, et al: Effects of cyclosporine therapy on plasma lipoprotein levels. *JAMA* 262:53–56, 1989.

35. Van Thiel DH, Iqbal M, Jain A, Fung J, Todo S, Starzl TE: Gastrointestinal and metabolic problems associated with immunosuppression with either CyA or FK506 in liver transplantation. *Transplant Proc* 22:37–40, 1990.

36. Penn I: Cancer complicating organ transplantation. *New Engl J Med* 323:1767–1769, 1990.

37. Swinnen LJ, Costanzo-Nordin MR, Fisher SG, et al: Increased incidence of lymphoproliferative disorder after immunosuppresion with the monoclonal antibody OKT3 in cardiac transplant recipients. *New Engl J Med* 323:1723–1728, 1991.

38. Luketic VA, Schiffman ML, McCall JB, Posner MP, Mills AS, Carithers, Jr, RL: *Ann Intern Med* 114:212–213, 1991.

39. Kusne S, Dummer JS, Singh N, et al: Infections after liver transplantation. An analysis of 101 consecutive cases. *Medicine (Baltimore)* 67:132–143, 1988.

40. Markin RS, Stratta RJ, Woods GL: Infection after liver transplantation. *Am J Surg Pathol* 14(Suppl 1):64–78, 1990.

41. Tollemar J, Ericzon BG, Holmberg K, Andersson J: The incidence and diagnosis of invasive fungal infections in liver transplant recipients. *Transplant Proc* 22:242–244, 1990.

42. Colonna JO, Winston DJ, Brill JE, et al: Infectious complications in liver transplantation. *Arch Surg* 123:360–364, 1988.

43. Boon AP, Adams DH, Buckels J, McMaster P: Cerebral aspergillosis in liver transplantation. *J Clin Pathol* 43:114–118, 1990.

44. Dodd LG, Nelson SD: Disseminated coccidioidomycosis detected by percutaneous liver biopsy in a liver transplant recipient. *Am J Clin Pathol* 93:141–144, 1990.

45. Castaldo P, Stratta RJ, Wood RP, et al: Clinical spectrum of fungal infections after orthotopic liver transplantation. *Arch Surg* 126:149–156, 1991.
46. Sayage LH, Gonwa TA, Goldstein RM, Husberg BS, Klintmalm GB: Cytomegalovirus infection in orthotopic liver transplantation. *Transplant Int* 2:96–101, 1989.
47. Bronsther O, Makowka L, Jaffe R, et al: Occurrence of cytomegalovirus hepatitis in liver transplant patients. *J Med Virol* 24:423–434, 1988.
48. Stratta RJ, Shaefer MS, Markin RS, et al: Clinical patterns of cytomegalovirus disease after liver transplantation. *Arch Surg* 124:1443—1449, 1989.
49. Alexander JA, Cuellar RE, Fadden RJ, Genovese JJ, Gavaler JS, Van Thiel DH: Cytomegalovirus infection of the upper gastrointestinal tract before and after liver transplantation. *Transplantation* 46:378–382, 1988.
50. Paya CV, Hermans PE, Wiesner RH, et al: Cytomegalovirus hepatitis in liver transplantation: prospective analysis of 93 consecutive orthotopic liver transplantations. *J Infect Dis* 160:752–758, 1989.
51. Paya CV, Holley KE, Wiesner RH, et al: Early diagnosis of cytomegalovirus hepatitis in liver transplant recipients: role of immunostaining, DNA hybridization and culture of hepatic tissue. *Hepatology* 12:119–126, 1990.
52. Stein DS, Verano AS, Levandowski RA: Successful treatment with ganciclovir of disseminated cytomegalovirus infection after liver transplantation. *Am J Gastroenterol* 83:684–686, 1988.
53. Haagsma EB, Klompmaker IJ, Grond J, et al: Herpes virus infections after orthotopic liver transplantation. *Transplant Proc* 19:4054–4056, 1987.
54. Singh N, Dummer JS, Kusne S, et al: Infections with cytomegalovirus and other herpesviruses in 121 liver transplant recipients: transmission by donated organ and the effect of OKT3 antibodies. *J Infect Dis* 158:124–131, 1988.
54a. Kusne S, Schwartz M, Breinig MK, et al: Herpes simplex virus hepatitis after solid organ transplantation in adults. *J Infect Dis* 163:1001–1007, 1991.
54b. Allen KA, Markin RS, Rennard SI, et al: Bronchoalveolar lavage in liver transplant patients. *Acta Cytol* 33:539–543, 1989.
54c. Alexander JA, Brouillette DE, Chien MC, et al: Infectious esophagitis following liver and renal transplantation. *Dig Dis Sci* 33:1121–1126, 1988.
55. Randhawa PS, Markin RS, Starzl TE, Demetris AJ: Epstein-Barr virus-associated syndromes in immunosuppressed liver transplant recipients. Clinical profile and recognition on routine allograft biopsy. *Am J Surg Pathol* 14:538–547, 1990.
56. Langnas AN, Castaldo P, Markin RS, Stratta RJ, Wood RP, Shaw BW, Jr: The spectrum of Epstein-Barr virus infection with hepatitis following liver transplantation. *Transplant Proc* 23:1513–1514, 1991.
56a. Scully RE, Mark EJ, McNeely WF, McNeely BU: Hepatic failure after liver transplantation. *New Engl J Med* 326:547–559, 1992.
57. Langnas AN, Marujo W, Stratta RJ, Wood RP, Shaw BW, Jr: Vascular complications after orthotopic liver transplantation. *Am J Surg* 161:76–82, 1991.
58. Hesselink EJ, Klompmaker IJ, Grond J, Gouw AS, van Schilfgaarde R, Sloof MJ: Hepatic artery thrombosis (HAT) after orthotopic transplantation (OLT)—the influence of technical factors and rejection episodes. *Transplant Proc* 21:2468–2468, 1989.
59. Lynch SV, Strong RW: Primary biliary cirrhosis: does it recur after transplantation? *J Gastroenterol Hepatol* 4:109–110, 1989.
60. Editorial: Is PBC cured by liver transplantation? *Lancet* 337:272–273, 1991.

61. Polson RJ, Portmann B, Neuberger J, Calne RY, Williams R: Evidence for disease recurrence after liver transplantation for primary biliary cirrhosis. Clinical and histologic follow-up studies. *Gastroenterology* 97:715–725, 1989.

62. Van Thiel DH, Gavaler JS: Recurrent disease in patients with liver transplantation: when does it occur and how can we be sure? *Hepatology* 7:181–183, 1987.

63. Herbener T, Zajko AB, Koneru B, Bron KM, Campbell WL: Recurrent cholangiocarcinoma in the biliary tree after liver transplantation. *Radiology* 169:641–642, 1988.

64. Higashi H, Yanaga K, Marsh JW, Tzakis A, Kakizoe S, Starzl TE: Development of colon cancer after liver transplantation for primary sclerosing cholangitis associated with ulcerative colitis. *Hepatology* 11:477–480, 1990.

65. Mora NP, Klintmalm GB, Poplawski SS, et al: Recurrence of hepatitis B after liver transplantation: Does hepatitis-B-immunoglobulin modify the recurrent disease? *Transplant Proc* 22:1549–1550, 1990.

66. O'Grady JG, Williams R: Liver transplantation for viral hepatitis. *Br Med Bull* 46:481–491, 1990.

67. Feray C, Zignego AL, Samuel D: Persistent hepatitis B virus infection of mononuclear blood cells without concomitant liver infection. The liver transplantation model. *Transplantation* 49:1155–1158, 1990.

68. Hart J, Busuttil RW, Lewin KJ: Disease recurrence following liver transplantation. *Am J Surg Pathol* 14(Suppl 1):79–91, 1990.

69. Bismuth H, Morino M: 134 liver transplants: experience of the group at the Paul Brousse Hospital. *G Chir* 9:561–564, 1988.

70. Davies SE, Portmann BC, O'Grady JG, et al: Hepatic histological findings after transplantation for chronic hepatitis B virus infection, including a unique pattern of fibrosing cholestatic hepatitis. *Hepatology* 13:150–157, 1991.

70a. Alexander JA, Demetrius AJ, Gavaler JS, Makowka L, Starzl TE, Van Thiel DH: Pancreatitis following liver transplantation. *Transplantation* 45:1062–1065, 1988.

71. Martin P, Munoz SJ, DiBisceglia AM, et al: Recurrence of hepatitis C virus infection after orthotopic liver transplant. *Heptology* 13:719–721, 1991.

72. Read AE, Donegan E, Lake J, et al: Hepatitis C in patients undergoing liver transplantation. *Ann Intern Med* 114:282–284, 1991.

73. Letter: Aplastic anemia after liver transplantation for non-A, non-B hepatitis. *New Engl J Med* 320:122—123, 1989.

74. Stock PG, Steiner ME, Freese D, Sharp H, Ascher NL. Hepatitis-associated aplastic anemia after liver transplantation. *Transplantation* 43:595–597, 1987.

75. Rizzetto M, Macagno S, Chiaberge E, et al: Liver transplantation in hepatitis delta virus disease. Lancet 2:469–471, 1987.

76. Penn, I. Hepatic transplantation for primary and metastatic malignancies of the liver. *Surgery* 110:726–734, 1991.

76a. Bird GL, O'Grady JG, Harvey FA, Calne RY, Williams R: Liver transplantation in patients with alcoholic cirrhosis: selection criteria and rates of survival and relapse. *BMJ* 301:15–17, 1990.

76b. Campbell DA, Jr, Rolles K, Jamieson N, et al: Hepatic transplantation with perioperative and long term anticoagulation as treatment for Budd-Chiari syndrome. *Surg Gynecol Obstet* 166:511–518, 1988.

77. Penn I: Transmission of cancer with donor organs. *Transplant Proc* 18:471, 1986.

78. Dzik WH, Arkin CF, Jenkins RL: Transfer of congenital factor XI deficiency from a

donor to a recipient by liver transplantation letter. *New Engl J Med* 316:1217–1218, 1987.

79. Friend PJ, McCarthy LJ, Filo RS, et al: Transmission of idiopathic (autoimmune) thrombocytopenic purpura by liver transplantation. *New Engl J Med* 323:807–811, 1990.
80. Pereira BJG, Milford EL, Kirkman RL, Levey AS: Transmission of hepatitis C virus by organ transplantation. *New Engl J Med* 325:454–460, 1991.
81. Henne Bruns D, Kremer B: Manifestation of Gilbert's syndrome after orthotopic liver transplantation: a rare cause of postoperative hyperbilirubinemia. *Clin. Transpl* p 309, 1989.
82. Morse JH, Turcotte JG, Merion RM, Campbell DA, Jr, Burtch GD, Lucey MR: Development of a malignant tumor in a liver transplant graft procured from a donor with a cerebral neoplasm. *Transplantation* 50:875–877, 1990.

—15—

THE TRANSPLANT COORDINATOR: A NEW BREED OF HEALTH PROFESSIONAL

Margaret M. Kadian

Liver transplantation is no longer experimental; it is the accepted therapy for end-stage liver disease. Since the initial cases done by Starzl beginning in 1963 and the advent of cyclosporine in 1978, the number of liver transplants in the United States has grown exponentially. Technical advances, including the use of the venovenous bypass and Viaspan preservation fluid, have greatly improved the outcome; one-year actuarial survival rates now approach 80%. In 1990, 2656 liver transplants were done in the United States, and there are an average of 1500 people waiting for livers during any given month. As a result of the increased number of transplants, the needs of this complex and diverse group of patients have grown proportionately, encompassing medicosurgical, psychosocial, financial, and educational areas.

The need to integrate these activities led to the development of the transplant coordinator. These professionals, at first working as nurses, social workers, or physicians' assistants, defined their own roles in response to their local situations, which varied with the hospital and surgeon. Initially, most coordinators worked in both the procurement and clinical areas. The system of organ allocation that is used today evolved from the practice established by the first coordinators. As the coordinator position developed, a division of roles between the procurement and clinical specialties occurred.

As the field expanded, a national organization, NATCO (North American Transplant Coordinators Organization), was established. NATCO recently formulated Standards of Excellence for the education, role development, and certification of transplant coordinators. The American Board of Transplant Coordinators has been established under the auspices of NATCO and is responsible for certification. Qualification to sit for the exam is established by the board's review of the applicant's education and professional experience. Professional women and men are certified as either Certified Clinical Procurement Coordinators (CCPCs) or Certified Clinical Transplant Coordinators (CCTCs). Certification based on skill and education led to the recognition of transplant coordination as a distinct health care profession.

Procurement coordinators work for either hospital-based or independent organ procurement agencies. Clinical transplant coordinators work in hospitals in both inpatient and outpatient settings, taking a pivotal role in the entire transplant process. Although certification is not currently required for practice in the field, NATCO has taken specific steps toward the eventual certification of all coordinators. While coordinators in different hospitals and organ procurement organizations have a variety of roles, the establishment of a national certification system and of practice standards has reinforced the role of the coordinator as integral to the success of a transplant program.

This chapter is designed to explain the transplant process and patient services in transplant centers by detailing the role of both procurement and clinical coordinators.

TRANSPLANT TEAM MEMBERS

The transplant team, which by definition is multidisciplinary, is one of the most holistic health care teams today. Transplant centers have designated personnel to address particular patient issues. This team includes, but is certainly not limited to hepatologists, gastroenterologists, pediatricians, nutritionists, social workers, surgeons, intensivists, nurses, administrators, ethicists, psychiatrists, cardiologists, pulmonologists, infectious disease specialists, nephrologists, and, of course, the transplant coordinator. The transplant coordinator's role is particularly diverse and has been compared to that of a producer, a quarterback, or a conductor. However, the job description varies from center to center. The coordinator is the liaison between the team members, working to ensure that all systems are functioning smoothly. The coordinator has both direct and indirect patient care responsibilities.

REFERRAL PROCESS

Most patients enter the transplant center's care by referral from the primary care physician, gastroenterologist, or hepatologist. Transplant centers have 24-hr accessibility to provide phone consultation on potential candidates. The referral may be made to the surgeon, hepatologist, or transplant coordinator. Appropriateness and timing for referrals are discussed at length in other chapters of this book; however, as a general rule, the earlier a patient is referred, the better. This allows enough time to evaluate the patient in detail and, where possible, to establish an etiology of the patient's liver disease and reevaluate the appropriateness of transplantation as a treatment modality. In nonurgent cases, patients and families are given the opportunity to receive instruction and meet other patients.

This lessens the anxiety about the transplant process and helps patients to be better prepared to participate in their care. Transplant evaluations may be handled in either the inpatient or outpatient setting, depending on the severity of the patient's disability and the distance of the patient from the center, and occasionally the insurance coverage.

Sometimes patients or family members will self-refer to a transplant center for evaluation. Their medical conditions may or may not warrant consideration for transplantation. These cases are best handled by initial consultation with one of the hepatologists or through the liver clinic.

Patient services at the initial stage of referral are to provide guidance as to the appropriateness of the referral, to assist with inquiries to insurance carriers, to refer to community support groups, to educate, and to make arrangements for initial consultation. During the initial discussion with the referring physician, plans are made for intake. Patients may also come for initial consultation as interhospital transfers or as outpatients.

Insurance coverage varies widely, and individual policies must be investigated. The transplant centers provide guidance for the patient and family with regard to third-party payers since financial stress adds to the anxiety of facing a life-threatening illness.[1] It first must be established that the policy is active, and will cover liver transplantation for the patient. The policy should also cover inpatient and outpatient care and medications. Other conditions of the policy to clarify include the annual or lifetime cap on monies available, the expiration date of the policy, and the requirements for renewal.

At the time of referral and initial consultation, psychological support systems must be identified. One of the greatest sources of anxiety for patients is the fear of death.[2,3] Myths about transplantation abound, and are very unsettling to patients and family members. The transplant coordinator provides information to begin to allay anxiety. Every patient is then referred to a primary social worker who follows the case from initial consultation and onward. The role of the social worker is detailed in Chapter 9. The American Liver Foundation (ALF) and the Transplant Recipients International Organization (TRIO) also provide information and telephone hotlines for patients and families. Patients and family members are encouraged to attend center-based support groups. Meeting patients who are going through the same stress is enlightening and helps the patient make an informed decision about transplantation.

Education begins with answering the questions most pressing for the patient and the family. A pretransplant manual is provided, and an initial discussion about the evaluation period and transplantation is held. Honesty and empathy demonstrated at this time help in establishing a trusting relationship between the patient and the transplant team. The most commonly asked patient questions are as follows:

How long is the wait for a liver donor?
How long is the surgery?
Where do most of the donors come from?
Can I get a disease from the donor?
How is the donor and the recipient matched?

Will I have enough time to get to the transplant center when a liver is available?

Can my family and/or friends store blood for me?

EVALUATION PERIOD AND RECIPIENT SELECTION

The evaluation is guided by protocol. However, the specific needs of each patient necessitate tailoring the workup to the individual. Potential recipient evaluations routinely include a history and physical examination, laboratory tests, radiologic studies, and subspecialty consultations. The transplant coordinator facilitates the evaluation and participates in data collection. Once the evaluation is completed, the coordinator works with the hepatologist to organize the data for presentation to the Recipient Review Committee. This committee provides team decisions about the appropriateness and timing of transplantation in accordance with policies previously established by the transplant center.

WAITING LIST FOR LIVER TRANSPLANTATION

When a potential candidate is accepted, that person is listed with the United Network for Organ Sharing (UNOS). Under the National Organ Transplant Act of 1984, it was mandated that a regulatory body be utilized to provide a fair system of organ allocation. UNOS is the agency currently contracted by the government to handle this process. Organs are shared, using a point system based on medical urgency, length of time on the list, and blood type matching. Consideration is not given to the etiology of the liver disease or age of the patient. For example a 65-year-old recovering alcoholic is not given lower priority than a 20-year-old with the Budd-Chiari syndrome. The goal of the system is to provide fair and equitable access to organs for all patients. The transplant coordinator maintains each center's list with UNOS.

Patients and families often have more needs during the waiting period than after the transplant. Patients on the waiting list are ill and often require complex medical care. While the patients remain in the care of their referring physicians, they are in constant touch with the transplant center. The transplant coordinator acts as a liaison between the patient, the transplant center, and the referring physician. The coordinator must monitor each candidate's condition closely since this may change that an individual's status on the UNOS list. It is essential that the coordinator be able to contact the patient when a liver becomes available. To facilitate this, a beeper is usually provided.

Support groups are particularly helpful at this stage for several reasons. First, the patient can be overwhelmed by "waiting for the phone to ring or the beeper to go off." Second, the family and patient are dealing with the very real possibility of death if a liver does not become available in time. Hope and fear coexist in the hearts of patients and their family members. A support group decreases anxiety by reassuring patients that they are not alone.[4] People cope with this stage differently. Some patients or families even become active in organ donor awareness programs. Some patients feel guilty because they "hope someone will die so they can get a liver." One way to help is to point out that we are not wishing for someone to die but hope that their families will consider the option of organ donation. Support groups also educate patients by introducing them to other people who have received transplants. This helps patients and their families to prepare for potential complications and to make them realize that transplantation is not without risk.

Patients and families also develop a support network outside these formal meetings. They may meet at clinic visits, talk on the phone, or share rides to the hospital. The pediatric population has special support needs. Parents need the most information during the pretransplant and recovery phases.[5] Both adult and pediatric patients use information gathering as a positive coping mechanism.[6] TRIO has chapters in many states and counties that provide support and education. They also work to formulate and influence health policy on the local, national, and international levels. This is further discussed by Klion and Miller in Appendix A.

TRANSPLANTATION

Emotional responses at the moment a liver becomes available and the patient is notified vary among different patients and their families, but they all are in need of continued support. Arrangements should previously have been made with the help of the coordinator and social worker to assure swift transportation of the patient to the hospital.

At this time a chain of events is also set into motion by phone calls initiated by the recipient coordinator. At any hour of the day or night a team of hospital staff must be availabe to begin the perioperative process, which involves transporters, x-ray technicians, nurses, residents, and other personnel.

In other than fulminant cases, preoperative teaching has already begun, but there is still a need for questions to be answered. This may be handled by the coordinator either in person or over the phone, or by the bedside nurse. This highlights the important role of the coordinator in educating all staff members.

Patient and family are kept abreast of estimated timing for the recipient surgery based on the progress of the donor surgery and donor team travel time.

The patient is brought to the holding area, where a team of nurses, anesthesiologists, surgeons, and perfusionists are preparing for a 10–24-hr procedure. A well-established routine with the blood bank is essential because of the large amount of blood and blood products required.

INTENSIVE CARE UNIT

In the waiting area, or from miles away, the family awaits information about the progress of the operation. An approximate schedule is shared with the family, including times they can expect updates. This avoids unnecessary anxiety for the family and reenforces, the role of the family as part of the team. Clear and accurate information not only reduces anxiety but also allows family participation.[1] "Supportive family members" who have been identified in the selection process, should continue to have a significant role in allaying anxiety and providing information to the rest of the family. After conveying surgical information, the coordinator prepares the family for the "postoperative look." Describing the ventilator, nasogastric tube, cardiac monitoring, etc. as "routine" is a good way to decrease the initial shock of seeing the postoperative patient. They should be told that the patient will be cool to touch, edematous, and probably not completely recovered from anesthesia. Flexible visiting privileges in the intensive care unit are helpful. While the patient is in the intensive care unit the coordinator should establish easy communication with the family, since many patients and families feel a loss of control and need to at least feel free to ask questions. An unhurried manner at this time will probably mean only a few extra moments from the transplant team and will go a long way in maintaining a good relationship with the family. Although the patient's underlying disease, which was the presenting reason for transplantation, may no longer be a problem, the patient will have to deal with a new set of medical issues. One hazard to patient–family communication, although unintentional, is too many team members talking to too many family members. The conversations are never identical, nor are they retold with accuracy. Therefore, having the family identify a spokesperson will maintain good communication. We have found that speaking with family members in the waiting area after rounds is best because it is a time when the coordinator and surgeon are together and rounds are made at a predictable time. This enables the coordinator to reinforce the surgeons' comments and elicit concerns to avoid frantic calls from family members.

IN-HOUSE POSTOPERATIVE PERIOD

Discharge planning starts when the patient leaves the intensive care unit and is on the surgical transplant floor. By this time the patient is stable and responsive to teaching. This is also the time when the patient's anxiety is the least.[7,8,9] Patient education, that began in the preoperative phase, now continues. For most adults, written material should be presented first, followed by discussion. The rate of teaching should be individualized. Successful teaching must address specific patient needs.

Clinical care is the major thrust of the acute postoperative period. However, a holistic approach to patient care is essential for complete recovery. Patients and their families are consumers and demand an array of services. The transplant coordinator has the background and education to identify and fulfill these needs and act as a liaison among the team, patient and family.

The coordinator, who is a knowledgeable member of the team, as well as a patient advocate, should take additional time with the patient and family to explain postoperative issues and ensure that the patient and family have direct access to the attending surgeon.

Once the patient is transferred to the surgical transplant unit, the inpatient coordinator should make rounds separately from the rest of the team in order to provide detailed patient education as well as to identify areas of need.

The exchange of information and thoughts builds trust between surgeon, coordinator, patient, and family. This trust allows patients to express their fears, discontentment with hospital personnel and services, and encourage constructive suggestions. A critique of the program by patient and family is a necessary part of quality assurance.

To integrate the multiple services required by the newly transplanted patient, we have established weekly discharge planning rounds. This is a 45-min session moderated by a coordinator and attended by the primary care nurse or senior clinical nurse, pharmacist, social worker, physical therapist, and nutritionist. Discharge planning is started as early as possible, to check on the patient's education process, to make arrangements for home care, visiting nurse service, discharge medication, and transportation. After having systematically addressed all needs, and after duplication of services is avoided, the patient is ready for discharge. This forum builds teamwork, and results in improved patient care.

The patients are all provided with a postoperative teaching manual, a medicine administration chart, and discharge reminders. Since patients and families are supersaturated with information during the stressful postoperative period, miscommunication can occur. In addition to the concepts presented in a postoperative manual, a two-page sheet of discharge reminders are handed out separately. This reminder sheet includes information, including drug schedule and directions, date and instructions for next clinic appointment, and reminder of other follow-up, e.g., ordering a "med alert" bracelet and a 24-hr telephone number for the transplant team. The medical administration record is clearly written in large print with specific instruction and a simple grid of a time schedule to record medicine administration.

OUTPATIENT PERIOD

Patients are encouraged to bring their manual and medical administration record to clinic with them, so that teaching can be reinforced and medical changes can be entered. As patients return to a more routine lifestyle, they are provided with a wallet-size medical record to carry with them at all times.

Handling a busy postoperative clinic is a constant challenge. For effective medical care, the clinic is staffed by a surgeon and/or surgical fellow, two transplant coordinators, a social worker, a nutritionist, and three medical assistants. Enough staff time should be available to provide empathetic, unhurried, and accurate care.

Because time and space are limited in our center, two preparatory methods are used to expedite care. A monthly meeting of key team members is held to review postoperative cases and issues. This is moderated by the postoperative coordinator and surgeon. A database on a laptop computer of all postoperative patients actively followed is utilized during this meeting. This table lists the date of transplant, the preoperative diagnosis, the postoperative complications, participation in studies and where applicable, current immunosuppression therapy and comments. Although it is not necessary to discuss in detail each patient biweekly, each patient is briefly reviewed to see if any team members have updates. Patients with specific issues are discussed. This enables a plan to be formulated for either implementation at the next clinic visit or to be conveyed to the referring physician. In addition to specific cases, this working meeting is a forum for new policies to be discussed with the team, such as current transplant protocols for hypertension, osteoporosis, and PCP prophylaxis. Since many practitioners care for patients, protocols are needed to provide continuity of care.

To streamline clinic hours, the postoperative coordinator or a study coordinator reviews charts before office hours and posts notes on the front of each chart for consideration or implementation. This includes issues such as the need for vaccination or tests or medical changes needed to follow study protocols. The coordinator and a surgeon review laboratory values and the notes from the clinic to adjust immunosuppression and/or to implement care or tests as indicated.

Patients seen in clinic know that their cases are reviewed again after clinic, and expect the coordinator's phone call the next day if medication changes or admission is needed. The transplant coordinator, in most cases, is a nurse clinician with advanced training, knowledge, and expertise. Many times a routine clinic visit or patient call will be handled by the coordinator. Physicians are, therefore, afforded more time to deal with the more complex clinical issues. A team that establishes the patient as a member understands each person's role and limitations, and trusts that team care does not necessarily mean being seen by the entire team each visit.

RETURN TO CARE OR REFERRING PHYSICIAN

At approximately 3 months postoperatively, patients in stable condition have their primary care returned to their referring physician. The coordinator or physician sends a summary letter to the referring physician detailing the hospital course, the patient's current condition, and a plan of care. It is the responsibility of the coordinator to be sure laboratory data are obtained and reviewed on an agreed-on schedule and that follow-up care is planned. Referring physicians handle an increasing share of the patient care; however, the transplant center remains involved, particularly to monitor immunosuppression.

It seems that a patient never really leaves the "loop" of care from the transplant center. The coordinator always remains the primary liaison between patient, primary care physician, and transplant team.

ROLE OF THE SENIOR COORDINATOR

As a clinician, researcher, and patient advocate, the accomplished transplant coordinator is involved in issues other than patient care. Public and professional education must be promoted through seminars and the media. Hospital boards and government agencies must be reached to promote organ donation. To improve the day-to-day care of transplant patients, coordinators must participate in planning health care and UNOS policy concerning issues ranging from organ allocation to health insurance and ethics in research.

It has become common practice to establish the position of a Senior or Chief Nurse Coordinator as a transplant program grows and subspecialties and more coordinators and other staff members are added.[10] The senior coordinator must devote less effort to clinical matters to allow time to coordinate the changing operations of a dynamic program. The chief coordinator must define the responsibilities of team members and assure that there is an adequate number of social workers, physicians, coordinating researchers, and other personnel and that their roles do not overlap. The Senior Coordinator's role as a core member of the health care team is (1) to ensure participants quality patient care, (2) to act as a patient advocate, (3) to coordinate personnel and departments in unified patient care, (4) to advocate and develop policies and procedures that are patient-driven, and (5) to participate in data collection and research. Therefore, the role of the Senior Coordinator is primarily in program development, education, operations, and quality assurance.

SETTING UP A NEW PROGRAM

As the field of transplantation involves more organs and multiorgan transplants and more centers in more states and more countries are established, coordinators will be called on to play a pivotal role in the development of new programs. This presents its own peculiar benefits and challenges.

Once a medical center elects to be a transplant center, a Certificate of Need (CON) is filed with the State Department of Health to obtain approval for performing a specific type of transplant. In addition to a lengthy application, the need for a transplant service for the population of the area has to be proven and key team members will need to be identified. Selection and training of staff and developing a team is the first step in establishing a successful transplant center. Under the direction of a Surgical Director, with both administrative and clinical expertise, the team of various professionals becomes a cohesive unit. Several factors are of critical importance: administrative support, an adequate referral base, and a strong working relationship with the local organ procurement agency.

CONCLUSION

The future of transplantation will be shaped by the needs of our patients. Continued research and development will mean implementing changes into transplant center routines. The role of the coordinator will inevitably affect and/or adapt to functioning of a transplant center.

The continued support of organizations like NATCO to standardize the role of coordinators will help in ensuring that the growing needs of this population are met.

REFERENCES

1. Sigardson-Poor K, Haggarty M: *Nursing Care of the Transplant Patient,* Philadelphia, Saunders, 1990.
2. Christopherson LK: Cardiac transplantations; a psychological perspective. *Circulation* 75:57–62, 1987.
3. O'Brien V: Psychological and social aspects of heart transplantation. *Heart Transplant* 4:229, 1985.
4. Hyler BJ, Conley MC, McMahon D: The role of nursing in a support group for heart transplant recipients and their families. *Heart Transplant* 4:453, 1985.
5. Weichler NK: Information needs of mothers and children who have had liver transplants. *J Ped Nurs* 5:88–95, 1990.
6. Lynn MR: Mothers' reactions to their children's hospitalizations. *J Ped Nurs* 1:274–277, 1986.
7. Griesbach, EH: Anxiety and the timing of diabetes teaching in the hospital: a literature review. *Diabetes Educator* 20:43, 1985.
8. Allender J, Shisslak C, Kasniak A, and Copeland J. Stages of psychological adjustment associated with heart transplantation. *Heart Transplant* 2:228–231, 1983.
9. Castelnouvo-Tedesco P: *Psychiatric Aspects of Organ Transplant,* New York, Grune & Stratton, 1971.10.
10. Williams L, Wood RP, Shaw BW: Role of nursing in the establishment of liver transplant program: impact on nursing or nursing impact? *Transplant Proc* 19:3367–3374, 1987.

—16—

PEDIATRIC LIVER TRANSPLANTATION

Joel R. Rosh and Keith J. Benkov

Pediatric patients have been important in the development of human orthotopic liver transplantation. The first human transplant performed by Thomas E. Starzl, in 1963, was a 3-year-old child with extrahepatic biliary atresia who died shortly after the operation.[1] Similar attempts failed in Boston and Paris.[2] It was not until July 23, 1967, that the first long-term survival was achieved by Starzl's team.[3] The recipient was an 18-month-old girl with a hepatoma who survived 13 months and died of metastatic disease.

The increased ability to treat rejection with the introduction of cyclosporine A in 1979,[4] combined with several technical improvements, made liver transplantation practical. In fact, in 1983, the NIH consensus statement declared that liver transplantation had become the accepted form of therapy for end-stage liver disease and was no longer an experimental procedure.[5]

By January 1989, more than 7000 transplants had been performed[6] at more than 120 centers. Refinements in surgical techniques, such as split livers,[7] live donors,[8] and reduced-volume grafting[9] had been a particular benefit to the pediatric patient.

The cost of pediatric liver transplantation has varied from an original cost of $23,000[10] to $500,000[11] more recently. The average cost is about $150,000 with the major determinant being the length of stay in the intensive care unit.[12] The liver is the costliest organ to transplant, compared to a heart transplant, which is about one-half the expense, and a kidney, which is about one-third the expense.

The price of a liver transplant actually compares quite favorably to the cost of medical therapy of caring for children with end-stage liver disease. One study from Boston, for example, found the average cost of medically treating an episode of variceal bleeding to be $35,000, and this rose to $53,000 when surgical intervention was required.[13]

TABLE 16-1. Recipient Selection Criteria in Pediatric Patients

Decreased hepatic synthetic function
Intractable complications of portal hypertension (GI bleeding, ascites, SBP, encephalopathy)
Malnutrition
Intractable pruritus
Rapidly rising bilirubin
Delayed growth and development
Metabolic bone disease

RECIPIENT SELECTION

Optimal timing of the transplant is one universally accepted reason for the increase in survival seen over the last decade.[12] The operation itself is a long procedure followed by an involved postoperative course. The NIH consensus statement expressed this concern as follows:

> An ideally timed liver transplantation procedure would be in a late enough phase of disease to offer the patient all opportunity for spontaneous stabilization or recovery, but in an early enough phase to give the surgical procedure a fair chance of success.[5]

The most important step toward an appropriately timed transplant is an early referral to the transplant center. The center's task of quantifying the optimal moment of transplantation is still an area of much laboratory[18-20] and clinical investigation.[21-24] Various clinical markers are currently used to decide which patients should be transplanted and when the procedure should be performed (Table 16-1).

The first clinical criterion used is an assessment of the natural history of the child's liver disease in the context of three broad classifications of hepatobiliary disorders. The first includes those diseases that are known to be irreversible and that have a progressive course of deteriorating liver function, as in extrahepatic biliary atresia with a Kasai procedure (hepatoportoenterostomy) that failed to provide biliary drainage. The next subset includes those diseases that have a variable natural history but can lead to progressive hepatic decompensation, such as intrahepatic bile duct hypoplasia and neonatal hepatitis. The last group of patients are those with acute fulminant disease, whether from acute viral or autoimmune hepatitis, or a metabolic disease such as Wilson's disease. The question in such patients is whether the native liver can be expected to recover from the acute episode. The specific disorders that are included within these three broad categories of childhood liver disease are dealt with in detail later in this section.

Along with considering the natural history of the child's liver disorder, an assessment of the degree of liver failure must be made. Potential transplant

TABLE 16-2. Contraindications to Pediatric Orthotopic Liver Transplantation

Absolute	
	Sepsis
	Extrahepatic malignancy
	Crippling nonhepatic disease
Relative	
	Severe malnutrition
	Cyanotic pulmonary AV shunting
	Poor social situation
	HIV infection
	Hepatitis B infection

recipients should be carefully monitored for a decrease in their hepatic synthetic function as manifested by a falling serum albumin or the development of coagulopathy. In addition, the level of serum bilirubin and its rate of rise should be observed. The development of symptomatic portal hypertension heralded by ascites, variceal bleeding, or encephalopathy indicates significant clinical deterioration.

As in any chronic illness, the growth and development of children with liver disease must be carefully monitored. Since malnutrition severely decreases the chances of postoperative recovery, its earliest manifestation should be considered as an indication for transplantation. The critical role of the liver in protein synthesis puts these children at extreme nutritional risk. Cholestasis with its attendant fat malabsorption also predisposes to metabolic bone disease, which can result in pathologic fractures and poor growth.

In addition to the indications for transplantation, several absolute as well as relative contraindications to transplantation exist. Patients with severe extrahepatic medical or neoplastic disease that will not respond to liver replacement (Table 16-2) should not be transplanted. The list of other contraindications has become smaller as surgical techniques have improved. Anatomic anomalies such as portal vein thrombosis or congenital absence were once considered contraindications, but can now be transplanted with a vascular graft.[25]

In a true sense, therefore, the most important aspect of the recipient selection process at the primary-care level is the actual referral to the transplant center. Early referral leads to transplantation before multiorgan failure occurs. It also allows for earlier aggressive intervention and support that may help prolong a relatively stable condition.[27] A longer wait before transplantation puts the child at risk for the complications of liver disease as well as growth failure,[28] increased developmental delay,[29] emotional lability,[30] and even sudden death.[31]

As has already been described, the actual disease entities that come to transplant can be subdivided into three main categories based on the time course: (1) chronic liver diseases that are slowly progressive with a decline in liver function, (2) diseases that are more stable but at risk for an irreversible complication, and (3) those children with acute fulminant disease.

Chronic Liver Disease

Chronic liver diseases in children that may result in a potential need for transplant include extra- and intrahepatic biliary atresia, certain familial cholestatic syndromes, idiopathic forms of cirrhosis, and chronic active hepatitis. These children are often relatively stable until they present with a sudden catastrophic event such as a variceal hemorrhage or peritonitis.

Extrahepatic Biliary Atresia

Extrahepatic biliary atresia is clearly the most common cause for transplantation at large pediatric centers, composing roughly 60% of the total pediatric cases performed.[32-34] Biliary atresia affects one in every 15,000 live births and accounts for about one-third of all cases of neonatal cholestasis.[35] Early portoenterostomy or the so-called Kasai procedure establishes bile flow in 40–80% of children.[5,36] Despite this, prior to liver transplantation, 5-year survival was roughly 25% and portal hypertension remained very common in those surviving.[37]

The 5-year survival rate in children transplanted for extrahepatic biliary atresia is similar to that of patients transplanted for other liver diseases. Initially there was some indication that frequent reoperation of these patients after a failed Kasai procedure increased the morbidity and mortality of transplantation. However, it is now felt that the major technical problems in these children arise from the congenital anomalies of the vasculature associated with biliary atresia and the small size of vessels.[38]

The general consensus is that all infants with biliary atresia should undergo one surgical attempt at a portoenterostomy as long as it is done before 3 months of age.[39] This allows a number of children to clear their jaundice and achieve a period of linear growth. In this way most children can grow to a larger size and have an increased chance of matching with a suitable donor liver,[12,32] while some may even avoid transplantation. Children with unsuccessful portoenterostomies should be referred for early evaluation but not necessarily immediate transplantation. Those children with initial drainage from the Kasai who then go on to manifest jaundice with or without portal hypertension, should be referred when synthetic function, decline in growth rate, or any of the previously discussed complications develop.

Intrahepatic Paucity of Bile Ducts

In a large series of 111 patients with paucity of interlobular bile ducts, 80 manifested the syndromatic form of arteriohepatic dysplasia, or Alagille's syndrome.[39] Only 5% of this large series died from liver disease. It is generally believed that Alagille's syndrome has a better overall prognosis than the nonsyndromatic form of intrahepatic biliary atresia.[39] This syndrome consists of intrahepatic paucity of bile ducts, typical facies, congenital heart disease that most commonly includes peripheral pulmonic stenosis, vertebral anomalies, and the persistence of posterior embryotoxon on slit-lamp examination. These patients can be a challenging group to transplant because of the concomitant congenital heart disease. Their 5-year actuarial survival rate is 54%.[40] The outcome for liver transplantation for nonsyndromatic intrahepatic paucity of bile ducts is hard to determine as these children are often lumped with Alagille's syndrome or under the heading of "biliary atresia."[32]

Metabolic Diseases

The next large category of liver disease that has been transplanted includes patients with metabolic conditions of the liver. Patients with some diseases, such as α-1-antitrypsin deficiency, Wilson's disease, and even hereditary tyrosinemia, are frequent liver transplant recepients. Other conditions such as galactosemia, Crigler-Najjar syndrome type I, hyperlipidemia types I and IV, protoporphyria, glycogen storage disease, and sea-blue histiocyte syndrome remain rare indications for transplantation.

α-1-Antitrypsin Deficiency

This condition is found in one in every 2000 newborns. It is defined by the serologic absence of this protease inhibitor that is produced in the liver. A variable number of children will progress to cirrhosis, while other young adults will present first with emphysema.[41] Of those who present with liver disease, 25% will recover without evidence of liver disease, while up to 50% will die by early adulthood if not transplanted.[27]

Liver transplantation corrects the deficiency of the protease inhibitor, giving the recipient the phenotype of the donor liver.[42] The indications for liver transplantation in this condition are similar to those of other chronic liver diseases. The effect of transplantation on existing or potential pulmonary disease is not yet known. In one series, 29 children underwent transplantation, 80% of whom had ascites and 60% had active gastrointestinal bleeding. The 5-year actuarial survival rate reached 83% compared to 60% in adults with the same condition.[43]

Wilson's Disease

Wilson's disease is a rare autosomal recessive disorder of copper metabolism with a worldwide prevalence of one in 30,000 despite a carrier frequency of one in 90. The disease results in an accumulation of copper in various tissues due to an inability to excrete biliary copper.[47] A low serum ceruloplasmin level is another frequently seen clinical feature. The typical triad of hepatic disease, neurologic involvement, and Kaiser-Fleisher rings facilitates the diagnosis but frequently, in children, the only presentation is liver disease.[48] There appears to be a tendency for presentation in adolescents with fulminant hepatic failure, which is a clear indication for transplantation. When the diagnosis is made prior to the onset of liver failure, chelation therapy is the first line management with transplantation reserved only for those who fail medical treatment.[49]

Tyrosinemia

There are several forms of tyrosinemia, but here we will discuss only the more common, but still extremely rare, congenital hereditary tyrosinemia. This is the acute form that generally presents in infancy with progressive liver dysfunction and Fanconi syndrome. There is deficiency of the enzyme fumarylacetoacetate and micronodular cirrhosis can develop quickly with early hepatoma formation.[44] Liver transplantation offers the best hope of treatment; however, it appears that the renal disease may not be corrected.[45] In the largest series of patients with hereditary tyrosinemia, 5 of 10 transplanted patients had hepatocellular carcinoma at the time of transplant; 4 of these 5 were alive and well at an average of 56 months posttransplant.[46]

Hypercholesterolemia

Several disorders that are characterized by extremely high serum cholesterol levels secondary to metabolic defects have been treated with transplantation. These include familial hypercholesterolemia and cholesterylester storage disease. The major defect appears to be a deficiency of LDL (low-density lipoprotein) receptors within the liver, which can be corrected by transplantation. The main indication for such aggressive therapy has been severe coronary heart disease in early childhood. There has been a varying degree of success with the combination of liver and heart transplantation in these children.[50,51] In a case of cholesterylester storage disease serum cholesterol returned to normal following transplant.[52] Other therapeutic options include bile acid sequestrants, 3-hydroxy-3-methylglutaryl coenzyme A (HMG CoA) reductase inhibitors, and portacaval shunts.[50]

Urea Cycle Defects

The more severe defects usually present in the neonatal period and result in neurologic impairment as well as rapid death.[53] Three cases of carbamyl phosphate synthetase deficiency have been transplanted,[54] with normalization of the ammonia levels but persistence of the abnormal aminoacid profiles.[55] Another girl with ornithine transcarbamylase deficiency has been successfully transplanted.[56]

Miscellaneous Disorders not Limited to Liver

Several cases of glycogen storage disease have been transplanted. These must be performed prior to any neurologic damage and the outcome is dependent on the metabolic defect as well as the other tissue deficiencies present.[12] In metabolic disease, such as glycogen storage type I, the question remains whether transplant and lifelong immunosuppression should be primarily offered or reserved for patients who failed dietary therapy. Patients with both hemophilia A[57] and B[58] have been successfully transplanted with subsequent normal factor levels. There has even been a child transplanted with cystic fibrosis, which is not corrected with transplantation.[59]

TABLE 16-3. Pretransplant Evaluation[a]

Diagnostic workup
Clinical assessment and intervention
Assessment of anatomy
Psychosocial assessment and support
Education

[a]Best performed on inpatient basis.

RECIPIENT EVALUATION

The recipient evaluation at the liver transplant center has multiple objectives (Table 16-3). The first is to confirm the patient's diagnosis. In adult patients a revised diagnosis is made in as many as 20% of referred cases.[12] This is less frequent in children, where congenital anatomic defects are the most common cause for referral. Next the severity and rate of progression of the liver disease is determined. Assessment of nonhepatic medical problems and nutrition form an important part of the evaluation. Finally, various imaging studies are used to define the patient's anatomic requirements for transplantation. In addition, an integral part of the recipient evaluation is a psychosocial evaluation of the child and family.

Recipient evaluation includes structured as well as informal patient education and is best accomplished through an inpatient hospital stay.[14] By having the child and family members at the center for several days, a rapport can be established that may otherwise not be possible. The family can spend time with all members of the transplant team while also being able to tour the intensive care and postoperative units. In this way, all staff that will be caring for the child can be met while questions and concerns of the entire family can be identified and addressed. An additional advantage of an inpatient evaluation is to give the families of other pre- and posttransplant patients a chance to meet and share common concerns.

To meet the above objectives, the evaluation consists of four major components: laboratory tests, imaging studies, consultant visits, and patient as well as family education.

Laboratory Testing

A full listing of the laboratory tests performed during the recipient evaluation is provided in Table 16-4. To confirm the patient's diagnosis, serologic tests for hepatitis A, B, and C viruses and markers for metabolic and autoimmune liver disease are measured.

Liver function tests, especially those of synthetic function (serum albumin, PT/PTT, fibrinogen), are included to determine the degree of liver cell dysfunction. If a coagulopathy is present, correction with parenteral vitamin K should be attempted. If such correction does not occur, a mixing coagulation study may help to differentiate between a circulating anticoagulant and a deficiency of liver-derived clotting factors. If the clinical picture so dictates, measurement of

TABLE 16-4. Laboratory Tests Performed during Recipient Evaluation

Blood	
Complete blood counts and differential	Serum electrolytes
Complete liver function panel	BUN and creatinine
Total protein and albumin	PT/PTT and fibrinogen
Factor levels and mixing studies as indicated	Serum vitamins A, E
Rickets screening: serum calcium and phosphorous, parathyroid hormone, vitamin D	Blood type
Hepatitis A, B, and C serology	HIV
Immune serology for measles, rubella, rubeola, and varicella	EBV and CMV titers
Imaging	
Abdominal ultrasound with Doppler of the portal and hepatic vasculature	Bone age
Constrast abdominal CT scan to include liver volume	Angiogram as needed

the levels of liver-derived factors (e.g., V and IX) in comparison to liver independent factors (e.g., VIII) will help to differentiate a consumptive coagulopathy from decreased hepatic synthesis. A nutritional assessment of the child is also part of the clinical evaluation. Serum protein, albumin, and levels of the fat-soluble vitamins A, D, and E are measured. The prothrombin time serves as a clinical vitamin K level. Additionally, an arterial blood gas or transcutaneous oxygen saturation is obtained to rule out pulmonary compromise from arterio-venous shunting.

The child's blood type is determined for purposes of organ matching. As is discussed elsewhere in the text, HLA matching is not required in liver transplantation. Serum antibody levels to cytomegalovirus (CMV), varicella, Epstein-Barr virus (EBV), and measles are determined to assess immunity and exposure status. Exposure to tuberculosis is also looked for with PPD and an anergy screen. Presence of HIV (human immunodeficiency virus) antibody is determined as well. Currently, each center decides its own policy as to the allocation of the resource of a new liver to HIV-positive patients.[15] These policies are sure to evolve with advances in treatment of HIV-positive individuals.

Imaging Studies

Several imaging studies are obtained as part of the recipient evaluation. An abdominal ultrasound with a Doppler duplex exam of the hepatic and portal vasculature is included to ensure patency. If there is any question regarding the patency or anatomy of the liver's vasculature, an angiogram is performed. A contrast CT scan of the abdomen allows for an estimation of the volume of the native liver and hepatic fossa while also evaluating the extent of varices and the possibility of a hepatic tumor. The bone age is determined to document the potential for linear growth after hepatic replacement.

Consultations

A major advantage of the inpatient recipient evaluation is that it provides an opportunity for the patient and family to meet with the entire transplantation team as well as with members of consultation services. All members of the transplant team, including pediatric gastroenterologists, transplant surgeons, anesthesiologists, intensivists, and the transplant nurse coordinators, evaluate the patient and meet with the family. Any nonhepatic medical condition such as a congenital cardiac anomaly or respiratory compromise should prompt a consultation from the appropriate medical service.

In addition to the medical visits, a full nutritional evaluation including anthropometric measurements and indirect calorimetry is performed by the team nutritionist. Specific guidelines for maximizing the nutritional support of the patient are made. This may include enteral[16] as well as parenteral therapies.[17] The most beneficial intervention prior to the actual transplant is improvement of the child's nutritional status.

The psychosocial assessment team is the final group to meet with the potential recipient. An evaluation by a child psychologist and, as needed, a psychiatrist, is used to establish the developmental status of the child. They also identify the stressors and any potential pathology that should be addressed before, during, and after the transplant. The team social worker is also called in to help in these areas as well as to aid the family with the finances required for the transplant and posttransplantation care. Since the potential recipient is a child, the report of the psychosocial team includes an assessment of the patient's family. In this way, a final decision is made as to whether the whole family unit can be expected to undergo the rigors of liver transplantation as well as comply with the posttransplant regime.

After the evaluation of the potential recipient is completed, the final decision to place a patient on the transplant waiting list is made by the transplantation selection committee. This is a multidisciplinary group that includes pediatric hepatologists, transplant surgeons, nurse coordinators, nutritionists, psychiatrists, social workers, and ethicists.

The committee reviews both the selection criteria for appropriateness for transplantation and the results of the evaluation to determine the patient's ability to undergo transplantation and cope with the posttransplantation medical problems.

Once it is decided that a child should be "listed," the patient is given a priority ranking in accordance with the guidelines of the United Network for Organ Sharing (UNOS).[26] A patient's UNOS ranking can be changed whenever there is a significant change in clinical status. For this reason close monitoring of the patient's condition is an important part of the preoperative medical care.

Preoperative Care

While a child awaits liver transplantation, several important interventions are implemented to medically and psychologically prepare the patient and family (Table 16-5).

TABLE 16-5. Preoperative Care of the Child Awaiting Liver Transplant

Aggressive nutritional support
Stop medications that interfere with posttransplant care
Avoid unnecessary surgery (Kasai revisions, shunts)
Sclerotherapy for variceal bleed
Psychosocial support
Immunizations

As previously outlined, children with liver disease are at a high nutritional risk.[60] An aggressive nutritional support regimen, whether enteral or parenteral, is established by the transplant center in conjunction with the referring physician. This therapy can, at times, be carried out at home with appropriate visiting nurse services. If this is not possible, a course of in-hospital nutritional intervention is undertaken.

The next aspect of pretransplant care is really a caveat against abdominal surgery. Multiple revisions of a portoenterostomy and portal–systemic shunt procedures should be avoided if at all possible. The anatomic alterations and postoperative adhesions that follow such operations make a future transplant more difficult and increase the risk of failure.[61] Rather than resorting to such procedures, any clinical deterioration should advance the patient's status on the waiting list and push up the time of transplantation.

The immunization records of children awaiting transplant should be thoroughly reviewed and all immunizations brought up to date.[62] When appropriate, immunity should be confirmed by serology. This is especially true for the live viral vaccines, which are contraindicated after transplantation because of the immunosuppression. This has become increasingly important due to the recent measles outbreaks and the subsequent revision of the measles vaccination schedule.[63] The latest immunization series for *Haemophilus influenza*[64] should be given as should pneumococcal vaccine if age-appropriate. Finally, a series of recombinant hepatitis B vaccinations should be given and immunity confirmed by serologic tests.

DONOR SELECTION

Until the potential of living-related donation is fully realized or an artificial liver is developed, cadaveric transplantation will be the only hope for thousands with end-stage liver disease.

The current shortage of viable donations most keenly impacts on pediatrics, especially on infants and small children because the majority of pediatric liver disease patients require a transplant by age 2,[65] while accidental death occurs in older age groups.[66,67] This problem has not gone unrecognized by the lay public. Several state governments have passed legislation to ease the process of donation.[68] Public awareness of organ transplantation continues to grow. In addition, technical advances such as reduced-volume grafting has helped to ameliorate the shortage of donor organs for the infant and small child.[66,69]

A serologic screen is performed on all potential donors. This includes testing for the A, B, and C hepatitis viruses, CMV, and HIV. Meticulous medical care of the donor assures adequate perfusion of the liver through the time of the harvest. In addition to hemodynamic instability, the donor can be disqualified on the basis of an acute systemic infection, a malignancy other than brain tumor, or significant liver trauma. The status of the liver is monitored via liver function tests and the coagulation profile. The general state of the donor is monitored with blood gases, electrolytes, and blood counts as well as the hemodynamic profile and urine output. The final criterion used is the gross appearance of the liver at the time of the harvest. We have recently been coupling this with a frozen-section biopsy when possible. Thus, good medical care of the donor as well as an experienced harvest team is critical to the overall success of the transplant procedure.

Which candidate on the waiting list receives the donation is a decision that is based on several variables, including blood grouping, liver size, and the recipient's clinical status.

It was found early on in the evolution of liver transplantation that the liver was resistant to the antibody mediated hyperacute rejection seen in renal transplantation.[10] As a result, it is not necessary to perform a crossmatch between donor lymphocytes and recipient serum.[70,71] HLA matching has also proved not to be necessary.[72] In fact, one retrospective study demonstrated better long-term survival in cases of HLA mismatch.[73] Size and ABO compatibility are the only true crossmatches performed in liver transplantation.

The need to preferably transplant within the same blood group is much emphasized,[11] although there are many reports of successful liver transplantation across ABO blood types.[74,75] This is best performed with "compatible mismatches" such as an AB recipient with an O donor. Such mismatching results in postoperative hemolysis that has led some authors to recommend preoperative exchange transfusion.[12]

Once the blood type of the donor is known, the candidate list is reviewed. It is a well-accepted practice that the sickest patient for whom a given liver is suitable should receive the organ.[24] The UNOS ranking system gives each transplant candidate a priority number based on the degree of liver dysfunction and need for pretransplantation hospital care. The patient with a compatible blood type and poorest short-term prognosis is selected as long as the donor liver is an apparent physical size match. In this way, a recipient is matched to the donor. Various other potential variables such as gender[76] and race[77] have been studied and shown not to impact on the matching process.

THE OPERATION

The technical aspects of both the donor and recipient operations are covered in detail elsewhere in this book. For the sake of completeness, and as a framework for problems pertinent to pediatrics, we will give a broad overview of these procedures.

Donor

The donor hepatectomy should include ample vascular resections to aid in the recipient operation. The celiac axis is dissected down to and resected at the aorta. The portal vein is usually divided at its retropancreatic origin at the confluence of the splenic, coronary, and superior mesenteric veins. The inferior vena cava is divided above the level of the renal veins, and the bile duct is transected at the level of the duodenum. The donor iliac artery is harvested as a potential vascular graft. Prior to its removal, the donor liver is infused with preservation solution. Once removed, the organ is stored in an ice bath of preservative solution. The solution currently in use is the University of Wisconsin (UW) solution,[78] which allows for a preservation time of >20 hr.[79] Thus, the organ may be harvested in the donor's hospital anywhere in the country, and the recipient operation can be performed back at the transplant center with a new surgical team, usually the next morning.[80]

Recipient

The recipient operation involves four vascular anastomoses: the suprahepatic vena cava, infrahepatic vena cava, portal vein, and then the hepatic artery. Biliary continuity is also established. If there is no recipient bile duct, as in biliary atresia, or if the duct is too small, as for infant recipients, a Roux-en-Y limb is established and a choledochojejunostomy is fashioned as the biliary conduit. If a Kasai procedure had been performed in the past, the same loop of jejunum is utilized. If there is an adequate recipient bile duct, then an end-to-end choledochocholedochostomy is performed. This anastomosis is often performed over a T-tube to allow postoperative bile flow monitoring as well as to give easy access for cholangiography. Recently, the possibility has been raised that this practice may contribute to biliary complications such as stricture.[81]

Technical Issues

Several other technical options have been developed for the operative problems encountered in liver transplantation. During the recipient hepatectomy and the subsequent anhepatic phase, the inferior vena cava is cross-clamped, thereby impeding venous flow. This can lead to hemodynamic and metabolic changes as well as intestinal congestion and renal impairment. Venovenous bypass, the use of an external bypass system to establish blood flow from a large vein in the lower to another in the upper half of the body, prevents these changes while allowing for decompression of the congested portal system and its collaterals.[82,83] This in turn decreases the degree of bleeding and the transfusion requirement of as much as 5–10 L in the average adult-sized patient.[7]

Establishing venovenous bypass is usually technically infeasible in pediatric patients weighing < 15 kg.[2] The use of a cell saver and rapid infusion systems are some of the other techniques now used to deal with intraoperative blood loss. Many pediatric patients have dense adhesions from a Kasai procedure or other previous surgery. Although this may make the recipient surgery and subsequent hemostasis more challenging, a recent study revealed no difference in mean anesthesia time, overall operative time, or mean intraoperative blood product requirement[84] between patients with and without a Kasai unless the portoenterostomy was created with a stoma.[85]

Vascular grafts are frequently required in children with congenital liver disease and anomalous vasculature. Whereas many of these anomalies were once considered to be contraindications to a transplant, they have now been overcome by creative grafting. Such grafts, however, are not without potential complications.[86]

Reduced-volume grafting,[87] which is the use of several segments or a lobe rather than the whole donor liver, is one of the most important technical advances in pediatric transplantation. The two most commonly used variants are the use of a left lobe (Couinaud segments II–IV and VIII_i) and a left lateral segment (Couinaud segments II and III) hepatic graft. There are several excellent reviews of the surgical technique involved.[69,87-89] Briefly, the volume reduction is performed in cold storage on the back table. The amount of reduction required is determined by inspecting the recipient's hepatic fossa intraoperatively.

Reduced-size transplants allow for the use of a liver from a donor that may weigh as much as 6–9 times more than the recipient.[69] Since whole-liver grafts usually are not recommended when the donor's body weight is greater than 200% that of the recipient,[90] this technique greatly increases the donor pool size for infants and small children. As has been discussed previously in this chapter, it is this population that most severely suffers from a donor shortage. Reduced-size grafting has lowered the waiting list mortality for such children from 25% to 2–14%.[27,67,69] This technique, a great boon to pediatric liver transplantation, does require skill and experience and should not be undertaken lightly.[91]

Skills acquired through reduced-size grafting have led to several other variations. Split-liver transplantation, or the use of one liver in two patients, has had limited use with variable success,[92-95] as have auxiliary liver implants.[92,96-99] Finally, using the left lateral segment of a family member's liver as the graft has been introduced recently.[100] Such living-related donation is being performed, in this country, at the University of Chicago on an experimental, protocol basis.[92,101]

POSTOPERATIVE CARE

The immediate postoperative care of the liver transplant patient involves careful monitoring of the patient's hemodynamics, electrolyte balance, and new-graft function. Therapy is directed toward fluid and electrolyte balance, prophylaxis of infection, and the continuation of the immunosuppression that was begun in the operating room. In small infants and children, prevention of a vascular thrombosis is a major concern as well.

Monitoring

Routine monitoring in the Mount Sinai pediatric intensive care unit (PICU) includes a cardiac monitor, transcutaneous pulse oximetry, and a variety of inva-

TABLE 16-6. Laboratory Studies Performed in Postoperative Period

Blood	
Complete blood counts and differential	Serum electrolytes
Complete liver function panel	BUN and Creatinine
Total protein and albumin	PT/PTT and fibrinogen
Arterial blood gas	Serum lactate
Serum ammonia	Cyclosporine trough level
Imaging	
Daily chest x-ray while intubated	
Daily abdominal sonogram with Doppler until postoperative day 4	

sive monitoring. An arterial catheter allows for continuous blood pressure evaluation and frequent blood gas, electrolyte, coagulation, and liver function studies. The laboratory exams performed appear in (Table 16-6). These are repeated at least every 8 hr for the first 24 hr and whenever clinically indicated. In larger children and adolescents, a Swann-Ganz catheter is used to monitor the central pressures and cardiac output. In infants and small children, a double-lumen indwelling or percutaneous central venous catheter is placed. This allows for central venous pressure (CVP) readings while providing a reliable infusion port for fluids, electrolytes, blood products, and pressors if required. Additionally, at least two large-bore peripheral intravenous lines are present to allow for rapid volume expansion if needed.

An indwelling Foley catheter measures urine output. A nasogastric tube placed to gravity allows for decompression as well as for early detection of upper gastrointestinal bleeding. Three Jackson-Pratt drains are also present, located in the right and left subdiaphragmatic spaces and at the biliary anastomosis. If a choledochocholedochostomy was performed, a T-tube may be present, allowing continuous bile flow monitoring.

Fluids and Electrolytes

Fluid administration should replace losses while providing adequate hydration to maintain perfusion. Urine output may be an unreliable measure of the fluid required since many patients undergo a phase of relative oliguria in the first 24–48 postoperative hours. The etiology of the oliguria is probably multifactorial and includes such insults as venous cross-clamping and nephrotoxic medications such as cyclosporine. The amount of fluid given, therefore, is adjusted to maintain the CVP in the 6–8-mmHg range. This assures an adequate circulating volume without undue hepatic venous congestion. To achieve this goal, we begin our patients on 100 mL/metabolic kg per day of intravenous fluid and adjust according to the CVP reading. If volume expansion is required, colloid solutions such as blood products or albumin is preferable to crystalloid solutions (e.g., Ringer's, normal saline).

The composition of the maintenance fluid given is also of critical importance. Surgical stress and high-dose steroids often cause hyperglycemia after a liver transplant. Bedside serum glucose determinations are taken hourly until stable in the immediate postoperative period. No glucose is administered until the serum glucose level begins to fall by >100 mg/dL per hour or reaches 250 mg/dL. After that point, solutions of >5% dextrose are rarely required. It should be remembered that hypoglycemia is indicative of graft dysfunction until proven otherwise.

The intravenous fluid composition is also tailored to any electrolyte disturbances that are encountered after transplantation. The most common derangements are a metabolic alkalosis, hypernatremia, hypocalcemia, and delayed hypokalemia. Low serum magnesium and phophorous levels may also be seen.

The metabolic alkalosis is not related solely to the citrate received via blood product administration[102,103] and is, in part, due to preoperative, chronic diuretic use. We have yet to have a patient with a pH >7.60 for which a 0.1*N* hydrochloric acid drip is recommended.[102]

Hypernatremia is also frequently seen, most likely because of the mobilization of the large total-body store of sodium from the preoperative cirrhotic state.[102] Since rapid fluctuations in serum sodium may contribute to neurologic complications such as seizures and central pontine myelinolysis,[104] high-sodium-containing solutions are avoided. It is preferred to start with a 0.5*N* saline solution in most patients.

Hypokalemia can be attributed to total-body depletion secondary to preoperative chronic diuretic therapy as well as the hyperaldosteronism of cirrhosis. Immediately after surgery, serum potassium levels may be normal or even elevated due to potassium released when preservative solution is flushed from the graft. Since urine output is expected to decrease during the early postoperative period, potassium is seldom added to the intravenous solution until the serum level falls below the normal range.

Hypocalcemia is another frequently encountered electrolyte disturbance. It is probably secondary to chelation from the preservatives in the blood products. Since acid–base disturbances are common and patients are often profoundly hypoalbuminemic immediately after a liver transplant, the ionized rather than the total calcium level is measured. Intravenous or enteral calcium is given as needed to normalize the ionized level. Low serum magnesium levels are frequently seen in cirrhosis[105] and cyclosporine-induced magnesium wasting[106] probably contributes to this after the transplant. Hypophosphatemia is postulated to occur secondary to the replenishing of adenosine triphosphate stores in the new graft.[102]

Hematologic Status

Our pediatric patients are maintained at a hematocrit of 30–35% to ensure tissue oxygenation without increasing serum viscosity. Thrombocytopenia is commonly seen, especially in patients with preoperative splenomegaly, and probably represents sequestration in the spleen and new graft. Platelets are rarely given unless there is clinical bleeding or a total count of <20,000 mm^3.

The coagulation status of the liver transplant patient is important for several reasons. The balance of coagulation and lysis factors has to be maintained to avoid bleeding and thrombosis. Clotting factors, therefore, are given only for clinical bleeding. In the infant and small child, we maintain a state of relative anticoagulation for the first 7–14 postoperative days with intravenous heparin titrated to keep partial thromboplastin time at 1.5 times greater than the control. Additionally, all our patients are anticoagulated with low-dose aspirin therapy initiated rectally immediately postop and then orally when feedings are reinstituted.

Infection Prophylaxis

We prophylax against bacterial infection with the administration of a broad-spectrum third-generation cephalosporin (cefotaxime) and vancomycin in the perioperative period.

We also use intravenous acyclovir (5 mg/kg per dose to a maximum of 100 mg IV q12h) and convert to 12.5 mg/kg per dose qid orally to prophylax against viral infection, primarily herpes and cytomegalovirus (CMV). High-dose, pooled intravenous immunoglobulin is added to the prophylactic regime if the recipient has negative CMV serology. When enteral feeding becomes possible, nystatin, and trimethoprim/sulfamethoxazole are added to prophylax against fungus and *Pneumocystis carinii,* respectively.

Respiratory Care

Our patients are returned to the PICU intubated. Most are extubated on the first postoperative day. On arrival and daily while in the PICU, a chest radiograph is obtained to check placement of tubes and catheters, assess the lung fields, and detect effusions. Right pleural effusions are common after liver transplant[107] and usually need no intervention. Exceptions are diagnostic tap as part of a fever evaluation or therapeutic drainage in case of respiratory compromise.

Vigorous pulmonary toilet is performed with incentive spirometry. This is important because of the pleural effusions already mentioned and splinting from the abdominal incision. In addition, infants and small children can have a temporary right hemidiaphragmatic paralysis postoperatively.[107] Bronchoscopy is readily used diagnostically and therapeutically if an infiltrate or persistent atelectasis is seen on the radiograph. If bronchoscopy is not diagnostic in cases of infection, an open-lung biopsy is performed. In addition to pneumonia and atelectasis, pulmonary edema and ARDS (acute respiratory distress syndrome) have been reported with azathioprine and cyclosporine after liver transplantation.[108,109]

Cardiovascular Status

Issues of hemodynamics and urine output have already been discussed. Systemic hypertension is commonly seen postoperatively and may be due to several factors, among them fluid overload, a high output cardiac state, increased levels of renin and catecholamines,[120] and cyclosporine-induced renal dysfunction. Although many authors have reported the need for postoperative nitroprusside drips,[27] we have usually been able to maintain adequate blood pressure control with a combination of diuretics, hydralazine, and, if required, either $beta_2$ receptor or calcium channel blockade. We have not had to lower our cyclosporine levels solely for blood pressure management in the postoperative period.

Graft Status

Of most importance is the level of function of the new graft. The coagulation profile, liver function tests—including the serum level of albumin, hepatocellular and cannulicular enzymes, and bilirubin are frequently sampled. If a T-tube is present, the color and flow of bile are also monitored. Hypoglycemia is considered ominous. The patient's mental status is carefully watched and always considered before any analgesia is administered.

Frequent investigations of the surgical anastomoses are also performed. A daily Doppler exam of the hepatic vasculature is conducted on the first 3 postoperative days to assure vessel patency. This can be performed via a transabdominal or an endoscopic, transgastric approach if needed.[110] If a T-tube is present, a T-tube cholangiogram is performed to rule out an anastomotic leak before enteral feeding is begun. If there is no T-tube, such a leak can sometimes be seen with a radionuclide scan.[111]

Gastrointestinal Status

Gastrointestinal bleeding is not uncommon after a liver transplant with several potential etiologies, including the Roux-en-Y anastomosis if one is present.[112] As a result, all our patients are begun on prophylactic H_2 antagonist or antacid therapy. The liver transplant patient also receives a host of medications that are potentially toxic to the pancreas and postoperative pancreatitis is a real concern. Serum amylase levels are monitored frequently and, since cyclosporine is delivered in a fat-based medium, pancreatic insufficiency should be considered in the patient in whom it is difficult to achieve adequate cyclosporine levels.

Renal Status

Oliguria, hypertension, and the hepatorenal syndrome have already been discussed. It is also frequent to see protein, glucose, and blood in the postoperative urine sediment. The urinary sediment reflects the renal insults of postoperative oliguria.

Neurologic Status

The mental status of the recipient is considered a crucial sign of new-graft function. We have seen patients in stage IV hepatic coma preoperatively wake up rapidly after a successful transplant. Encephalopathy can also accompany graft dysfunction. Analgesia is therefore titrated to relieve pain without oversedating the patient. A narcotic such as fentanyl is preferred since it is rapidly reversed and has a relatively short half-life.

There are a variety of commonly seen neurologic complications after a liver transplant.[113] Seizures can be seen in as many as a third of patients and usually occur during the first week.[114] In addition to electrolyte disturbances, some have implicated cyclosporine and hypocholesterolemia,[115] although this has been recently called into question.[116]

Nutrition

As with all stressed and postoperative patients, especially those who are already debilitated, adequate nutrition is of crucial importance for a good outcome. Surprisingly, in most patients who have an uncomplicated postoperative course, bowel function returns by the third postoperative day and oral nutrition can begin. We have used nasogastric supplementation in those children whose postopertive caloric requirements cannot be orally met.[117] We have often used elemental diets in the immediate postoperative period for the more debilitated recipients. These children have a great deal of bowel edema attributable to pre- as well as postoperative hypoalbuminemia and intraoperative venous cross-clamping. This last problem is exacerbated in the infant and small child who cannot undergo venovenous bypass during the transplant.

Unfortunately, a complicated posttransplant course often is accompanied by poor renal function, which imposes a significant fluid restriction on the patient. It becomes extremely difficult to deliver adequate calories to these patients who need it the most.

IMMUNOSUPPRESSION

The ability to modulate the recipient's immune system to ward off rejection of the graft is the key to long-term survival in organ transplantation (Table 16-7). The earliest attempts at immunosuppression included surgical intervention such as splenectomy and thoracic duct externalization. These were both ineffective and resulted in numerous complications.[10]

The first medical immunosuppression involved high-dose steroid therapy, usually in conjunction with azathioprine or cyclophosphamide. Antilymphocyte globulin was used as rescue therapy. Liver transplantation series utilizing such regimes reported only 20–30% long-term survival rates.[11]

TABLE 16-7. Immunosuppressive Agents Used in Organ Transplantation

ALG	Cyclosporine
OKT3	FK-506
Azathioprine	IL-2 Monoclonals
Steroids	Prostaglandins (?)

The late 1970s brought the introduction of cyclosporine A (CsA).[118,119] This powerful cyclic undecapeptide fungal derivative revolutionized the field of organ transplantation and made long-term survival a reality for scores of thousands of transplant recipients. Today, various combinations of immunosuppressive agents are used and each of these are discussed at length elsewhere in this book. We will therefore focus our discussion on aspects of these medications that are critical to the caregivers of pediatric liver transplant recipients.

Cyclosporine

Cyclosporine has been shown to interfere with the immune response at the level of interleukin-2 (IL-2) and its receptors.[119,120] It can be administered orally or intravenously. It is metabolized by the cytochrome p450 system of the liver and largely excreted in the bile. The gastrointestinal absorption of cyclosporine is variable, especially in children. It has been suggested that some of this variability may correlate with the length of the child's small intestine.[121] The presence of the Roux-en-Y biliary anastomosis may also play an influential role.[122] Since cyclosporine is hydrophilic and carried in an oil base, it is poorly absorbed in patients with fat malabsorption. This can become clinically relevant in the presence of cholestasis due to rejection. We have also seen poor CsA absorption in a child with chronic pancreatitis.

In addition to altered absorption, children also metabolize cyclosporine more rapidly than do adults. As a result, we often dose infants on an 8-hr[1] rather than 12-hr[1] basis. The initial daily dose is 3 mg/kg as a continuous infusion. When oral medication is instituted postoperatively, we start at 15–20 mg/kg daily orally and adjust the oral and intravenous dose to obtain a level of 800–1200 ng/mL by radioimmunoassay.[123] This level of immunosuppression is maintained for the first 4–6 months after transplantation, at which time the overall level of immunosuppression is reduced and CsA levels of 600–800 ng/mL are accepted.

The numerous side effects of cyclosporine are outlined elsewhere in the text. Of note in pediatrics is the hirsutism and hypertrichosis, which can be marked, but seem to become less pronounced with age. Hypertension as well as the nephrotoxicity of CsA are also notable concerns.[124] Early studies showed that the majority of children regain normal renal function and are off all antihypertensives within 2 years.[125] This observation has recently been challenged.[126]

Steroids

Corticosteroids act synergistically with cyclosporine and the other immunosuppressive agents. In addition to decreasing IL-2 levels, steroids affect lymphocyte expression, resulting in fewer CD_4 or helper T-cells.[127,128] The initial dose we use is 20 mg/kg, with a maximum dose of 1 g of methylprednisolone administered as an intraoperative pulse. The steroid dose is then tapered daily to an eventual oral dose of 0.2–0.3 mg/kg per day of prednisone. This dose is continued through one year of good hepatic function, at which time alternate day steroids are used to allow for improved linear growth.[129]

Azathioprine

Azathioprine is the third immunosuppressant routinely used in our pediatric recipients. This purine analog interferes with DNA synthesis and the proliferation of rapidly dividing cells. Myelosuppression is the drug's main side effect. The drug is introduced at 1.5–2 mg/kg per day. The dose is reduced if there is a significant fall in the absolute neutrophil count. Of note is that azathioprine is known to cause cholestasis and hepatic fibrosis[130] as well as hepatic venoocclusive disease.[131] It can also induce pancreatitis and the serum amylase is routinely monitored.

OKT3

OKT3 is a pan-T-cell monoclonal antibody produced by murine plasmacytomas. Its repeated use, therefore, is potentially limited by the recipient's elaboration of antimurine antibodies. Although there is now good evidence to support the use of OKT3 as the initial immunosuppressant,[132-134] we have reserved it for severe, steroid-unresponsive rejection in our pediatric patients.[135-137] The administration of OKT3 can be complicated by pulmonary edema; therefore, meticulous correction of fluid overload is done prior to the administration of the drug. A flu-like illness including fever and diarrhea is frequently seen early in the course of OKT3. Because of the risk of anaphylaxis, we pretreat all our pediatric OKT3 recipients with corticosteroids and diphenhydramine.

Immunosuppression—The Future

Currently, there is research being performed with more specific monoclonal antibodies such as those that recognize IL-2 receptors. These antibodies would bind only to the subgroups of T-cells involved in rejection.[138]

A new experimental immunosuppressant is FK-506. This macrolide antibiotic is about 100 times more biologically active by weight than cyclosporine.[139] Early clinical use of FK-506, primarily at the University of Pittsburgh, has been quite encouraging.[140] The drug is currently being evaluated as the primary source of immunosuppression in liver transplantation in a prospective randomized fashion by our center and 11 others.

SURGICAL COMPLICATIONS

The major complications of liver transplantation in the immediate postoperative period can be broadly divided into those that are surgical, infectious, and immunologic (Table 16-8). The problems of infection and rejection will be dealt with in separate sections of this chapter.

The postoperative surgical complications include bleeding, primary nonfunction, and anastomotis-related problems such as a vascular thrombosis.

TABLE 16-8. Postoperative Complications

Technical
Bleeding
Primary nonfunction (5–7%)
Hepatic artery thrombosis (10–30%)
Portal vein thrombosis (2%)
Infection
Bacterial
Opportunistic
Rejection
Acute
Chronic

Bleeding

Postoperative bleeding was more common in the early days of liver transplantation, but is still a major concern despite improvements in surgical technique. Up to one-third of the mortality occurring within the first postoperative week can be attributed to bleeding.[141] The vascularity of the liver and the peritoneum secondary to longstanding portal hypertension makes bleeding a real threat.[142] Of special concern is the increased risk of graft bleeding in children who receive reduced-volume rather than whole-organ transplants.[90]

Primary Nonfunction

Another surgical or technical complication is primary nonfunction, that is, a graft that does not function after reperfusion. Primary nonfunction occurs in about 5–6% of transplants at large centers when the UW preservative solution is used.[141] The etiology of this entity is not fully understood but is felt to occur during the harvest, from either donor hemodynamic instability or poor preservation technique.[143] Traditionally it was taught that few, if any, of these grafts would be viable if nonfunction persisted for more than 48 hr. Recent experience has shown that the administration of prostaglandin E_1 for approximately one week may help salvage a nonfunctioning graft.[144]

Anastomotic Complications

Leakage can occur at any of the four vascular or the biliary anastomosis.[145] Vascular thrombosis, especially hepatic artery thrombosis (HAT), with an incidence of 10–40%,[146,147] is of special concern in the smallest patients. Increased hepatic vascular resistance during rejection may lead to sluggish flow through the hepatic artery and subsequent thrombosis.[146]

The clinical presentation of HAT is varied and includes acute graft failure, delayed biliary leak, and recurrent fever with bacteremia.[148] A Doppler ultrasound study,[149] which is part of the evaluation of fever or hepatic dysfunction, may suggest the HAT. If the Doppler exam fails to demonstrate flow, an angiogram is necessary to confirm the diagnosis.

The management of HAT is dependent on the clinical picture. If the diagnosis is made early, the child can be brought back to the operating room for thrombectomy or bypass grafting. Since the hepatic artery is the primary source of blood to the extrahepatic biliary tree, biliary leak or stricture is a common complication of HAT, and surgical reconstruction of the biliary system may be required. If significant hepatic necrosis has occurred, then retransplantation becomes necessary.

The other major vascular complication is portal vein thrombosis (PVT). This is seen less commonly than HAT with an incidence of about 2%.[150] PVT may present in the postoperative period with a picture similar to that of HAT or later with manifestations of extrahepatic portal hypertension, variceal bleeding, and splenomegaly despite normal hepatic function.[102] The diagnosis again can be suggested by Doppler ultrasound[151] and confirmed by angiography.[152] Management is dictated by the clinical status of the patient. Surgery is performed if hepatic function is compromised, and can include shunting[153] as well as thrombectomy and bypass grafting. If hepatic function is good, nonsurgical management of the extrahepatic portal hypertension may be attempted.[154] We follow a child with PVT and excellent long-term graft function who has undergone successful sclerotherapy for variceal bleeding.

Other vascular complications such as thrombosis of the vena cava are less common and are reported in patients who have undergone liver transplantation for the Budd-Chiari syndrome.[155] We have also seen the disruption of the vascular anastomotic suture line with devastating results in association with mycotic infection.

REJECTION

Rejection is reviewed elsewhere in this text. In addition, there are many well-written reviews of the immunology,[156,157] which is the same in adult and pediatric recipients.[158]

The clinical picture of rejection is similar in pediatric and adult patients. Unexplained fever, malaise, headache, abdominal pain, and jaundice are all common signs and symptoms. The clinical findings may be more subtle in infants and young children who cannot verbalize such complaints, but the clinical findings are generally accompanied by increased serum levels of hepatic enzymes. In severe rejection, a sudden fall in synthetic activity is seen. The differential diagnosis should include sepsis, biliary leak or stricture, vascular compromise as in a thrombosis of the hepatic artery or portal vein, and possible drug hepatotoxicity.

Historically, rejection was diagnosed on clinical findings in the early days of liver transplantation. By the early 1980s, percutaneous liver biopsy was commonly employed to confirm the diagnosis.[159-162] The histopathology of rejection has become a well-described entity. Severity is graded as mild, moderate, or severe, depending on the degree of bile duct damage and portal inflammation as well as the presence of venous and arterial endothelialitis. The liver biopsy has allowed for the more judicious use of antimicrobials and a directed regime of immunosuppression. Some centers now use fine-needle aspiration and cytology as a means of diagnosing rejection of the graft.[163]

Rejection remains a common problem in liver transplantation. An estimated 80% of patients have some degree of rejection, usually in the early weeks after the transplant.[12] In its most severe and chronic form, rejection may lead to a decrease in the number of intrahepatic bile ducts, the so-called vanishing bile duct syndrome (VBDS).[164] An accelerated progression to this lesion has been described.[165] VBDS has traditionally been considered to be irreversible and always an indication for retransplant. It has recently been shown that VBDS in children can reverse after as long as one year if these patients remain clinically stable with the damaged graft.[166]

INFECTION

The liver transplant patient is subject to a significant risk of postoperative infection. Invasive vascular lines, postoperative drains, and potent immunosuppression are some of the risk factors faced by all recipients. In addition, many patients are transplanted while debilitated and malnourished. Many are also transplanted as part of a long hospitalization that frequently involves antibiotic administration. The transplant recipient is, therefore, at risk for infection by common as well as opportunistic organisms. It is no surprise that infection is seen in as many as 60–90% of liver transplant recipients[6] and is the cause of death in up to 50% of those who die within the first 6 months after transplantation.[141]

Bacterial Infection

The most common bacterial organisms encountered are gram-negative rods and gram-positive *Staphylococcus* species. Gram-positive infections are usually catheter-related, while biliary or vascular compromise predispose toward gram-negative infections.[167,168]

Since the most commonly encountered organisms are actually from the patient's native flora, we do not routinely use protective or reverse isolation. The appropriateness of this practice has been confirmed in other immunocompromised patients.[169]

Early pediatric liver transplants showed a significant incidence of bacterial and fungal sepsis.[170-172] While such infections remain a real concern, more judicious use of antibiotics, improved surgical technique, and better-tailored immunosuppression have lowered their rate of occurrence.[173] As a result, viral infections have gained relative importance.

Viral Infections

Cytomegalovirus (CMV) has long been recognized as the "troll" of organ transplantation.[174] In addition to actual CMV disease, it has been implicated in decreased graft survival[175] and suprainfections.[176] As a result, many centers have adopted aggressive protocols of surveillance for the virus. These often include weekly throat swabs, urine and buffy coat cultures, serial serologies, and even serial fine-needle liver aspirate cultures.[177] Published data from centers that have such protocols have added much to the understanding of CMV infection and disease in the pediatric liver transplant recipient.

The overall rate of CMV infection has varied from 48% to 85% and that of disease, from 33% to 50% in pediatric series.[177,178] Viremia usually occurs within 27–43 days after the transplant.[177] The incidence and extent of actual disease appears to be influenced by an early viremia[177] and the serologic status of the donor and recipient. There is good evidence that a seropositive donor is the single greatest risk factor for infection.[179] Cases involving seropositive donors and seronegative recipients run the highest rates of infection and disease.[179,180] The earlier belief[181] that seropositive recipients are at risk for only mild reactivation disease rather than reinfection by a donor's CMV strain has been convincingly refuted.[182,183] In fact, severe CMV disease has been observed in seropositive recipients,[178,184] and methods such as restriction endonuclease typing have shown such cases to be caused by reinfection by the donor's CMV, rather than reactivation of the recipient's CMV strain.[185]

The incidence of CMV infection and disease underscores the need for effective prevention and treatment. The use of organs from CMV seropositive donors is unavoidable. The current organ shortage and prevalence of CMV seropositivity in the general population precludes the exclusion of such donors. Prophylactic regimes of postoperative CMV hyperimmune[186-188] or pooled gammaglobulin[179] have been shown to at least ameliorate the extent of disease. Prophylaxis with the antiviral agent acyclovir has also been shown to be efficacious in reducing the incidence of symptomatic CMV disease in bone marrow[189] and renal transplant[190] recipients. There are also data to suggest that the same result can be achieved in pediatric liver transplant recipients.[178]

Although prophylaxis does seem possible, the need for an effective treatment remains. The antiviral, ganciclovir [DHPG or 9-[1-3-dihydroxy-2-propoxymethyl]guanine], usually used in combination with CMV hyperimmune or gammaglobulin, has been shown to be an effective treatment of invasive, disseminated CMV disease.[191-194] The usual dose of DHPG in children is 5 mg/kg per dose intravenously every 12 hr for 14–21 days. We have arranged for home intravenous therapy to complete the course in patients who are clinically stabile. When defined as the resolution of fever, the response to DHPG can be slow. One study revealed the range to be 2–9 days with a mean of 5.3 days.[195] Our experience has confirmed this observation. The main side effect of DHPG is usually a mild and transient myelosuppression. We have not seen significant renal impairment in our pediatric patients receiving DHPG.

Several other viruses have been shown to infect pediatric liver transplant recipients. Adenovirus has had a range of disease from a benign febrile illness to pneumonia and even loss of the graft.[196,197] Epstein-Barr virus (EBV) has also had a spectrum of disease. EBV usually produces an infectious mononucleosis-type disease, but may present as jaw pain, arthritis, encephalitis, pneumonitis, and systemic lymphoproliferative disease that can be fatal.[198-201] EBV disease is almost always characterized by circulating atypical lymphocytes and pancytopenia. Most forms of EBV disease respond to a reduction in immunosuppression.[198-202]

There has also been much experience with varicella infection in pediatric liver transplant recipients.[203] Such infections have been reported only in children who were seronegative for the virus. Prophylaxis with varicella immunoglobulin or treatment of active varicella with intravenous acyclovir has been very effective. However, there have been reports of mortality from varicella pneumonia and hepatitis.[203,204]

SURVIVAL AFTER PEDIATRIC LIVER TRANSPLANTATION

During the early years of liver transplantation, many surgeons stated that it was improper to offer the surgery to children.[205] The poor operative survival, coupled with the unwanted effects of high-dose steroids, made the quality of life for these children unacceptable. The introduction of cyclosporine is credited with an almost overnight increase in long-term pediatric survival from 34% to 74%.[206] In addition to more effective immunosuppression, early referral and better selection of recipients have allowed for greater overall survival[207] (Table 16-9). Current data show that children can now expect a long-term survival rate of 70–90% after a liver transplant.[208]

In general, pediatric liver transplant recipients tend to fare better than adults. The largest proportion of deaths occur within the first 6 months after surgery with survival curves plateauing at about one year after transplantation.[2] While it has been shown in adult patients that the preoperative creatinine level is the single most prognostic laboratory value,[22] this has not been the case in children.[209] Rather, the levels of indirect bilirubin, cholesterol, and partial thromboplastin time are most predictive of survival in children.[24] In addition, the presence of ascites, deep hepatic coma, and the child's nutritional status are the only clinical findings shown to impact on the outcome of liver transplant.[24,208,210]

Early reports from pediatric centers cautioned against transplantation in small infants due to a higher morbidity and mortality, often from hepatic vascular compromise. The small hepatic artery and threat of thrombosis in these patients has led many centers to begin the use of routine postoperative anticoagulation with agents such as aspirin, heparin, and Dextran 40.[211] Another vascular problem is the portal vein hypoplasia that is found in many of these children,[24] espe-

TABLE 16-9. Factors in Increased Survival

Better timing of transplantation
Improved preservation solution (UW)
Refinements in surgical technique
Judicious use of antibiotics
Recognition and control of rejection
Cyclosporine

cially those with extrahepatic biliary atresia. This has led to our routine use of a portal vein graft in small children. Such refinements in surgical technique have made it possible to obtain reasonable results in even very small infants. Recent authors have stated that liver transplantation should be considered in infants who weigh >3 kg.[33]

Retransplantation may be required by as many as 30% of pediatric recipients and was considered to be a poor prognostic indicator.[206] It should be noted, however, that this was relatively early data that may have been confounded by the surgical technique of the time. Later series have shown that the overall survival is related to the reason for the failure of the original graft rather than simply the performance of a second transplant.[32]

QUALITY OF LIFE AFTER PEDIATRIC LIVER TRANSPLANTATION

As liver transplantation has become the accepted therapy for pediatric end-stage liver disease, greater emphasis has been placed on the assurance of good medical care and quality of life for the thousands of liver graft recipients.

Growth

The pediatric patient with liver disease fails to thrive for numerous reasons. Liver failure itself is responsible for disordered protein synthesis and calorie utilization. Chronic cholestasis leads to fat malabsorption, while poor intake is common secondary to chronic illness.[60,212] Successful hepatic replacement eliminates these causes of growth failure, and should therefore result in improved growth.[213] Short-term studies have shown that at least 50% of pediatric recipients continue on the growth curve they were on at the time of transplant.[214,215] Longer follow-up periods have demonstrated that with alternate-day steroid dosing and continued well-being, as many as 76% achieve an acceleration in growth velocity.[215,216]

Development

Children with liver disease have shown delayed mental development that is correlated to the age of onset of the illness.[217] The etiology of this delay is probably multifactorial, relating to protein-calorie malnutrition[218] as well as other nutritional deficiencies, most notably vitamin E.[219,220] The chronicity of the illness[217] and its metabolic effects,[221] especially if accompanied by encephalopathy,[222] contribute to this delay as well.

In order to be considered completely efficacious, liver transplantation should have a positive effect on the developmental delay caused by pediatric liver disease. As with linear growth, improvement in cognitive skills is not immediate, although preliminary follow-up data are suggestive of a positive trend.[125,223] In both these reports, all children whose developmental scores were significantly below age level preoperatively, tested within the normal range after transplantation. However, recent data suggest that liver transplant recipients have neuropsychologic deficits when compared to other chronically ill children.[224] Therefore, careful testing and remediation are required in order to maximize the effect of hepatic replacement on mental development.

Lifestyle

The improvement in the quality of life for a child with end-stage liver disease after liver transplantation is readily apparent. As already noted, this was not always the case. An early study of 27 pediatric recipients noted a low survival rate and a poor quality of life. Numerous medical problems, growth retardation, and unwanted side effects of medications were listed as the major problems.[225] The psychiatric profile of pediatric recipients in the precyclosporine era was dismal.[226]

Cyclosporine brought objective improvement in lifestyle for pediatric liver transplant recipients.[227] Most patients return to school. They are usually in standard, age-appropriate classes or only one year behind grade level—as a result of illness and missed classes prior to the transplant.[125,228] A survey of 65 pediatric recipients and their families found these children to spend fewer days in the hospital, take fewer medications, and have improved gross motor and social behavior after transplantation.[125,223] The social rehabilitation and physical well-being has ultimately led to normal family life and even successful pregnancy after liver transplantation.[229,230]

Parental Effects

The emotional and financial stress that liver transplantation places on the entire family can be formidable. The most stressful periods are immediately before the surgery and during the postoperative recovery period.[231] It is during these times that families require the most support by staff, family, and friends. Parental fears and concerns, however, frequently persist after the transplant. These usually center around issues of rejection, side effects of chronic medications, and continued medical expenses.[14]

As has been seen in other families of chronically ill children,[232] the divorce rate in liver transplant families falls far below the national average,[233] with a range of 12–17%.[14,125]

Medical Follow up

The long-term follow-up of a child with a liver transplant is an area in pediatrics that is just beginning to bloom. Careful survey of these children will ultimately demonstrate the long-term utility of the procedure, its effect on the growth and development of the child, and its impact on the family and society as a whole. Such study will have to be combined with an ever-vigilant assessment for infection, rejection, malignancy, and other long-term effects of chronic immunosuppression, while providing routine well-child care appropriately modified for these special children.

REFERENCES

1. Starzl TE, Marchioro TL, von Kaulla KN, et al: Homotransplantation of the liver in humans. *Surg Gynecol Obstet* 117:659–676, 1963.
2. Starzl TE, Esquivel C, Gordon R, Todo S: Pediatric liver transplantation. *Transplant Proc* 19:3230–3235, 1987.
3. Starzl TE, Groth CT, Breltschneider L, et al: Orthotopic homotransplantation of the human liver. *Ann Surg* 168:392–415, 1968.
4. Calne RY, Rolles K, White DJG, et al: Cyclosporine A initially as the only immunosuppressant in 34 patients of cadaveric organs: 32 kidneys, 2 pancreases, and 2 livers. *Lancet* 2:1033–1036, 1979.
5. Salans LB, Roth HP, Kraut JR, et al: National institutes of health consensus development conference statement. Liver transplantation. *Hepatology* 4:107S–110S, 1984.
6. Hockerstadt K: Review: liver transplantation today. *Scand J Gastroenterol* 25:1–10, 1990.
7. Starzl TE, Iwatsuki S, Esquivel CO, et al: Refinements in the surgical technique of liver transplantation. *Semin Liver Dis* 5:349–356, 1985.
8. Starzl TE, Iwatsuki S, Shaw BW, Jr, et al: Immunosuppression and nonsurgical factors in the improved results of liver transplantation. *Semin Liver Dis* 5:334–343, 1985.
9. DeHemptine B, DeVille JG, Kestens PJ, Otte JB: Volume reduction of the liver graft before orthotopic transplantation: report of a clinical experience in 11 cases. *Transplant Proc* 19:3317–3322, 1987.
10. Starzl TE, Iwatsuki S, Van Thiel DH, et al: Evolution of liver transplantation. *Hepatology* 2:614–636, 1982.
11. Kleinman RE, Vacanti JP: Liver transplantation. In Walker WA, Durie PR, Hamilton JR, et al: *Pediatric Gastrointestinal Disease,* p 1109, Philadelphia, Decker, 1991.
12. Paradis KJG, Freese DK, Sharp HL: A pediatric perspective on liver transplantation. *Pedi Clin N Am* 35:409–433, 1988.
13. O'Donnell TF, Gembarowica RM, Callow AD, et al: The economic impact of acute variceal bleeding: cost-effectiveness implications for medical and surgical therapy. *Surgery* 88:693–701, 1980.
14. Gold LM, Kirkpatrick BS, Fricker FS, Zitelli B: Psychosocial issues in pediatric organ transplantation: the parents' perspective. *Pediatrics* 77:738–744, 1986.
15. Starzl TE, Demetris AJ, van Thiel D: Liver transplantation—Part I. *New Engl J Med* 321:1014–1022, 1989.
16. LeLeiko NS, Murray C, Munro HN: Enteral support of the hospitalized child. In Suskind RM: *Textbook of Pediatric Nutrition,* p 357, New York, Raven Press, 1981.
17. Weisdorf S, Lysne J, Lersa F: TPN in hepatic failure and transplantation. In Lebenthal E: *TPN: Indications, Utilization, Complications and Pathophysiological Considerations,* p 463, New York, Raven Press, 1986.
18. Jenkins RK, Clowes GHA, Jr, Bosari S, Pearl RH, Khettry U, Trey C: Survival from hepatic transplantation. *Ann Surg* 204:363–374, 1986.
19. Nikkila K, Hockerstedt K, Miettinen T: Serum cholesterol, plant sterols and lathosterol indicate severe damage and transplantation. *J Hepatol* 9(Suppl 1):198, 1989.
20. Hockerstedt K, Risteli L, Salmela K, Risteli J: Serum Type III procollogen peptide as a marker in liver transplantation. *Transplant Proc* 22:1574–1575, 1990.

21. Groth CC, Duborig RS, Corman J, et al: Metabolic effects of hepatic replacement in Wilson's disease. *Transplant Proc* 5:829–833, 1973.

22. Cuervas-Mans V, Millan I, Gavaler JS, Starzl TE, van Thiel DH: Prognastic value of preoperatively obtained clinical and laboratory data in predicting survival following orthotopic liver transplantation. *Hepatology* 6:922–927, 1986.

23. Zitelli BJ, Malatack J. Gartner J, Jr, et al: Evaluation of the patient for liver transplantation. *Pediatrics* 78:559–565, 1986.

24. Malatack JJ, Schaid DJ, Urbach AH: Choosing a pediatric recipient for orthotopic liver transplantation. *J Ped* 4:479–489, 1987.

25. Woodle ES, Thistlethwaite JR, Emond JC: Successful hepatic transplantation in congenital absence of recipient portal vein. *Surgery* 107:475–479, 1990.

26. United Network for Organ Sharing: *UNOS Policies, UNOS Update* 6:18, 1990.

27. Shaw BW, Jr, Wood RP, Kaufman SS, Williams L, Antonson DL, Vanderhoof J: Liver transplantation therapy for children: Part I. *J Ped Gastroenterol Nutr* 7:157–166, 1988.

28. Burgess DB, Martin HP, Lilly JR: The developmental status of children undergoing the Kasai procedure for biliary atresia. *Pediatrics* 70:624–629, 1982.

29. Perrin EC, Gerrity SP: Development of children with a chronic illness. *Ped Clin N Am* 31:19–31, 1984.

30. Sabbeth B: Understanding the impact of chronic childhood illness on families. *Ped Clin N Am* 31:47–57, 1984.

31. Gartner JC, Jaff R, Malatack JJ, et al: Hepatic infarction and acute liver failure in children with extra hepatic biliary atresia and cirrhosis. *J Ped Surg* 22:360–362, 1987.

32. Esquivel CO, Iwatsuki S, Gordon RD, et al: Indications for pediatric liver transplantation. *J Ped* 111:1039–1045, 1987.

33. Kalayoglu M, Stratta RJ, Sollinger HW: Liver transplantation in infants and children. *J Ped Surg* 24:70–76, 1989.

34. Otte JB, Yandza T, de Ville de Goyet J, Tan KC, Salizzoni M, de Memptinne B: Pediatric liver transplantation: report on 52 patients with a 2-year survival at 86%. *J Ped Surg* 23:250–253, 1988.

35. Balistreri WF: Neonatal cholestasis: medical progress. *J Ped* 106:171–184, 1985.

36. Alagille D: Liver transplantation in children: indications in cholestatic states. *Transplant Proc* 19:3242–3248, 1987.

37. Sokal EM, Veyckemans F, de Ville de Goyet J, et al: Liver transplantation in children less than 1 year of age. *J Ped* 117:205–210, 1990.

38. Alagille D, Estrada A, Hadchouel M, et al: Syndromatic paucity of intralobular bile ducts (Alagille's syndrome or arteriohepatic dysplasia): review of 80 cases. *J Ped* 110:195–200, 1987.

39. Stewart BA, Hall RJ, Lilly JR: Liver transplantation and the Kasai operation in biliary atresia. *J Ped Surg* 23:623–626, 1988.

40. ChapChap P, Esquivel CO, Iwatsuki S, et al: Liver transplantation for arteriohepatic dysplasia (Alagille's syndrome). *Surg Gynecol Obstet* (in press).

41. Sharp HS: The current status of alpha-1-antitrypsin, a protease inhibitor, in gastrointestinal disease. *Gastroenterology* 70:611–621, 1976.

42. Hood J, Koep P, Peters R, et al: Liver transplantation for advanced liver disease with alpha-1-antitrypsin deficiency. *New Engl J Med* 302:272—275, 1980.

43. Esquivel CO, Vicente E, Van Thiel D, et al: Orthotopic liver transplantation for alpha-1-antitrypsin deficiency: an experience in 29 children and ten adults. *Transplant Proc* 19:3798–3802, 1987.
44. Weinberg AG, Mize CE, Worthen HG: The occurrence of hepatoma in the chronic form of hereditary tyrosinemia. *J Ped* 88:434–438, 1976.
45. Tuchman M, Freese DK, Sharp HL, et al: Contribution of extrahepatic tissues to biochemical abnormalities in hereditary tyrosinemia type I: study of three patients after liver transplantation. *J Ped* 110:399–403, 1987.
46. Esquivel CO, Mieles L, Marino IR, et al: Liver transplantation for heriditary tyrosinemia in the presence of hepatocellular carcinoma. *Transplant Proc* 21:2445–2446, 1989.
47. Scheinberg IH, Sternlieb I: *Wilson's Disease,* Philadelphia, Saunders, 1984.
48. Sternlieb I: Wilson's disease: transplantation when all else has failed. *Hepatology* 8:975–976, 1988.
49. Perman JA, Werlin SL, Grand RJ, Watkins JB: Laboratory measures of copper metabolism in the differentiation of chronic active hepatitis and Wilson's disease in children. *J Ped* 94:564–568, 1979.
50. Bilheimer DW: Portacaval shunt and liver transplantation in treatment of familial hypercholesterolemia. *Arteriosclerosis* 9(Suppl 1):I158–I163, 1989.
51. Starzl TE, Bilheimer DW, Bahnson HT, et al: Heart-liver transplantation in a patient with familial hypercholesterolemia. *Lancet* 1:1382–1383, 1984.
52. Hoeg JM, Starzl TE, Brewer HB, Jr: Liver transplantation for treatment of cardiovascular disease: comparison with medication and plasma exchange in homozygous familial hypercholesterolemia. *Am J Cardiol* 59:705–707, 1987.
53. Martinez-Ibanez V, Margarit C, Tormo R, et al: Liver transplantation in metabolic diseases. Report of five pediatric cases. *Transplant Proc* 19:3803–3804, 1987.
54. Starzl TE: personal communication.
55. Tuchman M: Persistent acitrullinemia after liver transplantation for carbamylphosphate synthetase deficiency (letter). *New Engl J Med* 320:1498–1499, 1989.
56. Largilliere C, Houssin D, Gottrand F, et al: Liver transplantation for ornithine transcarbamylase deficiency in a girl. *J Ped* 115:415–417, 1989.
57. Gibas A, Dienstag JL, Schafer AI, et al: Cure of hemophilia A by orthotopic liver transplantation. *Gastroenterology* 95:192–194, 1989.
58. Merion RM, Delius RE, Campbell DA, Jr, Turcotte JG: Orthotopic liver transplantation totally corrects factor IX deficiency in hemophilia B. *Surgery* 104:929–931, 1988.
59. Cox KL, Ward RE, Furgiuele TL, Cannon RA, Sanders KD, Kurland G: Orthotopic liver transplantation in patients with cystic fibrosis. *Pediatrics* 80:571–574, 1987.
60. Goulet OJ, deVille JG, Otte JB, Ricour C: Preoperative nutritional evaluation and support for liver transplantation in children. *Transplant Proc* 19:3249–3255, 1987.
61. Starzl TE, Gordon RD: Liver transplantation in children—a solution for biliary atresia? *Proc Am Coll Surgeons, Ann Clin Cong* 71:17–18, 1985.
62. Andrews A, Ginsburg C: Orthotopic hepatic transplantation for unimmunized children—a paradox of contemporary medical care. *Ped Res* 21:282A, 1987.
63. American Academy of Pediatrics: *Report of the Committee on Infectious Diseases: The Red Book, 1991,* p 313, Elk Grove Village, AAP, 1991.
64. American Academy of Pediatrics: *Report of the Committee on Infectious Diseases: The Red Book, 1991,* p 225, Elk Grove Village, AAP, 1991.

65. Vital statistics of the United States 1982: *Mortality, Parts A, B*, Vol 2, p 186, Hyattsville, MD, 1986.

66. Pichlmayr R, Broelsch CH, Wonigest K, et al: Experience with liver transplantation in Hannover. *Hepatology* 4:56S–60S, 1984.

67. Emond JC, Whitington PF, Thistlethwaite JR, Alonso EM, Broelsch CE: Reduced-size orthotopic liver transplantation: use in the management of children with chronic liver disease. *Hepatology* 10:867–872, 1989.

68. Iglehart JK: Transplantation: the problem of limited resources. *New Engl J Med* 309:123–128, 1983.

69. Otte JB, deVille JG, Sokal E, et al: Size reduction of the donor liver is a safe way to alleviate the shortage of size-matched organs in pediatric liver transplantation. *Ann Surg* 211:146–157, 1990.

70. Iwatsuki S, Rabin BS, Shaw BW, Starzl TE: Liver transplantation against T-cell positive warm crossmatches. *Transplant Proc* 16:1427–1429, 1984.

71. Gordon RD, Fung JU, Markus B, et al: The antibody crossmatch in liver transplantation. *Surgery* 100:705–715, 1986.

72. Shaw BW, Wood RP, Kaufman SS, et al: Liver transplantation therapy for children, Part 2. *J Ped Gastroenterol Nutr* 7:797–815, 1988.

73. Markus BH, Duquesnoy RJ, Gordon RD, et al: Association of HLA compatibility and decreased liver transplant survival. *Transplant Proc* 20:43–44, 1987.

74. Gordon RD, Iwatsuki S, Esquivel CO, et al: Liver transplantation across ABO blood groups. *Surgery* 2:342–348, 1986.

75. Iwatsuki S, Iwiki Y, Kano T, et al: Successful transplantation from cross-match positive donors. *Transplant Proc* 13:286–288, 1981.

76. Pillay P, Van Thiel DH, Gavaler JS, Starzl TE: Donor gender does not affect liver transplant outcome in children. *Dig Dis Sci* 35:686–689, 1990.

77. Pillay P, Van Thiel DH, Gavaler JS, Starzl TE: Effect of race upon organ donation and recipient survival in liver transplantation. *Dig Dis Sci* 35:1391–1396, 1990.

78. Wahlberg JA, Love R, Landegaard L, Southard JH, Belzer FO: Successful 72 hour preservation of the canine pancreas. *Transplantation* 43:5–8, 1987.

79. Kalayoglu M, Sollinger HW, Stratta RJ, et al: Extended preservation of the liver for clinical transplantation. *Lancet* 1:617–619, 1988.

80. Olthoff KM, Millis JM, Imagawa DK, et al: Comparison of UW solution and euro-collins solutions for cold preservation of human liver grafts. *Transplantation* 49: 284–290, 1990.

81. Rouch DA, Emond JC, Thistlewaite JR, Mayes JT, Broelsch CE: Choledochocholedostomy without a T-tube or internal stent in transplantation of the liver. *Surg Gynecol Obstet* 170:239–244, 1990.

82. Shaw BW, Martin DJ, Marquez JM: Venous bypass in clinical liver transplantation. *Ann Surg* 200:524–534, 1984.

83. Ringe B, Bornschener A, Blumhardt G, Bechstein WO, Wonigeit K, Pichlmayr R: Experience with veno-venous bypass in human liver transplantation. *Transplant Proc* 19:2416, 1987.

84. Lewis JH, Bontempo FA, Cornell FW, et al: Blood use in transplantation: liver, heart, artificial heart and heart-lung. *Transplant Proc* 20(Suppl 1):530–532, 1988.

85. Wood RP, Langnus AN, Stratta RJ, et al: Optimal therapy for patients with biliary atresia: portoenterostomy ("Kasai" procedures) versus primary transplantation. *J Ped Surg* 25:153–162, 1990.

86. Lerut J, Tzakis A, Bron K, et al: Complications of venous reconstruction in human orthotopic liver transplantation. *Ann Surg* 205:404–414, 1987.
87. Bismuth H, Houssin D: Reduced-size orthotopic liver graft in hepatic transplantation in children. *Surgery* 95:367–371, 1984.
88. Broelsch CE, Emond JC, Thistlethwaite JR, et al: Liver transplantation in children including the concept of reduced size liver transplantation in children. *Ann Surg* 208:410–420, 1988.
89. Broelsch CE, Emond JE, Thistlethwaite JR, et al: Liver transplantation with reduced-size donor organs. *Transplantation* 45:519–523, 1988.
90. DeHemptinne B, Salizzoni M, Yandza TC, deVille JG, Tan KC, Kestens PJ: Indication, technique, and results of liver graft volume reduction before orthotopic transplantation in children. *Transplant Proc* 19:3549–3551, 1987.
91. Stratta RJ, Wood RP, Langnas AN: Effect of extended preservation and reduced-size grafting on organ availability in pediatric liver transplantation. *Transplant Proc* 22: 482–484, 1990.
92. Broelsch CE, Emond JC, Whitington PF, Thistlethwaite JR, Baker AL, Lichter JL: Application of reduced-size liver transplants as split grafts auxiliary orthotopic grafts and living related segmental grafts. *Ann Surg* 212:368–377, 1990.
93. Shaw BW, Jr, Wood RP, Stratta RJ: Management of arterial anomalies encountered in split-liver transplantation. *Transplant Proc* 22:420–422, 1990.
94. Emond JC, Whitington PF, Thistlethwaite JR, et al: Transplantation of two patients with one liver. *Ann Surg* 212:14–22, 1990.
95. Otte JB, deVille JG, Alberti D, et al: The concept and technique of the split-liver in clinical transplantation. *Surgery* 107:605–612, 1990.
96. Fortner JG, Yeh SDJ, Kim DK, et al: The case for and technique of heterotopic liver grafting. *Transplant Proc* 11:269–275, 1979.
97. Tepstra OT, Reuvers CB, Schalm SW: Auxiliary heterotopic liver transplantation. *Transplantation* 45:1003–1007, 1988.
98. Tepstra OT, Schalm SW, Weimar W, et al: Auxiliary partial liver transplantation for end-stage chronic liver disease. *New Engl J Med* 319:1507–1511, 1988.
99. Jerusalem C, van der Heyde MN, Schmidt WJ, Tjebbes FA: Heterotopic liver transplantation: unfavorable outflow conditions as a possible cause for late graft failure. *Eur Surg Res* 4:187–197, 1973.
100. Strong RW, Lynch SV, Ong TH, Matsunami H, Koido Y, Balderson GA: Successful liver transplantation from a living donor to her son. *New Engl J Med* 322:1505–1507, 1990.
101. Singer PA, Siegler M, Whitington PF, et al: Ethics of liver transplantation with living donors. *New Engl J Med* 321:620–622, 1989.
102. Shaw BW, Stratta RJ, Donovan JP, Langnas AN, Wood RP, Markin RJ: Postoperative care after liver transplantation. *Semin Liver Dis* 9:202–230, 1989.
103. Marquez J, Martin D, Kang YG, et al: Cardiovascular depression secondary to citrate intoxication during hepatic transplantation in man. *Anaesthesia* 65:457–461, 1986.
104. Wszolek ZK, McComb RD, Pfeiffer RF, et al: Pontine and extrapontine myelinolysis following liver transplantation: relationship to serum sodium. *Transplantation* 48: 1006–1012, 1989.
105. Lim P, Jacob E: Magnesium deficiency in liver cirrhosis. *Q J Med* 41:291–300, 1972.
106. June CH, Thompson CB, Kennedy MS, et al: Correlation of hypomagnesemia with the onset of cyclosporine-associated hypertension in marrow transplant recipients. *Transplantation* 41:47–51, 1986.

107. Moulin D, Clement SC, Reynaert M, et al: Intensive care for children after orthotopic liver transplantation. *Intensive Care Med* 15(Suppl 1):S71–S72, 1989.

108. Krowka MJ, Cortese DA: Pulmonary aspects of chronic liver disease and liver transplantation. *Mayo Clin Proc* 60:407–418, 1985.

109. Powell-Jackson PR, Carmichael FJL, Calne RY, Williams R: Adult respiratory distress syndrome and convulsions associated with administration of cyclosporine in liver transplant recipients. *Transplantation* 38:341–343, 1984.

110. Rosh JR, Ritter S, Benkov KJ, et al: Endoscopic color Doppler examination of the hepatic and portal vasculature after orthotopic liver transplantation. *Gastrointest Endosc* 37:190–191, 1990.

111. Sharp HS, Snover D, Burke BA, et al: The role of clinical evaluation in graft rejection following liver transplantation in extrahepatic biliary atresia. In Daum F: *Extrahepatic Biliary Atresia,* p 119, New York, Marcel Dekker, 1983.

112. Koep LJ, Starzl TE, Weil R: Gastrointestinal complications of hepatic transplantation. *Transplant Proc* 11:257–261, 1979.

113. Martinez AJ, Estol C, Faris AA: Neurologic complications of liver transplantation. *Neurol Clin N Am* 6:327–348, 1988.

114. Adams DH, Benson B, Honigsberger L, et al: Neurological complications following liver transplantation. *Lancet* 1:949–951, 1987.

115. DeGroen PC, Aksamit AJ, Rakela J, Forbes GS, Krom RAF: Central nervous system toxicity after liver transplantation: the role of cyclosporine and cholesterol. *New Engl J Med* 317:861–866, 1987.

116. Hughes RL: Cyclosporine-related central nervous system toxicity in cardiac transplantation (letter). *New Engl J Med* 323:420–421, 1990.

117. Sharbhogue RLK, Bistrian BR, Jenkins RL, et al: Increased protein catabolism without hypermetabolism after human orthotopic liver transplantation. *Surgery* 101: 146–149, 1987.

118. Borel J, Feurer C, Magree C, et al: Effect of the new antilymphocytic peptide cyclosporine A in animals. *Immunology* 32:1017–1025, 1977.

119. Kahan BD: Cyclosporine: the agent and its actions. In Kahan BD: *Cyclosporine,* p 5, New York, Grune & Stratton, 1985.

120. Kahan BD. Cyclosporine: the agent and its actions. *Transplant Proc* 17(Suppl 1):5–18, 1985.

121. Whitington PF, Emond JC, Whitington SH, Broelsch CE, Baker AL: Small bowel length and the dose of cyclosporine in children after liver transplantation. *New Engl J Med* 322:733–738, 1990.

122. Kehrer BH, Whitington PF, Black DD: The effect of Roux-en-Y biliary enterostomy on the absorption of cyclosporine: relevance to poor drug bioavailability in children after orthotopic liver transplantation. *Transplant Proc* 20:523–528, 1988.

123. Sanghvi A, Seltman H, Diven W: Cyclosporine measurement in transplantation. *Arch Pathol Lab Med* 109:1072–1075, 1985.

124. Iwatsuki S, Esquivel C, Klintmalm G, et al: Nephrotoxicity of cyclosporine in liver transplantation. *Transplant Proc* 17(Suppl 1):191–195, 1985.

125. Zitelli BJ, Miller JW, Gartner JC, Jr, et al: Changes in lifestyle after liver transplantation. *Pediatrics* 82:173–180, 1988.

126. McDiarmid SV, Ettenger RB, Hawkins RA: The impairment of true glomerular filtration rate in long-term cyclosporine-treated pediatric allograft recipients. *Transplantation* 49:81–85, 1990.

127. Dupont E, Wybran J, Toussaint A: Glucocorticosteroids and organ transplantation. *Transplantation* 37:331–335, 1984.

128. Hockland M, Larsen B, Heron I, Plesner T: Corticosteroids decrease the expression of beta-2 microglobulin and histocompatibility antigens on human peripheral blood lymphocytes in vitro. *Clin Exp Immunol* 44:239–246, 1981.

129. Iwatsuki S, Starzl TE, Shaw BW Jr, et al: Pediatric liver transplantation. In Gips CH, Krom RAF: *Progress in Liver Transplantation*, Dordrecht, Martinus Nijhoff, 1985, p. 196.

130. Zimmerman HJ: *Heptotoxicity*, New York, Appleton-Century Crofts, 1978, p528.

131. Marubbio AT, Danielson B. Hepatic veno-occlusive disease in a renal transplant recipient receiving azathioprine. *Gastroenterology* 69:739–743, 1975.

132. Gordon RD, Tzakis AG, Iwatsuki S, et al: Experience with orthoclone OKT3 monoclonal antibody in liver transplantation. *Am J Kidney Dis* 11:141–144, 1988.

133. Esquivel CO, Fung JJ, Markus B, et al: OKT3 in the reversal of acute hepatic allograft rejection. *Transplant Proc* 19:2443–2446, 1987.

134. Millis JM, McDiarmid SV, Hiatt JR, et al: Randomized prospective trial of OKT3 for early prophylaxis of rejection after liver transplantation. *Transplantation* 47:82–88, 1989.

135. Goldstein G, Kremer AB, Barnes L, Hirsch RL: OKT3 monoclonal antibody reversal of renal and hepatic rejection in pediatric patients. *J Ped* 111:1046–1050, 1987.

136. Kremer A, Barnes L, Hirsch R, Goldstein G: Orthoclone OKT3 monoclonal antibody reversal of hepatic and cardiac allograft rejection unresponsive to conventional immunosuppressive treatments. *Transplant Proc* 19(Suppl 1):54–57, 1987.

137. Colonna JO II, Goldstein LI, Brems JJ, et al: A prospective study on the use of monoclonal anti-T3-cell antibody (OKT3) to treat steroid-resistant liver transplant rejection. *Arch Surg* 122:1120–1123, 1987.

138. Otto G, Thies J, Mannel M, Herfarth C, et al: Monoclonal antibody to interleukin-2 receptor in liver graft rejection (letter). *Lancet* 335:1596–1597, 1990.

139. Starzl TE, Makowka L, Todo S, et al: FK506: a potential breakthrough in immunosuppression. *Transplant Proc* 19(Suppl 6):3–104, 1987.

140. Starzl TE, Fung J, Venkataramman R, Todo S, Demetris AJ, Jain A: FK506 for liver, kidney and pancreas transplantation. *Lancet* 2:1000–1004, 1989.

141. Bismuth H, Lastaing D, Otte JB, Rolles K, Ringe B, Sloot M: Hepatic transplantation in Europe. *Lancet* 2:674–676, 1987.

142. Lewis J, Bontempo F, Cornell F, et al: Blood use in liver transplantation. *Transfusion* 27:222–225, 1987.

143. Kennedy EM, Wood RP, Shaw BW: Primary nonfunction: is there a contribution from the back table bath? *Transplantation* 49:739–743, 1990.

144. Greig PD, Woolf GM, Abecassis M, et al: Prostaglandin E_1 for primary nonfunction following liver transplantation. *Transplant Proc* 21:3360–3361, 1989.

145. Busuttil R, Goldstein L, Danovitch G, et al: Liver transplantation today. *Ann Int Med* 104:377–389, 1986.

146. Hiatt JR, Ament ME, Bergquist WJ, et al: Pediatric liver transplantation at UCLA. *Transplant Proc* 19:3282–3288, 1987.

147. Wozneg P, Zagko AB, Bron KM, et al: Vascular complications after liver transplantation. *Am J Radiol* 147:657–663, 1986.

148. Tzakis A, Gordon RD, Shaw BJ, et al: Clinical presentation of hepatic artery thrombosis after liver transplantation in the cyclosporine era. *Transplantation* 40:667–671, 1985.

149. Zemal G, Zajko AB, Skolnick NL, et al: The role of sonography and transhepatic cholangiography in the diagnosis of biliary complications after liver transplantation. *Am J Radiol* 151:943–946, 1988.

150. Larut J, Tzakis AG, Bron KM, et al: Complications of venous reconstruction in human orthotopic liver transplantation. *Ann Surg* 205:404–414, 1987.

151. Van Gunsbeke D, Avnie F, Delcour C, et al: Sonographic features of portal vein thrombosis. *Am J Radiol* 144:749–752, 1985.

152. Cardella JF, Castaneda-Zuniga WR, Hunter D, et al: Angiographic and interventional radiologic considerations in liver transplantation. *Am J Radiol* 146:143–153, 1986.

153. Rouch DA, Emond JC, Ferrari M, et al: The successful management of portal vein thrombosis after hepatic transplantation with a splenorenal shunt. *Surg Gynecol Obstet* 166:311–316, 1988.

154. Burke GW, Ascher NL, Hunter D, et al: Orthotopic liver transplantation: nonoperative management of early acute portal vein thrombosis. *Surgery* 104:924–928, 1988.

155. Portman B, O'Grady J, Williams R: Disease recurrence following orthotopic liver transplantation. *Transplant Proc* 18(Suppl 4):136–143, 1986.

156. Andres GA, Accini L, Ansell JD, et al: Immunopathologic studies of orthotopic human liver allografts. *Lancet* 1:275–280, 1972.

157. Bach FH, Sachs DH: Current concepts: immunology—transplantation immunology. *New Engl J Med* 317:489–492, 1987.

158. Tilney NL, Strom TB, Kupiec-Weglinski JW: Humoral and cellular mechanisms in acute allograft injury. *J Ped* 111:1000–1003, 1987.

159. Snover D, Sibley R, Freese DS, et al: Orthotopic liver transplantation: a pathologic study of 63 serial liver biopsies from 17 patients with special reference to the diagnostic features and natural history of rejection. *Hepatology* 4:1212–1222, 1984.

160. Demetris AJ, Lasky S, Van Thiel D, et al: Pathology of hepatic transplantation: a review of 62 adult allograft recipients immunosuppressed with a cyclosporine/steroid regimen. *Am J Pathol* 118:151–161, 1985.

161. Williams J, Peters T, Vera S, et al: Biopsy-directed immunosuppression following liver transplantation in man. *Transplantation* 39:589–596, 1985.

162. Snover DC, Freese DK, Sharp HL, et al: Liver allograph rejection. *Am J Surg Pathol* 11:1–10, 1987.

163. Kirby RM, Young JA, Hubscher SG, Elias E, McMaster P: The accuracy of aspiration cytology in the diagnosis of rejection following orthotopic liver transplantation. *Transplant Int* 1:119–121, 1988.

164. Donaldson P, Alexander G, O'Grady J, et al: Evidence for an immune response to HLA class I in the vanishing bile duct syndrome after liver transplantation. *Lancet* 1:945–948, 1987.

165. Ludwig J, Wiesner RH, Butts KP, Perkins JD, Krom RAF: The acute vanishing bile duct syndrome (acute irreversible rejection) after liver transplantation. *Hepatology* 7:4176–4183, 1987.

166. Hubscher SG, Buckles JA, Elias E, McMaster P, Neuberger JM: Reversible vanishing bile duct syndrome after liver transplantation: report of 6 cases. *Transplant Proc* 23:1415–1416, 1991.

167. Zitelli BJ, Gartner JC, Malatack JJ, Urbach AH, McGregor RS: Liver transplantation. In Balistreri WF, Stocker JT: *Pediatric Hepatology*, pp 371–372, New York, Hemisphere Publishing, 1990.

168. Hoffer SA, Teele RL, Lillehei CW, Vacanti JP: Infected bilomas and hepatic artery thrombosis in infant recipients of liver transplants—interventional radiology and medical therapy as an alternative to retransplantation. *Radiology* 169:435–438, 1988.

169. Nauseef WM, Maki DG: A study of the value of simple protective isolation in patients with granulocytopenia. *New Engl J Med* 304:448–453, 1981.

170. Georgri A, Wonegut K, Worck K: Infection after orthotopic grafting of the liver. *Transplant Proc* 18:146, 1986.

171. Ho M, Wajszezuk CP, Hardy A, et al: Infections in kidney, heart and liver transplant recipients on cyclosporine. *Transplant Proc* 15:2768–2772, 1983.

172. Zitelli BJ, Gartner JC, Malatack JJ, et al: Pediatric liver transplantation: patient evaluation and selection, infectious complications and lifestyle after transplantation. *Transplant Proc* 19:3309–3316, 1987.

173. Zitelli BJ, Malatack JJ, Urbach AH, et al: Pediatric hepatology—3 year experience with pediatric liver transplantation with cyclosporine and steroids. In Winter PM, Kany YG: *Hepatic Transplantation,* p 66, Philadelphia, Praeger Special Studies, 1986.

174. Balfour HH: Cytomegalovirus—the troll of transplantation. *Arch Int Med* 139:279–280, 1979.

175. Weichl JD, Pass RF, Diethelm AG, Whitely RJ, Alford CA: Effect of primary and recurrent cytomegalovirus infections upon graft and patient survival after renal transplantation. *Transplantation* 28:443–446, 1979.

176. Gorensek MJ, Stewart RW, Keys TF, McHenry MC, Babiak T, Goormastic M: Symptomatic cytomegalovirus infection as a significant risk for major infections after cardiac transplantation. *J Infect Dis* 158:884–887, 1988.

177. Barkholt LM, Ericzon BG, Ehrust A, Forsgren M, Andersson JP: Cytomegalovirus infections in liver transplant patients: incidence and outcome. *Transplant Proc* 22: 235–237, 1990.

178. King SM, Petric M, Superina R, Graham N, Roberts EA: Cytomegalovirus infections in pediatric liver transplantation. *Am J Dis Child* 144:1307–1310, 1990.

179. Gorensek MJ, Carey WD, Vogt D, Goormastic M: A multivariable analysis of risk factors for cytomegalovirus infection in liver transplant recipients. *Gastroenterology* 98:1326–1332, 1990.

180. Dussaix E, Wood C: Cytomegalovirus infection in pediatric liver recipients. *Transplantation* 48:272–274, 1989.

181. Pollard RB: Cytomegalovirus infections in renal, heart, heart-lung, and liver transplantation. *Ped Infect Dis J* 7(Suppl):97–102, 1988.

182. Rakela J, Wiesner RH, Tasuelli HF: Incidence of cytomegalovirus infection and its relationship to donor-recipient serologic status in liver transplantation. *Transplant Proc* 19:2399–2402, 1987.

183. Chou S: Acquisition of donor strains of cytomegalovirus by renal transplant recipients. *New Engl J Med* 314:1418–1423, 1986.

184. Fox AS, Tolpin MD, Baker AL, et al: Seropositivity in liver transplant recipients as a predictor of cytomegalovirus disease. *J Infect Dis* 157:383–385, 1988.

185. Grundy JE, Super M, Sweny P, et al: Symptomatic cytomegalovirus infection in seropositive kidney recipients: reinfection with the donor virus rather than reactivation of the recipient virus. *Lancet* 2:132–135, 1988.

186. Snydman DR, Werner BG, Heinze-Lacey B, et al: Use of cytomegalovirus immuno-

globulin to prevent cytomegalovirus disease in renal transplant recipients. *New Engl J Med* 317:1049–1054, 1987.

187. Salibe F, Gugenheim J, Samed D, Bismuth H: Incidence of cytomegalovirus infection and effects of cytomegalovirus immune globulin prophylaxis after orthotopic liver transplantation. *Trnasplant Proc* 19:4081–4082, 1987.

188. Salibe F, Arulnaden JL, Gugenheim J, et al: Cytomegalovirus hyperimmune globulin prophylaxis after liver transplantation: a prospective randomized controlled study. *Transplant Proc* 21:2260–2262, 1989.

189. Meyers JD, Reed EC, Shepp DH, et al: Acyclovir for prevention of cytomegalovirus infection and disease after allogenic marrow transplantation. *New Engl J Med* 318:70–75, 1988.

190. Balfour HH, Chace BA, Stapleton JT, Simmons RL, Fryd DS: A randomized, placebo-controlled trial of oral acyclovir for the prevention of cytomegalovirus disease in recipients of renal allografts. *New Engl J Med* 320:1381–1387, 1989.

191. Harbison MA, de Girolami PC, Jenkins RL, Hammer SM: Ganciclovir therapy of severe cytomegalovirus infections in solid-organ transplantation. *Transplantation* 46:82–88, 1988.

192. Gudnason T, Belani KK, Balfour HH: Ganciclovir treatment of cytomegalovirus disease in immunocompromised children. *Ped Infect Dis J* 8:436–440, 1989.

193. Salmela K, Hockerstadt K, Lautenschlayer I, et al: Ganciclovir in the treatment of severe cytomegalovirus disease in liver transplant patients. *Transplant Proc* 22: 238–240, 1990.

194. D'Alessandro AM, Pirsch JD, Stratta RJ, Sollinger HW, Kalaoglu M, Belzer FO: Successful treatment of severe cytomegalovirus infections with ganciclovir and cytomegalovirus hyperimmune globulin in liver transplant recipients. *Transplant Proc* 21:3560–3561, 1989.

195. Paya CV, Hermans PE, Smith TF, et al: Efficacy of ganciclovir in liver and kidney transplant recipients with severe cytomegalovirus infection. *Transplantation* 46:229–234, 1988.

196. Breinig MK, Zitelli BJ, Starzl TE, et al: Epstein-Barr virus, cytomegalovirus, and other viral infections in children after liver transplantation. *J Infect Dis* 156:273–279, 1987.

197. Salt A, Sutehall G, Sargaison M, et al: Viral and toxoplasma gondii infections in children after liver transplantation. *J Clin Pathol* 43:63–67, 1990.

198. Randhawa PS, Markin RS, Starzl TE, Demetris AJ: Epstein-Barr virus-associated syndromes in immunosuppressed liver transplant recipients. *Am J Surg Pathol* 14:538–547, 1990.

199. Ho M, Miller G, Atchison RW, et al: Epstein-Barr virus infections and DNA hybridization studies in posttransplantation lymphoma and lymphoproliferative lesions: the role of primary infections. *J Infect Dis* 152:876–886, 1985.

200. Penn I: Lymphomas complicating organ transplantation. *Transplant Proc* 15:2790–2797, 1983.

201. Nakazato P, Esquivel CO, Urbach AH: Lymphoma and hypercalcemia in a pediatric orthotopic liver transplant patient. *Transplantation* 48:1003–1006, 1989.

202. Starzl TE, Nalesnik MA, Porter KA, et al: Reversibility of lymphomas and lymphoproliferative lesions developing under cyclosporine-steroid therapy. *Lancet* 1:583–587, 1984.

203. McGregor RS, Zitelli BJ, Urbach AH, Malatack JJ, Gartner JC: Varicella in pediatric orthotopic liver transplantation recipients. *Pediatrics* 83:256–261, 1989.

204. Alonso EM, Fox AS, Franklin WA, Whitington PF: Postnecrotic cirrhosis following varicella hepatitis in a liver transplant patient. *Transplantation* 49:650–653, 1990.

205. Calne RY: *Liver Transplantation—the Cambridge/Kings College Hospital Experience*, p 61, Orlando, FL, Grune & Stratton, 1983.

206. Gartner J, Zitelli BJ, Malatack J, et al: Orthotopic liver transplantation in children: 2 year experience with 47 patients. *Pediatrics* 74:140–145, 1984.

207. Superina RA, Pearl RH, Roberts EA, et al: Liver transplantation in children: the initial Toronto experience. *J Ped Surg* 24:1013–1019, 1989.

208. Iwatsuki S, Starzl TE, Todo S, et al: Experience in 1000 liver transplants under cyclosporine-steroid therapy: a survival report. *Transplant Proc* 20(Suppl 1):498–504, 1988.

209. Clement SC, Moulin D, Reynaert M: Postoperative care in pediatric orthotopic liver transplantation. *Transplant Proc* 19:3338–3343, 1987.

210. Schmidt K, Burdelski M, Bernsau U, et al: Analysis of current results of liver transplantation in children. *Transplant Proc* 19:2449–2450, 1987.

211. Esquivel CO, Koneru B, Karrer F: Liver transplantation before one year of age. *J Ped* 110:545–548, 1987.

212. Kaufman SS, Murray ND, Wood RP, Shaw BW Jr, Vanderhoof JA: Nutritional support for the infant with extrahepatic biliary atresia. *J Ped* 110:679–686, 1987.

213. Hehir DJ, Jenkins RL, Bistrian BR, Blackburn GL: Nutrition in patients undergoing orthotopic liver transplant. JPEN 1985; 9:695–700, 1985.

214. Stewart S, Uaauy R, Belknap W, et al: One-year follow-up of mental/motor development and growth in children after successful liver transplantation. *Ped Res* 21:278A, 1987.

215. Urbach A, Gartner JC, Malatack J, et al: Linear growth following pediatric liver transplantation. *Am J Dis Child* 141:547–549, 1987.

216. Spolidoro JVN, Berquist WE, Pehlivanoglu E, et al: Growth acceleration in children after orthotopic liver transplantation. *J Ped* 112:41–44, 1988.

217. Stewart SM, Uauy R, Kennard BD, Waller DA, Benser M, Andrews WS: Mental development and growth in children with chronic liver disease of early and late onset. *Pediatrics* 82:167–172, 1988.

218. Dobbing J: Human brain development and its vulnerability. In Sinclair JC, Warshaw JB, Bloom RS: *Biologic and Clinical Aspects of Brain Development*, pp 3–12, Evansville, Mead Johnson & Co, 1975.

219. Sokol RJ, Guggenheim MA, Heubi JE, et al: Frequency and clinical progression of the vitamin E deficiency neurologic disorder in children with prolonged neonatal cholestasis. *Am J Dis Child* 139:1211–1215, 1985.

220. Stewart SM, Uauy R, Waller DA, Kennard BP, Andrews WS: Mental and motor development correlates in patients with end-stage biliary atresia awaiting liver transplantation. *Pediatrics* 79:882–888, 1987.

221. Msall M, Batshaw ML, Suss R, et al: Neurologic outcome in children with inborn errors of urea synthesis. *New Engl J Med* 310:1500–1505, 1984.

222. Jervis GA: Encephalopathy in infantile hepatic cirrhosis. *Acta Neuropathol* 48: 73–75, 1979.

223. Stewart SM, Uauy R, Waller D, Kennard BD, Benser M, Andrews WS: Mental and motor development, social competence and growth one year after successful pediatric liver transplantation. *J Ped* 114:574–581, 1989.

224. Stewart SM, Hiltebeitel C, Nici J, Waller DA, Uauy R, Andrews WS: Neuropsychological outcome of pediatric liver transplantation. *Pediatrics* 87:367–376, 1991.

225. Starzl TE, Koep LJ, Schroter GBJ, et al: The quality of life after liver transplantation. *Transplant Proc* 11:252–256, 1979.

226. Penn I, Bunch D, Olenik D, et al: Psychiatric experience with patients receiving renal and hepatic transplants. *Semin Psychiatr* 3:133–144, 1971.

227. Zitelli BJ, Gartner JC, Jr, Malatack JJ, et al: Orthotopic liver transplantation in children: two-year experience with 47 patients. *Pediatrics* 74:140–145, 1984.

228. Andrews WS, Wanek E, Fyock B, Gray S, Benser M: Pediatric liver transplantation: a three-year experience. *J Ped Surg* 24:77–82, 1989.

229. Cundy TF, O'Grady JG, Williams R: Recovery of menstruation and pregnancy after liver transplantation. *Gut* 31:337–338, 1990.

230. Penn I, Makowski EL, Harris P: Parenthood following renal and hepatic transplantation. *Transplantation* 30:397–400, 1980.

231. Weichler NK: Information needs of mothers of children who have had liver transplants. *J Ped Nurs* 5:88–96, 1990.

232. Sabbeth BF, Leventhal JM: Marital adjustment to chronic illness: a critique of the literature. *Pediatrics* 73:762–768, 1984.

233. National Center for Health Statistics: Provisional statistics. *Month Vital Statist Rep* 29:1–2, 1980.

—17—

HISTOPATHOLOGY OF LIVER TRANSPLANTATION

Swan Nio Thung and Michael A. Gerber*

INTRODUCTION

Hepatic allografts are susceptible to a wide variety of injuries. These include diseases common to nongrafted livers and those unique to grafts. Therefore, in contrast to the rule of "one specimen, one diagnosis" in nongrafted livers, there are often more than one process affecting the grafts. This can produce considerable differential diagnostic difficulties. An attempt must be made by the pathologist to identify the different diagnoses and to put them in order of clinical importance and treatability. The biopsy findings have to be incorporated into the overall patient care, and for this reason the pathologist must be familiar with the clinical problems and management of patients with orthotopic liver transplantation (OLT).

In this chapter, we summarize our experience with 820 liver biopsy specimens from 150 patients who underwent OLT at Mount Sinai Medical Center in a 2.5-year period.

BIOPSY SCHEDULES

At our institution, protocol biopsies of the donor liver are performed before transplantation (back table, preperfusion biopsy), at the end of transplantation procedure (day 0, postperfusion biopsy), after 1 week, after 12 months, and then yearly. Nonprotocol biopsies are performed to determine the cause(s) of allograft dys-

*We are grateful to Elizabeth Vargas for secretarial help and to Glenn Maffei for photographic assistance.

function or to evaluate the effectiveness of treatment for rejection. Preperfusion biopsy is done to record changes originally present in the donor liver, such as the amount of portal fibrosis in older donors, proliferation of bile ductules, and steatosis. Most biopsy specimens are essentially normal because prior donor disease is rare. Among the donor livers, we have seen one with unsuspected primary biliary cirrhosis and one with granulomas in portal tracts. Frozen sections, when indicated, are performed on donor livers. Livers with severe ischemic injury due to cardiac failure or hypotension resulting in centrolobular ballooning or necrosis of hepatocytes ("shock" livers) and severe steatosis are excluded. No consistent changes in donor livers have been identified by light microscopy that correlate with primary graft failure,[1] except for rare cases with severe diffuse macrovesicular steatosis.[2]

Postperfusion biopsies are done to evaluate harvesting and perioperative injury and to diagnose hyperacute rejection (see below).[3]

HANDLING OF TISSUE SPECIMENS

Needle Biopsy Specimens

All specimens are submitted in three parts: (1) in 10% neutral buffered formalin for routine light microscopy, (2) in 3% glutaraldehyde for electron-microscopic studies, and (3) fresh or in Michelle's solution for immunohistochemical studies of antigens otherwise destroyed during routine processing of formalin fixed tissue.[4] Fixed or fresh tissues may be used for the detection of nucleic acids using the polymerase chain reaction (PCR).[5] Appropriate clinical information must accompany the biopsy. This information should include the patient's original disease, the date of transplantation(s), the results of studies of vascular and bile duct patency (i.e., ultrasound, arteriography, cholangiography), graft functions at the time of transplantation, the levels of serum liver enzymes, current immunosuppressive treatment—particularly if additional immunosuppressives have recently been given, and the reason for the biopsy (to rule out rejection, viral disease, recurrent hepatitis, etc.). Different conditions tend to occur at different times posttransplant, and therefore the dates of OLT and liver biopsy are important. The biopsy specimens submitted in the morning are processed by a rapid technique and are available for review within 4 hr. All transplant biopsy slides are reviewed daily, in the afternoon by the pathologist and clinicians, before treatment decisions are made. In addition, interesting cases are reviewed weekly by the clinicians with their pathologist. In most instances, hematoxylin and eosin (H&E) stain of the formalin-fixed, paraffin-embedded sections are sufficient for diagnosis. Other special stains that are useful include periodic acid-Schiff stain with diastase digestion (D-PAS stain), trichrome stain to demonstrate connective tissue, and iron stain. Immunohistochemical studies for the identification of hepatitis B surface (HBsAg) and hepatitis B core (HBcAg) antigens, hepatitis delta (δ) antigen, cytomegalovirus (CMV), herpes simplex virus (HSV), adenovirus, α-1-antitrypsin, and cytokeratin are performed depending on the suspected diagnoses.[6,7] Immunofluorescence studies to detect immunoglobulins (IgG, IgA, IgM), complement components (C3 and C1q) and fibrinogen are performed on all postperfusion biopsies and biopsies with severe or treatment-resistant allograft rejection.

Specimens submitted for electron-microscopic studies are embedded in plastic and stored. Thin sections are cut and examined only when indicated.

Whole Livers

Whole-liver specimens are obtained at the beginning of transplantation when the recipient's (native) liver is excised, when the allograft is removed because of failure, and at autopsy. Material for microbiologic studies is obtained in the operating room. The liver specimen is examined, photographed, weighed, and measured. Gross examination of failed allografts and autopsy specimens should include a thorough inspection of the hilar region. Particular attention should be given to all biliary and vascular anastomosis sites. Pertinent information such as vascular patency should be obtained from the surgeons since this may not be obvious in the specimen or not part of it. After careful gross examination of the entire liver, parallel transverse sections across both lobes are made. Focal lesions such as infarcts and abscesses are identified and sectioned. In native livers, attention is paid to identify incidental hepatocellular carcinoma (HCC) and large regenerative nodules (macroregenerative nodules, MRN) that may harbor small HCC.[8]

Histologic sections are taken from the hilar region and from both lobes.[9] Bulk freezing of tissue for biochemical or gene cloning studies (e.g., metabolic, genetic, or viral disease), quick freezing for frozen sections, and glutaraldehyde fixation for electron-microscopic studies are carried out in all resected livers and autopsy specimens.

HISTOPATHOLOGY OF POSTTRANSPLANT LIVER

Donor Disease

In most instances, donor livers show no disease on light microscopy.[9,10] Nonspecific changes, such as focal portal fibrosis, mild proliferation of bile ductules, or the slight steatosis that may be seen in normal individuals[11] may be present in donor livers. Mild portal fibrosis is often found in livers from older donors. Electron-microscopic studies demonstrated preferential degeneration of sinusoidal lining cells. There is, however, no correlation between the ultrastructural sinusoidal integrity or other light-microscopic features and graft function.[1] Preperfusion biopsy is useful in documenting these changes and serves as the baseline in evaluating "preservation" or "harvesting" injury and other histopathologic changes in the grafts.

"Preservation" Injury

Histopathologic changes present in postperfusion but absent from preperfusion biopsy specimens are caused by "preservation" injury. The insults may occur

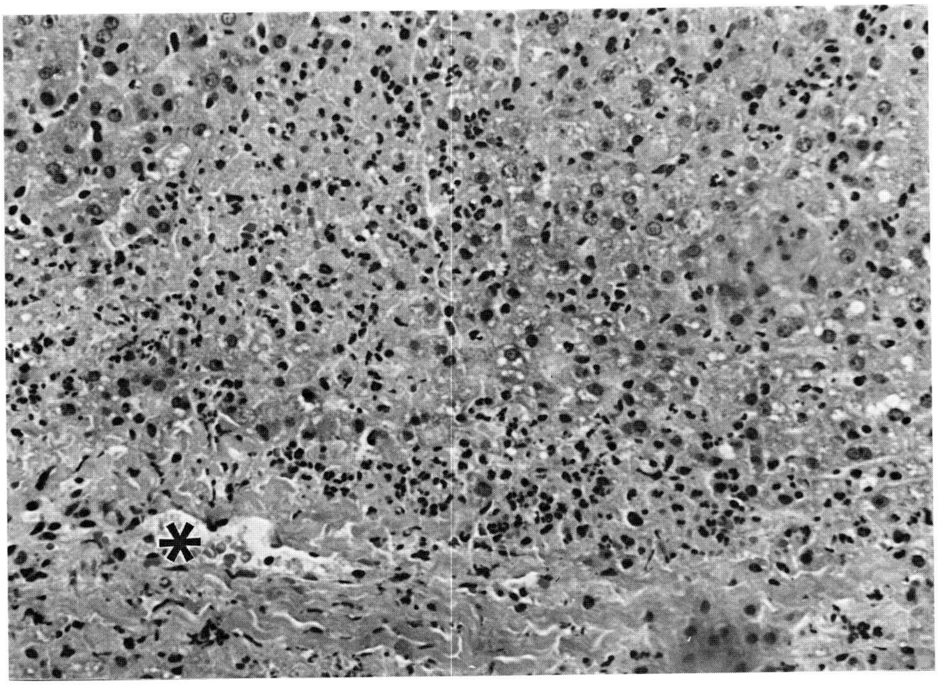

Figure 17-1. Harvesting injury seen in a 2-hr postperfusion biopsy specimen showing necrosis of hepatocytes and neutrophilic infiltration around the terminal hepatic venule (*), and neutrophilic aggregates within sinusoids (H&E, ×100).

between the time of organ harvest to shortly after reperfusion in the recipient. Most of the damage has been attributed to cold preservation or ischemic injury within the donor or recipient. The degree of severity ranges from accumulation of polymorphonuclear leukocytes (PMNs) in sinusoids and around terminal hepatic venules, as seen in "surgical" hepatitis,[11,12] to more extensive centrolobular necrosis of hepatocytes (Fig. 17-1). In our experience, the extent of centrolobular necrosis correlates well with the elevation of serum tranferase activities 48-hr posttransplantation, but does not seem to have any effect on the long-term survival of the graft. Although persistent elevation of bilirubin may last up to 1–2 months after OLT,[8] "preservation" injury accounts for only a subset of grafts that fail to function after transplantation.[1]

Follow-up biopsies on patients with "preservation injury" in initial specimens may show regenerative changes without residual lesions. If, however, the initial damage is accompanied by more severe bridging necrosis and proliferation of bile ductules, graft failure or residual damage such as pericentral and portal fibrosis may develop.

Biliary Tract Complications

Bile duct complications include acute or chronic obstruction, intrahepatic or anastomotic strictures, biliary leaks, cholangitis, and biliary–vascular fistulae.

Liver biopsy is not the best means to diagnose bile duct abnormalities. The diagnosis should be established by cholangiography.

The morphologic changes of large bile duct obstruction are characteristic: the portal tracts are edematous and contain dilated or tortuous ducts with marginal proliferation of bile ductules and infiltration by PMNs. Centrolobular cholestasis and bile infarcts or bile lakes are often seen.[13,14] These almost pathognomonic criteria used to diagnose mechanical biliary obstruction in nongrafted livers, are not frequently seen in grafts. The diagnostic features may be obscured considerably because (1) the obstruction is often incomplete or functional such as in bile duct leakage, (2) the portal changes may be combined with those of allograft rejection, (3) centrolobular cholestasis may be due to other conditions such as "functional cholestasis" or rejection, and (4) proliferation of bile ductules may be seen in other conditions such as severe "preservation" injury, nearby infarcts, or abscess formation. Differentiation of early bile duct obstruction or cholangitis from rejection, especially when biopsy is done after augmented immunosuppressive therapy has been given (partially treated rejection), can be difficult. In partially treated rejection, the mixed cellular infiltrate with predominantly mononuclear cells in portal tracts, which is characteristic for cellular allograft rejection, disappear, leaving only PMNs. Blood supply to the biliary tree in humans is derived only from the hepatic artery,[15,16] and therefore, any disturbance in hepatic artery bloodflow will affect the bile ducts. Although an increased number of bile ductular structures is a common phenomenon in diseased livers and may not be related to a specific cause or pathogenesis,[17,18] when observed in great numbers in liver grafts it should warrant studies of bile duct or vascular patency.

Cholestasis of Unknown Cause

Centrolobular cholestasis of varying degrees with or without feathery degeneration of hepatocytes is commonly seen in the early posttransplant period (color plate 1). This type of cholestasis, which is canalicular and hepatocellular, and occurs in the absence of known causes such as bile duct obstruction, viral hepatitis, or rejection, is called "functional cholestasis."[19] Functional cholestasis is transient and is found in about 25% of cases in the first 2 or 3 weeks after OLT.[9] Prolonged "functional cholestasis" occurs in grafts with severe "preservation" injury. In these livers, bile plugs and concretions are seen in the dilated bile canaliculi, and varying degrees of bile ductular proliferation and fibrosis are present in portal tracts. Multiplication or proliferation of bile ductular structures may be a reaction to facilitate bile flow from bile canaliculi within lobules to larger bile ducts.

Ischemic Lesions

The hepatic artery supplies approximately 30% of the oxygenated blood to the hepatic parenchyma, but is the major source of blood supply to the hilar and portal structures including bile ducts and branches of portal vein.[20-23]

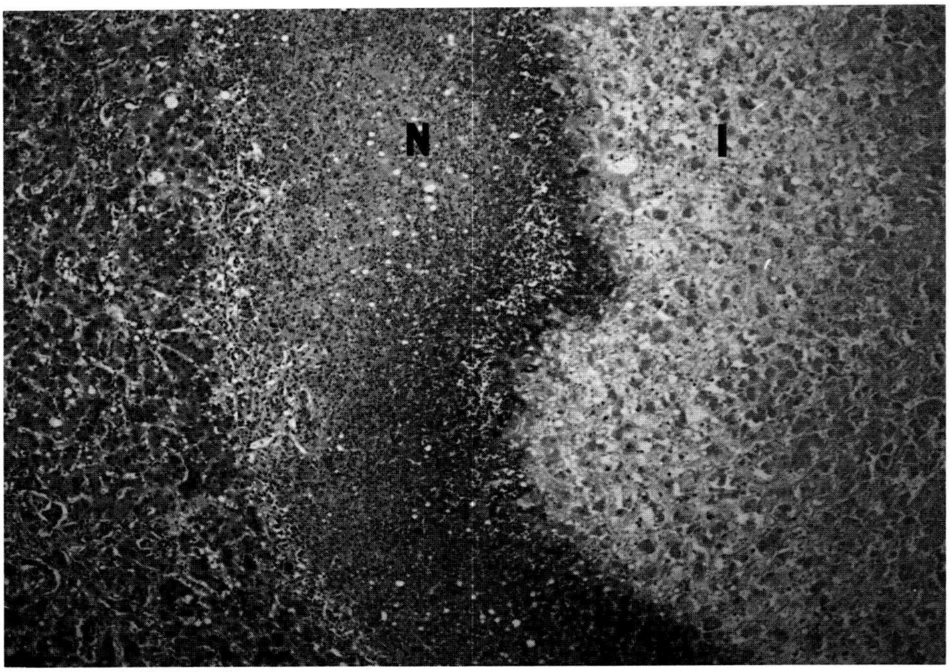

Figure 17-2. Ischemic infarction with loss of nuclear staining of hepatocytes (I). Dense neutrophilic infiltration is seen as a dark rim at the periphery of the lesion (N). Infarction was caused by thrombosis of hepatic artery 10 days after OLT (H&E, ×40).

Hepatic Artery Thrombosis

Hepatic artery thrombosis is more common in children than in adults. Signs of hepatic artery thrombosis include fever, sudden increase in serum transferase activities, recurrent septicemia from infected liver infarcts, and bile leaks.[24] Retransplantation is necessary in most of these cases. The incidence of hepatic artery thrombosis in our patients is approximately 5%. It occurred within the first 3 weeks after OLT. Examination of the removed failed allografts revealed areas of zonal infarction (Fig. 17-2).

Coagulative necrosis involving zone 3 or zones 3 and 2, leaving a rim of periportal hepatocytes intact may be observed focally in the noninfarcted parenchyma.

Microvesicular steatosis is sometimes seen in the cytoplasm of hepatocytes undergoing coagulative necrosis. Other areas may show centrolobular cholestasis, diffuse steatosis, ballooning of hepatocytes, or no changes.[8] Portal tracts may exhibit proliferation of bile ductules with a polymorphonuclear (PMN) infiltrate or changes consistent with rejection. Because of the uneven distribution of the ischemic injury in the liver, needle biopsy is a rather insensitive tool for diagnosing vascular thrombosis. In fact, the diagnosis of hepatic artery thrombosis in all our cases was based on a combination of clinical, operative, sonographic, and radiographic findings. In one case, a liver biopsy obtained 3 days before removal of the failed graft showed scattered individual hepatocytes undergoing eosinophilic degeneration. Zonal necrosis or infarction were not observed. On the other hand, biopsy evidence of infarcted liver tissue does not necessarily mean that the large vessels are thrombosed and that the graft will fail. Subcapsular liver necrosis is sometimes observed in allografts with patent extrahepatic arteries and portal and hepatic veins. Various etiologic possibilities are entertained for these focal lesions, particularly the role of hypoperfusion.[25] Focal subcapsular necrosis in superficial biopsy specimens should not be misinterpreted as being representative of the entire organ. Special stains for fungi and bacteria should be performed when ischemic necrosis or infarction are seen in liver biopsy specimens, since these lesions often become sources of infection.

Portal Vein Thrombosis

Portal vein thrombosis is less common than hepatic artery thrombosis. It is often seen complicating hepatic artery thrombosis. The manifestations are variable, ranging from severe acute hepatocellular injury to no abnormalities.[26] Portal vein thrombosis is seen in half of our cases with thrombosis of the hepatic artery.

Acute Massive Hepatic Necrosis

A syndrome of fulminant hepatic failure with distinctive clinical and pathologic features has been observed in patients with OLT.[10] The typical clinical presentation is that of an uneventful initial postoperative period, followed by a sudden deterioration in graft function, progressing rapidly to graft failure.[27] The pathologic changes are those of ischemic injury with typical coagulative necrosis involving zones 3 and 2 and sometimes the entire lobule, with only mild inflammation (Fig. 17-3). The portal tracts remain intact. Regenerative changes in the form of ductular hepatocytes and double-cell thick plates of the remaining periportal hepatocytes may be seen. The cause of this type of acute graft failure is not known. Occlusive lesions of large arteries and veins are absent. The histologic findings suggest, however, that at least the final pathway of the process leads to ischemic-type injury.[10] We encountered one such case with the typical clinicopathological features described above. Harvesting injury was not observed in the postperfusion biopsy specimen. Immunofluorescence studies to demonstrate immunoglobulins, complement, and fibrinogen in the postperfusion biopsy and the failed graft were negative. Antibody mediated rejection, therefore, could be excluded as possible etiology. The first allograft was replaced 3 days after OLT, and the patient is doing well 5 months after the second OLT.

Rejection

Hepatic allograft rejection is defined as a clinical and pathologic condition resulting from immunologic reactions of the host against the graft, which may lead to graft damage and graft failure. Rejection is the most common cause of posttransplantation liver dysfunction, and one of the major factors in graft loss. Approximately 80% of liver allografts experience one or more episodes of acute rejection.[28,29] The histopathologic findings in liver allograft rejection have been well described.[9,10,28-40] Unfortunately, difficulties still exist regarding terminology

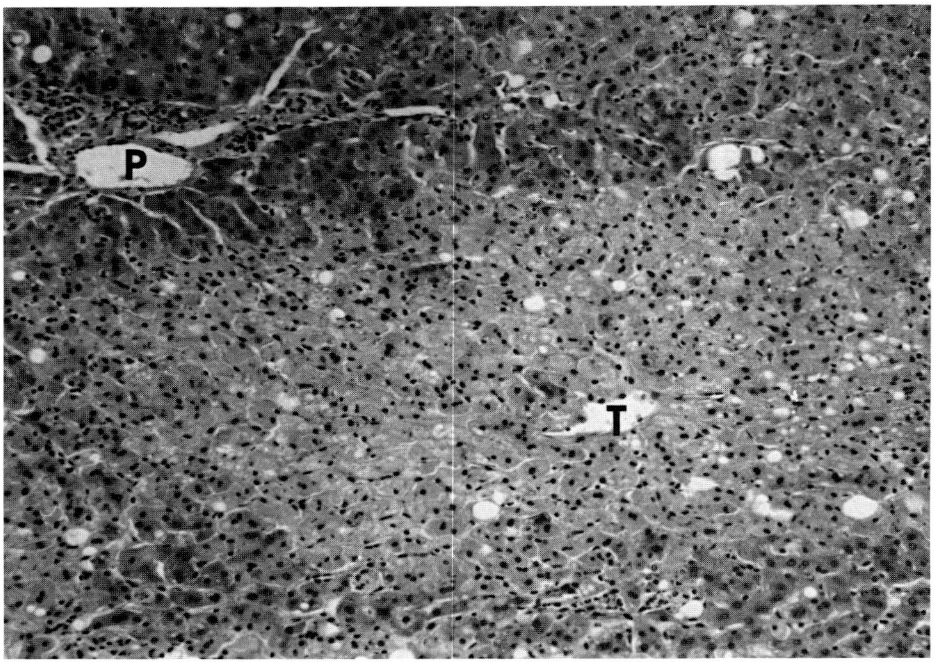

Figure 17-3. Coagulative necrosis involving zones 3 and 2 of the acini, sparing a rim of periportal hepatocytes (P = portal tract, T = terminal hepatic venule) in an allograft removed during retransplantation for poor function 3 days after the first OLT. The hepatic artery was patent (H&E, ×100).

such as "acute" versus "chronic" rejection, grading of severity, and markers for treatability and prognosis.[29,38] The separation of liver allograft rejection into acute and chronic forms may be somewhat artificial, since what is referred to as "chronic (noncellular) rejection" may be seen in the first several months posttransplantation and what is called "acute (cellular) rejection" may occur much later. As long as the chronologic inconsistencies are recognized, the terms "acute" and "chronic" rejection still appear useful, since they describe characteristic pathologic features that predict response to treatment and reversibility. The terms used by the pathologist, especially the ones that are treatment-relevant, should be well understood by the clinicians. Clinical signs of acute allograft rejection may include fever, fatigability, abdominal pain, hepatosplenomegaly, anorexia, decreased bile drainage from the T-tube, and increased liver enzyme activities. The clinical findings, however, do not always correlate with the histologic features.

Liver allograft rejection, as in other organ transplants, is subclassified into hyperacute, acute, and chronic rejection.

Hyperacute Rejection

Hyperacute rejection is mediated by preformed antibodies. This condition, which starts minutes after revascularization of the graft and causes rapid graft failure, has been observed frequently in renal and cardiac allografts,[41-44] but only rarely in hepatic allografts.[3,45-47] Furthermore, the process of hyperacute rejection of liver grafts develops more slowly than with kidney grafts. This was decribed by Starzl et al.[47] in 2 patients who received liver and kidney from the same donors. In hyperacute liver allograft rejection the preformed antibodies may be directed against ABO blood group antigens, major histocompatibility (MHC) antigens, or vascular endothelial cell (VEC) antigens. Hyperacute rejection resulting in hemorrhagic infarction occurred 5 times more frequently in ABO-incompatible than in ABO-compatible grafts.[46] Antibodies against MHC antigens can be detected by crossmatching the patient's serum with a panel of lymphocytes or with lymphocytes from the potential donor in a complement-dependent lymphocytotoxicity assay. Antibodies to VEC in hyperacute rejection are donor-specific.[48,49] The antigens on the VEC seem to be carried by monocytes as well.[50] A progressive and severe coagulopathy developing shortly after revascularization of the graft should arouse suspicion of an antibody mediated hyperacute rejection, even if the cytotoxic antibody crossmatch with the donor has been nonreactive. In these cases, the postperfusion liver biopsy taken hours after revascularization of the graft shows clustering of PMNs in sinusoids and single-cell necrosis of hepatocytes. The histologic changes are similar to those of "preservation" injury. Immunohistochemical staining of the postperfusion biopsy reveals diffuse deposition of immunoglobulins (IgG or IgM) and complement components (C_3 and/or C1q) in a granular pattern along the sinusoids (3) (color plate 2). Fibrinogen deposition is also seen within the sinusoids. We have observed such a case in a young woman who received an ABO-compatible liver allograft for autoimmune chronic active hepatitis and cirrhosis. The cytotoxic antibodies tested against a panel of lymphocytes [panel reactive antibodies (PRA)] were negative before transplantation. The allograft functioned poorly, and biopsy at day 8 revealed features of cellular rejection, dropout of centrolobular hepatocytes, and IgG and C_3 deposits within the sinusoids. Failure of the graft necessitated retransplantation at day 34. Similar granular deposition of immunoglobulins and complement components in the sinusoids have been observed in liver allografts in animals presensitized to donor antigens.[51] In hypersensitized inbred rat recipients, there seemed to be a marked decrease in the level of cytotoxic antibodies after liver, but not after heart transplantation. This may explain the privileged position of the liver in regard to rejection following ABO-incompatible or crossmatch-positive transplantations .[52]

Acute Cellular Rejection

Acute cellular liver allograft rejection occurs days to weeks posttransplantation. It can be observed as early as 2–3 days after OLT. It is uncommon after 2 months unless the patient is inadequately immunosuppressed. Acute cellular rejection, as the name indicates, is mediated predominantly by immune cells, although humoral components may also play a role. It is observed in about 60–65% of biopsy specimens obtained from our patients within the first 2 months. Prophylactic OKT3 given early to patients who were considered to be at high risk for rejection may have lowered its incidence in our patients. In this early posttransplantation period, the histologic diagnosis of rejection is not difficult. The histo-

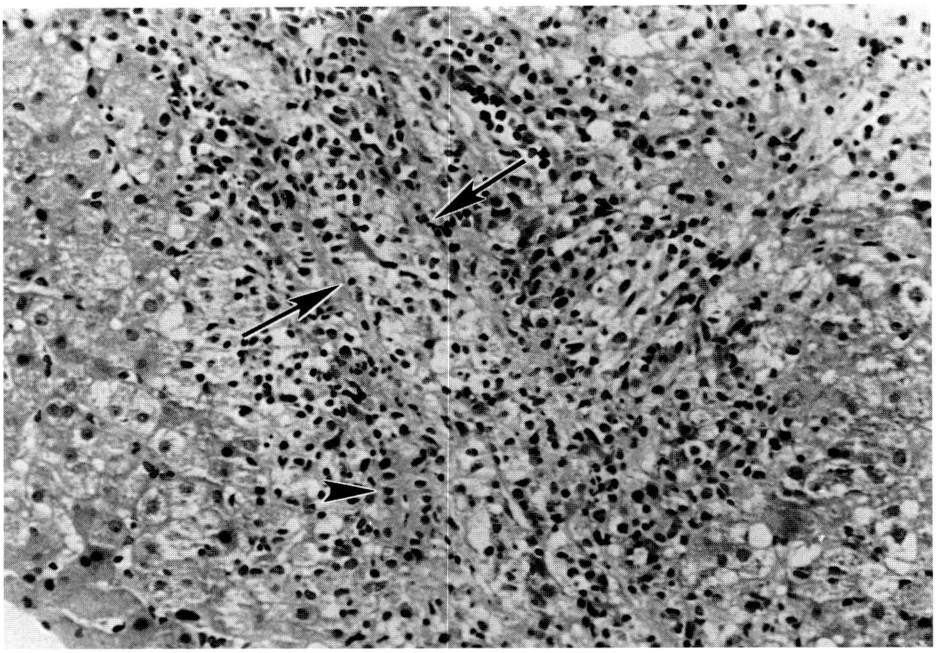

Figure 17-4. Portal tract with characteristic features of cellular rejection. It is edematous and contains mixed cellular inflammatory infiltrate. The portal vein with severe endothelitis (arrows) and the injured bile duct (arrowhead) are difficult to recognize. One week after OLT (H&E, ×100).

logic features are characteristic. The portal tracts are enlarged by edema and mixed-cellular infiltrate. The inflammatory infiltrate consists predominantly of mononuclear cells: immunoblasts, lymphocytes, plasma cells, and macrophages (Fig. 17-4, color plate 3).

Immunologic staining for phenotypic characteristics has shown that the majority of the cells are T-cells,[53] either predominantly T helper or mixed T helper and T suppressor/cytotoxic cells.[54] Neutrophils and eosinophils are also present admixed with the mononuclear cells. During the early phases, eosinophils may predominate in some cases. Although their presence may simulate an allergic drug reaction, eosinophils are helpful in diagnosing rejection, particularly when viral hepatitis is part of the differential diagnosis. The inflammatory cells are usually confined to the portal triads. Inflammatory cell infiltration beneath and adhering to endothelial cells of portal veins is particularly characteristic, so called *endothelitis*[10,37] (Fig. 17-4). The immunocytes in endothelitis consist mainly of helper and suppressor/cytotoxic T-cells as well as natural-killer (NK) cells.[37] Under the electron microscope, the endothelial cells often show evidence of cytoplasmic damage. Inflammatory cells may fill the lumen of portal veins and capillaries and obscure the vessels. In other conditions, the lumen of portal veins is usually open. Infiltration and damage to small interlobular bile ducts (*rejection cholangitis*), which is an important feature in acute cellular rejection, is often seen. Neutrophils and lymphocytes invade the bile duct epithelium (Fig.

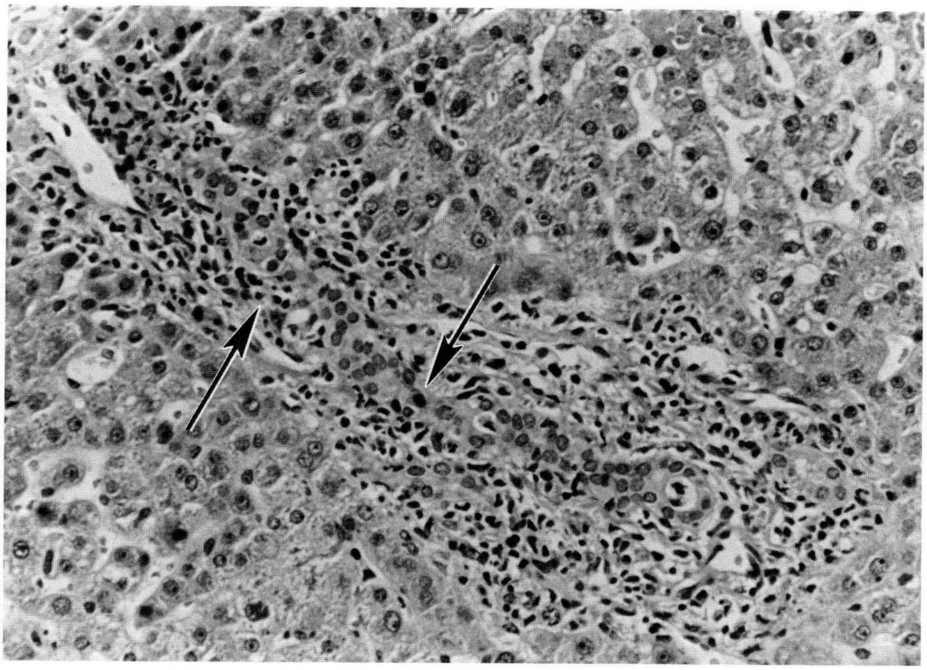

Figure 17-5. Interlobular bile duct with features of rejection cholangitis. The degenerative changes of the bile duct epithelial cells results in irregularity of the bile duct. Lymphocytic and neutrophilic infiltrations obscure the bile duct in some areas (arrows) (H&E, ×100).

17-5). The epithelial cells demonstrate degenerative alterations, e.g., vacuolization, ballooning, or eosinophilia of the cytoplasm and nuclear pyknosis, and regenerative changes, e.g., mitotic activity. Ducts with a diameter of 30–60 μm are preferentially affected, although larger bile ducts are occasionally also involved.[55] Hepatic artery branches may be infiltrated by inflammatory cells and difficult to recognize, but necrotizing arteritis is rare.[28,56,57] The parenchyma usually shows activation of sinusoidal lining cells and a slight increase in inflammatory cells. Scattered hepatocytes may undergo ballooning or eosinophilic degeneration. Cholestasis is often present. The terminal hepatic venules show similar changes as seen in portal veins (Fig. 17-6). These changes suggest that antigens predominantly displayed on endothelial cells and bile duct epithelium may represent the main targets in liver allograft rejection. Following, but not before, transplantation, the bile duct epithelium, as well as portal and central vein and hepatic artery endothelium, expressed HLA-DR antigens.[54,55] These HLA class II antigens may be one of the preferential targets for rejection. Difficulties in the diagnosis of rejection are experienced when (1) other conditions, particularly viral hepatitis coexist (see under "Hepatitis") or (2) liver biopsy is performed only after augmented immunosuppression therapy has been started (partially treated rejection). As a rule, cellular rejection except for rare cases, respond well to antirejection therapy.

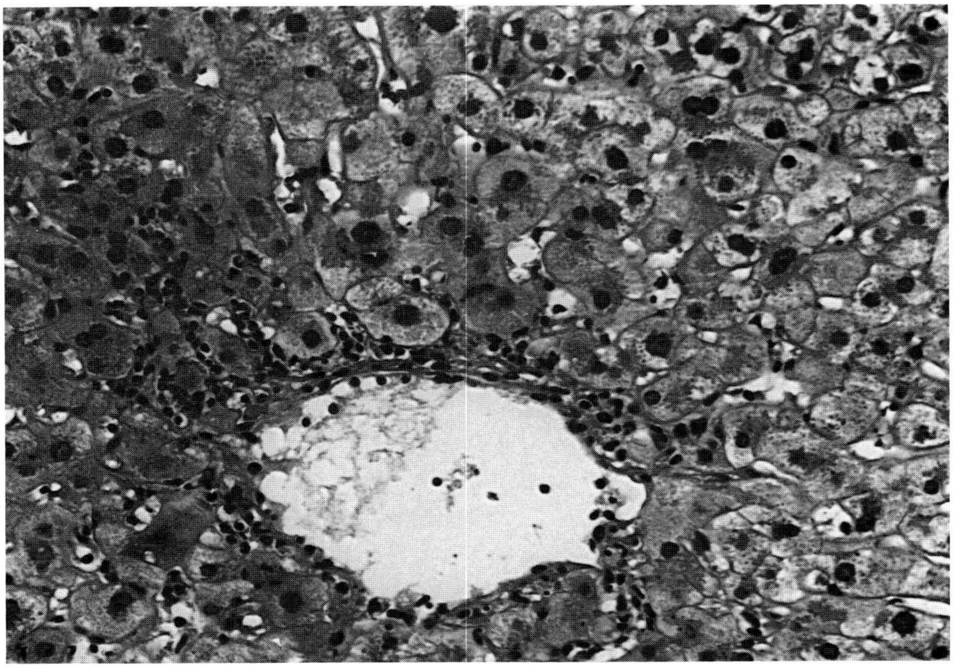

Figure 17-6. Terminal hepatic venule with characteristic features of rejection endothelitis. Lymphocytes invade the endothelium both from the luminal side and the subendothelial layer. One week after OLT (H&E, ×400).

Partially Treated Rejection

After 1 or 2 weeks of treatment for rejection, inflammatory cells, particularly the mononuclear cell fraction, usually decrease or disappear in biopsy specimens. Endothelitis may or may not improve. The portal tracts often remain edematous with residual neutrophils, plasma cells, and eosinophils (color plate 4). Mild fibrosis may be seen in portal tracts. The changes of partially treated rejection may resemble those of acute mechanical biliary obstruction. Proliferation of bile ductules is more prominent in bile duct obstruction, while degenerative changes of bile duct epithelium are seen in partially treated rejection (Fig. 17-7; color plate 5). For diagnostic purposes, it is critical to obtain information of recent antirejection therapy. In difficult cases, the diagnosis of rejection will be confirmed by evaluation of the histologic response to therapy in sequential biopsies. The histologic effect of antirejection treatment does not necessarily run parallel with the clinical picture. Thus, the histologic monitoring of antirejection therapy should always be combined with clinical monitoring.

Grading of Rejection

The histologic grading of acute cellular rejection for severity and response to therapy is still controversial.[38] Features such as arteritis, bile duct paucity, hepatocellular ballooning, dropout, or necrosis are thought to be significant predictors

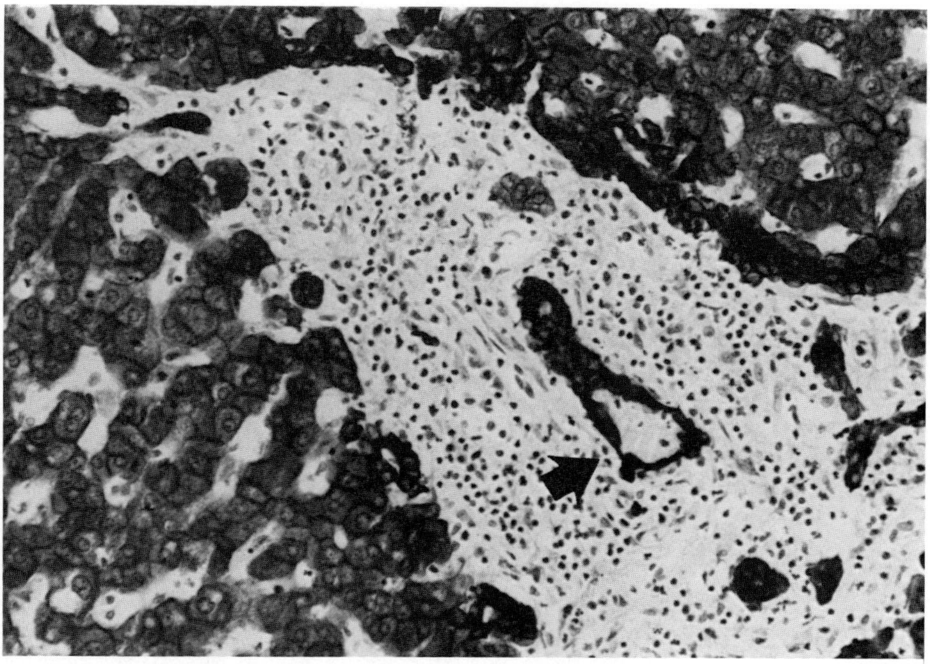

Figure 17-7. Bile duct injury (arrow) persists in a liver biopsy specimen showing partially treated rejection. The remaining inflammatory cells consist predominantly of neutrophils. (Immunoperoxidase stain using antibody to low-molecular-weight cytokeratin, counterstained with Harris' hematoxylin; ×100.)

for poor outcome.[29] The difficulties in using these criteria to predict severity of rejection are as follows: (1) arteritis involves mainly larger arteries, which are not included in needle biopsy specimens; (2) there are many possible histologic pictures of rejection; (3) hepatocellular ballooning, dropout, or necrosis may be unrelated to rejection and may result from other factors, e.g., viral hepatitis, drug toxicity, or ischemia due to severe "preservation" injury or disturbance in hepatic artery or portal vein bloodflow; and (4) it is important to stress that there is not always clinicopathologic correlation. We have seen in protocol biopsies taken 1 week after OLT, changes that we considered "severe" cellular rejection in patients with no clinical symptoms and very mild elevation of liver enzyme activities. Centrolobular ballooning, dropout, and necrosis of hepatocytes in liver biopsy specimens with cellular rejection or in rebiopsies following treatment, in our experience, were observed in patients who responded poorly to conventional rejection treatment. We have seen centrolobular hepatocellular degeneration (Fig. 17-8) in 2 cases who had treatment-resistant rejection and who were noted to have IgG and complement fixation in the sinusoids. These patients responded to subsequent treatment with cyclophosphamide and plasmapheresis, suggesting a combined humoral and cellular allograft rejection.[4] Other investigators suggested that endothelitis and/or phlebitis of hepatic vein branches may cause blockage of sinusoidal outflow, sinusoidal dilatation, and dropout of hepatocytes.

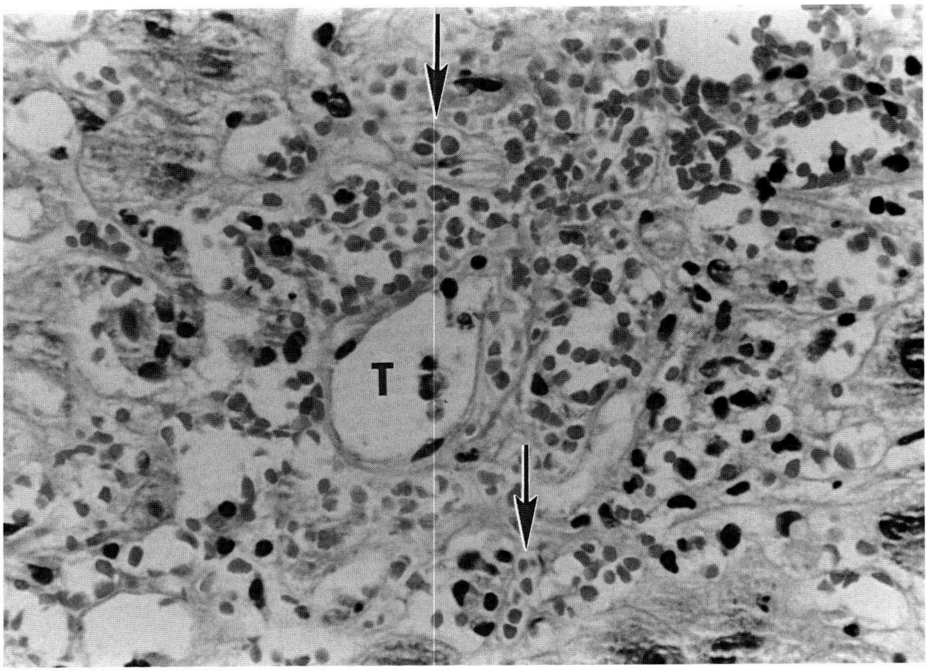

Figure 17-8. Necrosis of centrolobular hepatocytes (T = terminal hepatic venule) with red blood cells within the dilated sinusoids and spaces of Disse (arrows). Liver biopsy from a patient with severe allograft rejection, taken 7 days after OLT (H&E, ×400).

When this centrolobular necrosis persisted, ductopenia or vanishing bile duct syndrome (VBDS) often followed.[58]

Chronic Noncellular Rejection

Chronic noncellular rejection occurs weeks to months after transplantation. It is often seen 3 to 4 months after OLT, but has been observed as early as 7 weeks.[34] Chronic rejection (CR) may proceed from prolonged severe cellular rejection, multiple episodes of cellular rejection, or low-grade "ongoing" cellular rejection. The characteristic histologic changes[28-40,58-62] include (1) a decreased number of small bile ducts [vanishing bile duct syndrome, (VBDS); Figs. 17-9, 17-10]; (2) narrowing or obliteration of hepatic artery branches by subintimal accumulation of lipid-laden macrophages or foam cells (*rejection arteriopathy;* Fig. 17-11); (3) centrolobular necrosis, fibrosis, and cholestasis (Fig. 17-12); and (4) portal fibrosis with minimal inflammation.

The pathogenesis of rejection arteriopathy is not known. The presence of dendritic cells, with their important role in T-cell-dependent immune stimulation in the arterial wall, signals the occurrence of an ongoing immunologic reaction directed at native constituents of the artery or at exogenous antigens, which may permeate the damaged vessel wall.[59] While the pathogenesis is not clear, its consequences are obvious. It causes necrosis of centrolobular hepatocytes and subsequently fibrosis due to ischemia, as well as bile duct damage and loss, because bile ducts are supplied solely by the peribiliary plexus originating from

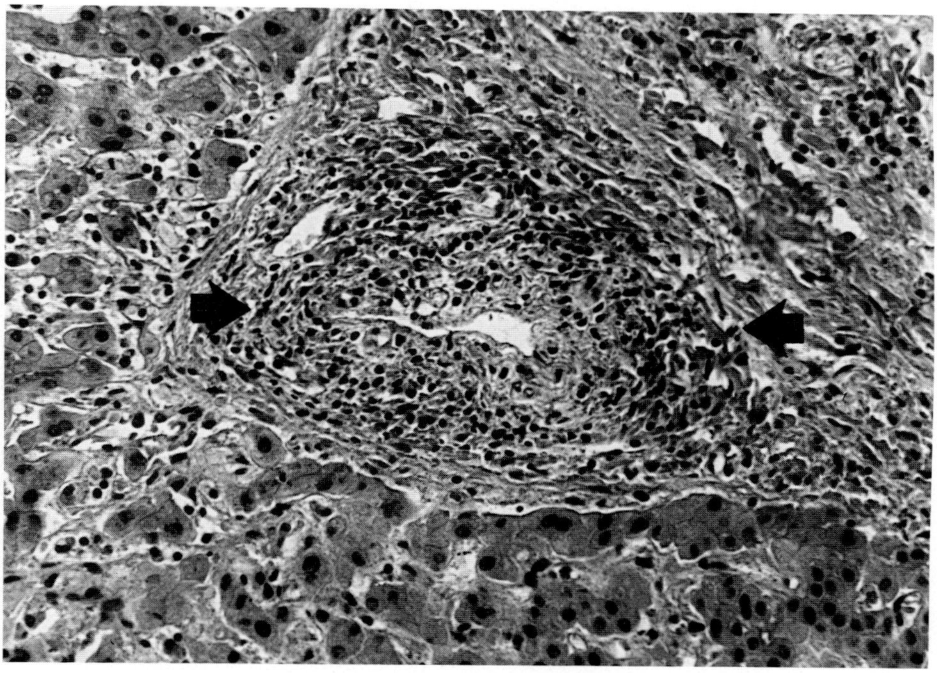

Figure 17-9. Fibroinflammatory lesion in the wall of a medium sized bile duct (arrows), resembling that seen in primary sclerosing cholangitis, in allograft removed for vanishing bile duct syndrome due to chronic rejection. (H&E, ×250).

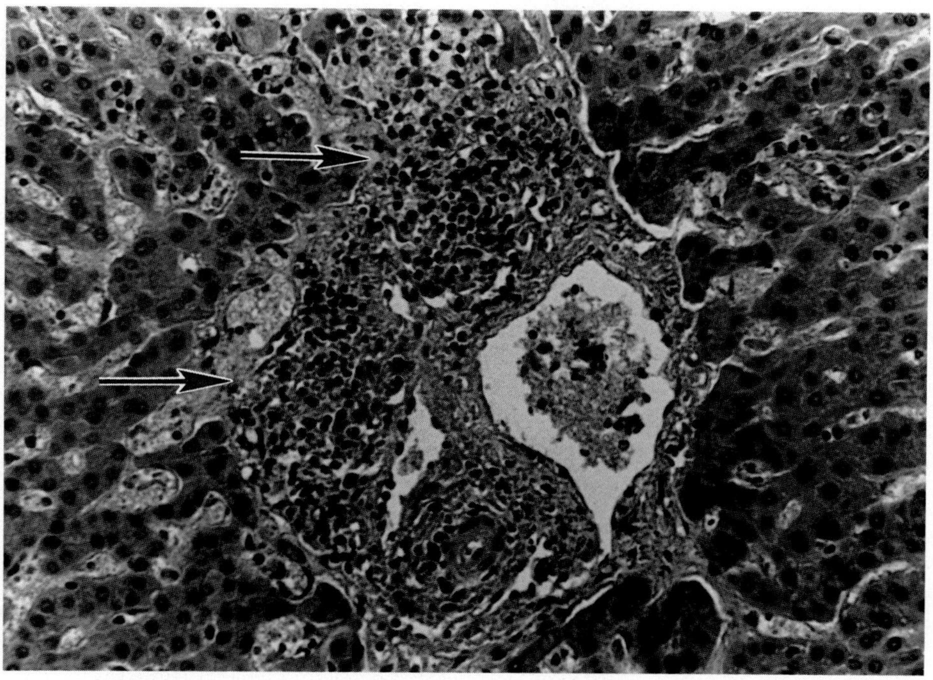

Figure 17-10. A portal tract showing lymphocytic infiltration in areas where the bile ducts were originally (arrows) in an allograft removed during retransplantation for vanishing bile duct syndrome. This inflammatory infiltrate will eventually disappear (H&E, ×100).

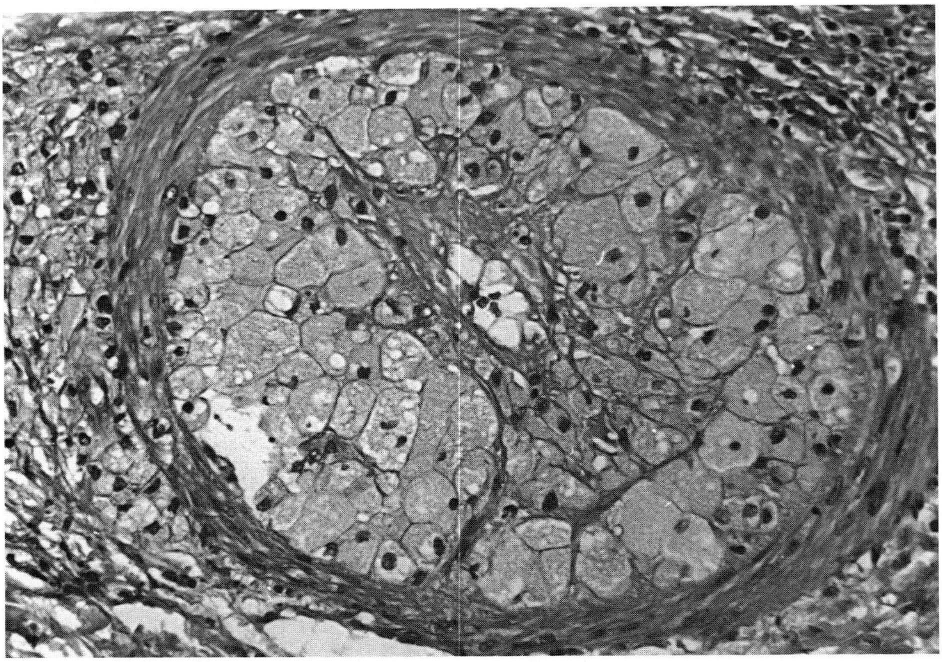

Figure 17-11. A medium-sized branch of hepatic artery showing subintimal accumulation of lipid-laden macrophages causing obliteration of its lumen. A few lymphocytic and lipid-laden cells are seen in the adventitia. Rejection arteriopathy, 4 months after OLT (H&E, ×250).

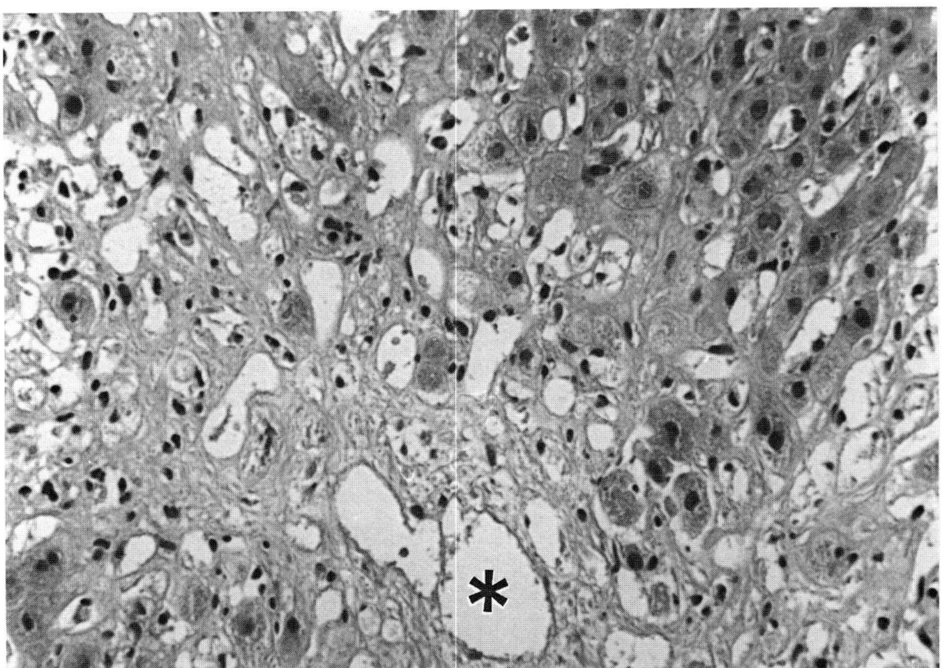

Figure 17-12. Centrolobular necrosis and fibrosis (* = terminal hepatic venule) with mild mononuclear cell infiltrate in a patient with chronic rejection and rejection arteriopathy (H&E, ×250).

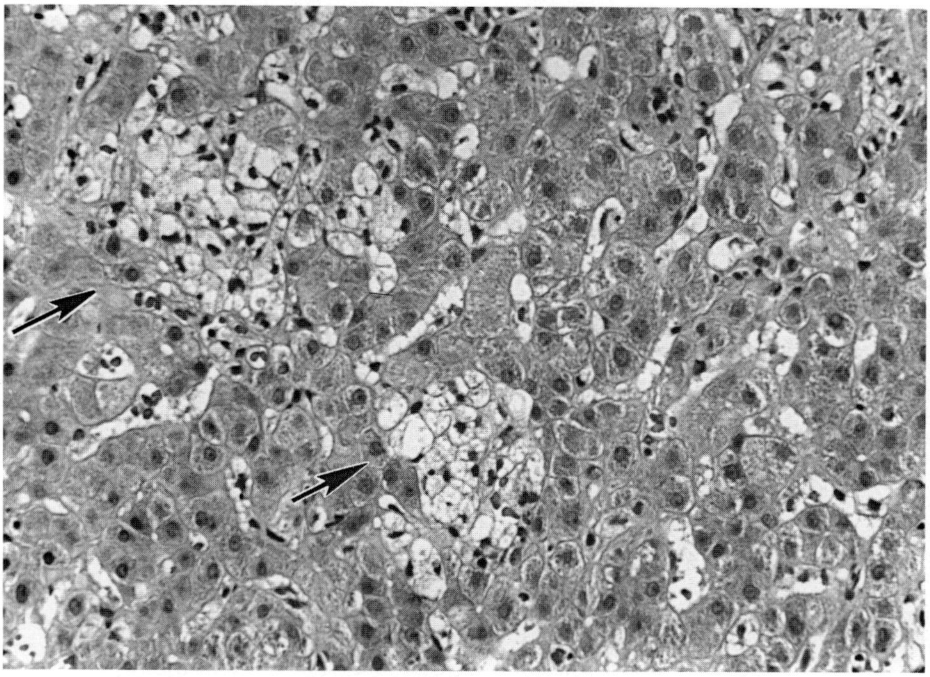

Figure 17-13. Clusters of lipid-laden macrophages in the sinusoids (arrows) of a patient with vanishing bile duct syndrome resulting from multiple episodes of severe acute cellular rejection. Four months after OLT (H&E, ×250).

the hepatic artery. This suggests that VBDS is due to ischemic injury. The similarity of bile duct lesions in CR and in graft-versus-host disease[28,35] suggests that immunologic injury is responsible for the destruction of bile ducts while histometric analysis of bile ducts supported both possible mechanisms.[60] In addition, fibroinflammatory lesions as seen typically in primary sclerosing cholangitis are observed in larger bile ducts. As the destruction continues, bile ducts become difficult to identify and special staining procedures such as trichrome or D-PAS and immunohistochemical staining such as for keratins are required to demonstrate any remaining bile duct structures.

In liver biopsy specimens, medium and large hepatic artery branches are not included, and therefore, rejection arteriopathy usually seldom contributes to the diagnosis of CR. Accumulation of these lipid laden macrophages within sinusoids (Fig. 17-13), however, is helpful in predicting the presence of rejection arteriopathy. These foam cells have also been observed within the adventitia of hepatic artery branches, in hilar nerves and lymph nodes, in the wall of large bile ducts, and within the Glisson's capsule beneath the mesothelial lining (Fig. 17-14).

Patients with CR experience an indolent asymptomatic rise in alkaline phosphatase and gamma glutamyl transferase activities and later become progressively jaundiced. The condition is usually refractory to immunosuppressive therapy and is the major cause of late graft failure. Retransplantation for CR was performed in 4 of our cases, 2 following severe, treatment-resistant acute cellular

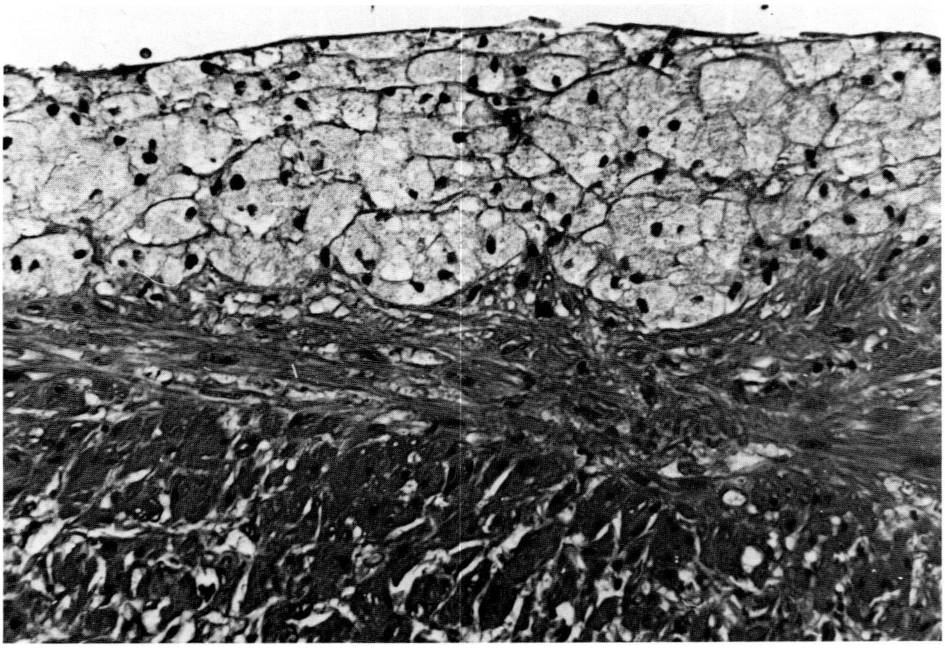

Figure 17-14. The same lipid-laden macrophages as seen in rejection arteriopathy being deposited within the Glisson capsule of an allograft with vanishing bile duct syndrome from chronic rejection. Four months after OLT (H&E, ×250).

rejection, 1 following reduction of immunosuppressive drugs due to cytomegalovirus (CMV) infection, and 1 following noncompliance of immunosuppressive drug intake. Two of these patients are still alive today.

Infection

Infections are common in the immediate posttransplantation period and frequently account for immediate postoperative mortality. In one study, infectious complications were present in 20 of 22 patients autopsied. The extrahepatic organs involved primarily by infections were lungs and brain.[63] While bacterial and fungal infections tend to involve other organ systems and rarely pose a diagnostic problem for the pathologist, viral infections often affect the allografts.

Bacterial Infections

Liver infarcts may be infected and may form abscesses, which may be seen in liver biopsy specimens. In ascending bacterial cholangitis, portal edema, proliferation of bile ductules, and PMNs around the bile ducts and within the wall and lumen of bile ducts are prominent findings. The main risk factor predisposing to bacterial infections appears to be the duration of the transplantation procedure.[64] Of all deaths resulting from infection, 81% were caused by bacterial infection.[64]

Fungal Infections

Intraabdominal fungal infections result from biliary leak, postoperative collections, perforated bowel, and wound abscesses. Systemic fungal infections may ensue and have been described in patients who succumbed.[9] The most common organisms were *Aspergillus fumigatus* followed by *Candida* species.[65] Fungal infection, however, was never encountered in liver biopsy specimens.

Viral Infections

"Opportunistic" Viruses

CYTOMEGALOVIRUS (CMV). CMV hepatitis was observed in 10 (6–7%) of our patients. Other centers have reported an incidence as high as 48%.[66] Occurring most frequently between 4 and 8 weeks posttransplantation, it represents either a primary infection or reactivation of a latent infection. Primary infection is often associated with more severe disease,[67] although we have not observed any differences pathologically. CMV infection in the liver may mimic rejection clinically and is almost invariably associated with clinical features such as fever, elevation of liver enzyme activities, leukopenia and thrombocytopenia. The characteristic histopathologic lesions, e.g., small collections (10–20 cells) of neutrophils (microabscess) or a mixed collection of inflammatory cells surrounding a necrotic hepatocyte ("microgranuloma"), and eosinophilic nuclear and basophilic cytoplasmic inclusions within enlarged mesenchymal or parenchymal cells[68,69] were seen as early as 9 days and as late as 92 days posttransplantation (Fig. 17-15). Although lobular necroinflammatory activity may be seen, extensive necrosis is rare. Immunohistochemical staining, which is performed on routine formalin-fixed, paraffin-embedded sections to localize the different CMV antigens is useful in confirming the diagnosis (Fig. 17-16). In a retrospective study, immunohistochemical staining as well as in situ hybridization for CMV-DNA (Fig. 17-17) detected CMV infection before the characteristic light-microscopic changes appeared.[70] Therefore, these sensitive techniques are used to study cases strongly suspected to have CMV infection in the absence of microabscesses or viral inclusions. It is important to confirm the diagnosis of CMV rapidly, now that an effective drug, ganciclovir is available.[71]

HERPES SIMPLEX AND VARICELLA ZOSTER VIRUSES. Herpes simplex I and II and varicella zoster have been identified as causes of allograft hepatitis. They occur earlier than CMV hepatitis, and may be diagnosed as early as 3 days posttransplantation. The clinical presentation mimic that of rejection or other type of hepatitis. In contrast to CMV hepatitis, herpes hepatitis when untreated may lead to submassive or massive hepatic necrosis.[8] Foci of circumscribed acidophilic necrosis of hepatocytes admixed with predominantly neutrophilic inflammatory cells are seen scattered within the lobules. In more severe hepatitis, these necrotic foci coalesce forming geographic areas of necrosis.[72] Viable hepatocytes in the periphery of these lesions may contain ground-glass nuclei (color plate 6). The characteristic Cowdry type A inclusions, however, are rarely seen. Multinucleated hepatocytes are sometimes present. Immunohistochemical studies are useful in detecting herpes virus antigens in the liver. Early recognition of

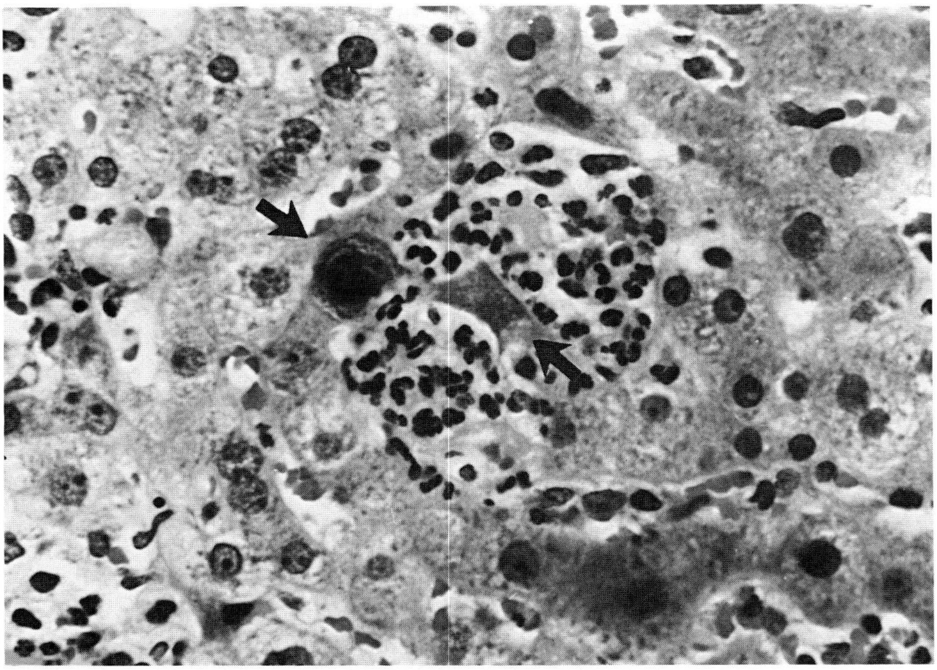

Figure 17-15. Two hepatocytes with nuclear and cytoplasmic cytomegalovirus inclusions (arrows) surrounded by a cluster of neutrophils, forming a microabscess. Twenty-five days after OLT (H&E, ×400).

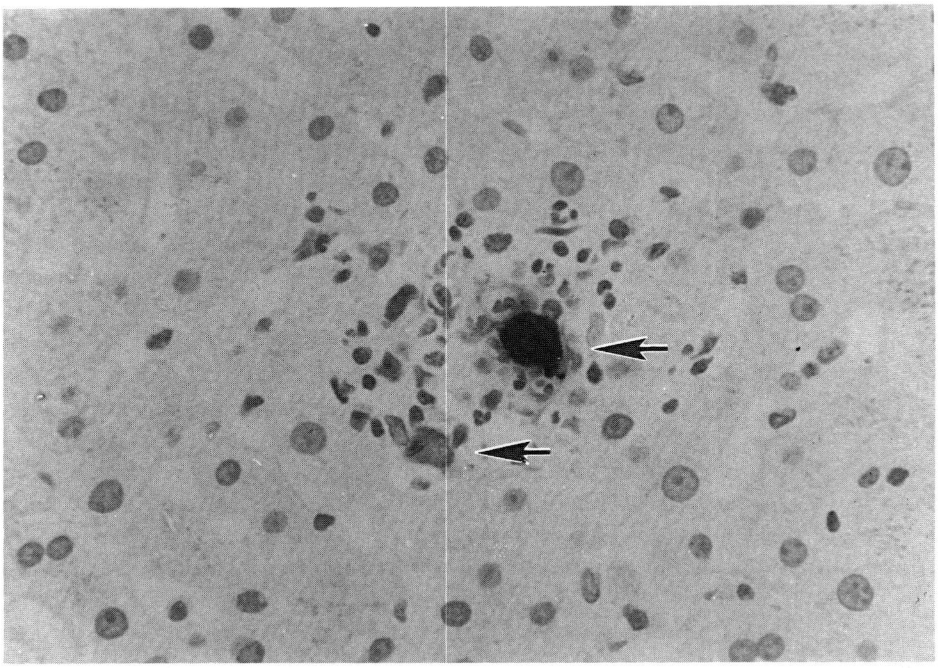

Figure 17-16. Two enlarged cells containing cytomegalovirus antigen (arrows) within a microabscess in a patient who developed CMV hepatitis 1 month after OLT (immunoperoxidase stain using monoclonal antibody to early CMVAg, counterstained with Harris' hematoxylin, ×400).

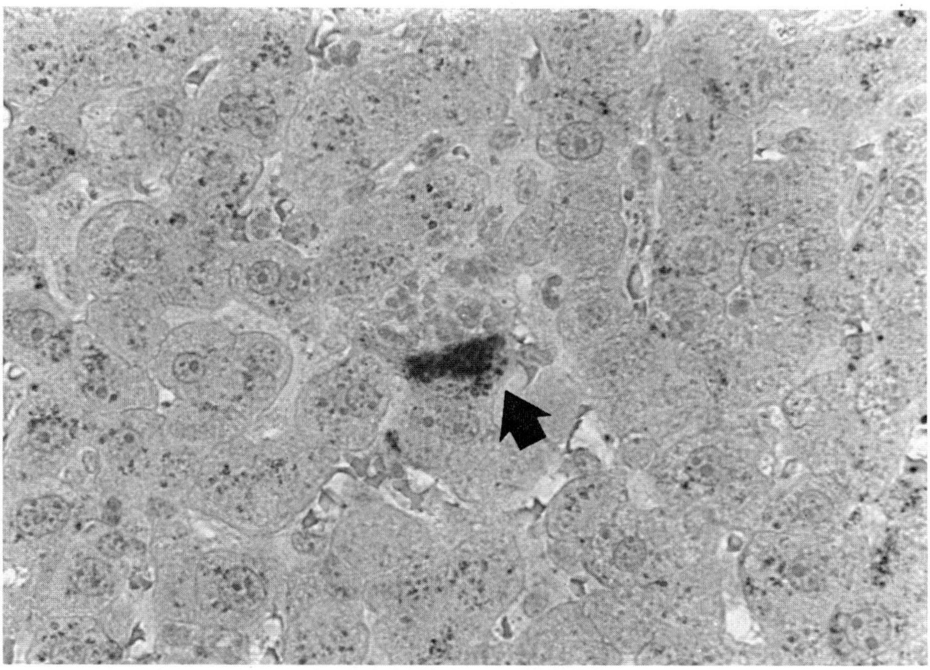

Figure 17-17. An enlarged cell containing cytomegalovirus-DNA within a microabscess (arrow) (in situ hybridization, biotin-labeled CMV-DNA probe, ×400).

the diagnosis is crucial since effective treatment is available. We have seen 3 cases of herpes hepatitis, 2 of them responded well to antiviral treatment (acyclovir) and 1 needed retransplantation for massive hepatic necrosis.

EPSTEIN-BARR VIRUS (EBV). EBV hepatitis in allografts is most commonly seen during the first 2–3 months posttransplantation. The clinical signs and symptoms are often similar to infectious mononucleosis. Mild elevations of liver enzymes are seen frequently. Circulating atypical lymphocytes constituting 10 50% of all lymphocytes in the peripheral circulation are invariably present.[73] The histopathologic alterations range from changes seen in infectious mononucleosis, i.e., infiltration of portal tracts and sinusoids by lymphocytes, some of them atypical, with only minimal hepatocellular injury[72] to a more extensive portal and sinusoidal mixed infiltrate containing atypical large noncleaved cells and immunoblasts as seen in immunoblastic lymphoma. Bile duct damage in these cases is mild, but may be difficult to differentiate from that seen in cellular rejection. Disproportionately heavy portal inflammation with mild bile duct damage favors the diagnosis of EBV infection. Immunophenotypic analysis of the infiltrate in EBV infection demonstrated predominantly B-cells in contrast to acute cellular rejection which contained mainly T-cells.[73] Immunohistochemical staining for EBV antigens and serological studies help to confirm the diagnosis.

There is an increased incidence of lymphoproliferative disorders in immunosuppressed organ transplant recipients. These tumors are most commonly of B-cell origin and are associated with active infection by EBV.[74-77] Lymphoproliferative disorders were diagnosed in 1.7% of patients from the Pittsburgh-Denver series with a median time of onset of 4.4 months after transplantation, the shortest interval between organ allograft and tumor diagnosis being 21 days.[75] The microscopic appearance of posttransplantation lymphoproliferative disorders (PTLDs) is that of a diffuse proliferation of lymphoid cells. Some lesions are polymorphic in appearance, containing varying proportions of small lymphocytes, small and large cleaved and noncleaved lymphocytes, immunoblasts, plasmacytoid and plasma cells, while others are monomorphic and composed of uniform lymphoid cells at one stage of differentiation. While the polymorphic appearance may be either nonclonal or clonal as determined by immunoglobulin gene rearrangement studies, the monomorphic appearance is often associated with clonality.[75] Both clonal and nonclonal lesions frequently regress if immunosuppression is reduced.[75,76,78]

We have seen a case of PTLD diagnosed 6 weeks after transplantation (color plate 7). The tumor occupied all portal tracts and extended into the surrounding parenchyma. The tumor was monomorphic and oligoclonal by immunoglobulin gene rearrangement studies. EBV infection was suspected in a liver biopsy specimen taken 3 weeks earlier. This diagnosis, however, was never confirmed. Retransplantation was performed for liver failure, but the patient died 4 days later. At autopsy, PTLD was found to involve other organs as well.

ADENOVIRUS. Adenovirus infection occurs in the first 4–5 weeks after transplantation. The patients often present with fever and elevation of aminotransferase activities. Histologically, foci of hepatocellular necrosis with collection of monocytoid cells are seen. Hepatocytes in the periphery of necrotic foci may contain the characteristic intranuclear inclusions.[79,80] The liver lesions are similar to those described for herpes hepatitis except for a lesser degree of hepatocellular necrosis and mononuclear inflammatory response with adenovirus infection.[8] Immunohistochemical staining for adenovirus can be performed on frozen sections to confirm the diagnosis. Under the electron microscope crystalline arrays of virions may be seen within the nuclear inclusions. We have not observed adenovirus infection among our liver allografts.

Hepatotropic Viruses. Viral hepatitis is defined as diffuse or focal hepatocellular injury, necrosis, and/or inflammation secondary to infection by a variety of viruses.[72] Viral hepatitis may be acute or chronic. Histologic features do not clearly distinguish acute from chronic hepatitis. Therefore, the two forms are separated primarily on the basis of duration of the disease, with 6 months generally being accepted for the separation.[81] The pathology of viral hepatitis in the allograft is similar to that seen in nongrafted livers.[82]

Among the hepatotropic viruses, [i.e., hepatitis A (HAV), hepatitis B (HBV), hepatitis C (HCV), hepatitis delta (HDV), and hepatitis E (HEV)], HBV and HCV are the two viruses known to infect liver allografts, either as intercurrent or recurrent infections (see below under "Recurrent Diseases").

HEPATITIS B. Intercurrent acute viral hepatitis (AVH) with the characteristic spotty necrosis can be observed a few weeks to months after liver transplantation. In the absence of acute cellular rejection, it is not difficult to make the diagnosis.

But in the presence of acute cellular rejection with its characteristic portal tract abnormalities, the diagnosis of AVH, especially when it is mild, can be easily missed, because lobular necroinflammatory changes of varying degrees may be present in rejection. Similar to nongrafted patients, liver allograft recipients with AVH may remain asymptomatic, or the disease may resolve or may progress to chronic hepatitis (either chronic persistent or chronic active hepatitis) and even to cirrhosis. Portal inflammation and fibrosis seen in chronic hepatitis B are also observed in chronic noncellular rejection. It may be difficult to differentiate or to separate these two entities. Bile duct damage and loss are more readily seen in chronic rejection. The diagnosis of hepatitis B can be confirmed by demonstration of hepatitis B viral markers and HBV-DNA in the serum and/or hepatitis B core (HBcAg) and surface (HBsAg) antigens in the liver biopsy specimens by immunohistochemical techniques.[83,84]

Intercurrent HBV infection was observed in 2 of our patients. One remained asymptomatic 2.5 years after OLT and the other developed severe acute hepatitis with extensive ballooning degeneration of hepatocytes and relatively mild lymphocytic infiltrate 2.5 months after transplant (color plate 8). In the latter patient, HBcAg was stainable in rare hepatocytic nuclei one month after OLT. Liver failure developed 4 months posttransplantation necessitating a second allograft. Hepatitis B recurred and diffuse ballooning degeneration affecting entire lobules, and bridging necrosis were observed. HBsAg remained undetectable in the liver, but HBcAg was demonstrable in many nuclei and cytoplasm of hepatocytes. The presence of HBcAg in cytoplasm is a marker for active viral replication and active liver disease.[85] Similar cases with fulminant course have been observed previously,[86] which raises the possibility that HBV in these patients may be cytopathic.

HEPATITIS C. The diagnosis of acute hepatitis C should be suspected in allograft recipients who develop rising serum aminotransferase activities 6–10 weeks posttransplantation. The histopathology of acute and chronic hepatitis C is similar, but not identical, to that of hepatitis B (see above under "Hepatitis B"). Unfortunately, it is difficult to substantiate the diagnosis. The currently available anti-HCV tests are often not helpful in confirming the diagnosis; for instance, allograft recipients with acute hepatitis C may still be negative for anti-HCV, while positive anti-HCV does not necessarily indicate hepatitis C in allografts. In a preliminary study, we confirmed the suspected pathologic diagnosis of acute hepatitis C in 8 out of 9 cases by demonstrating HCV RNA in frozen liver biopsy specimens following polymerase chain reaction (PCR). In three cases, the disease progressed to chronic hepatitis with significant activity and bridging fibrosis (Fig. 17-18). Hepatitis C may involve and damage bile ducts, and therefore, its differentiation from rejection, especially chronic noncellular rejection, is often very difficult. When both diseases are present concomitantly, difficulties arise in pointing out which process causes more liver damage.

Drug Toxicity

It is difficult to implicate a specific agent causing injury to the liver allografts because (1) the patient often receives several potential hepatotoxic drugs, (2) the

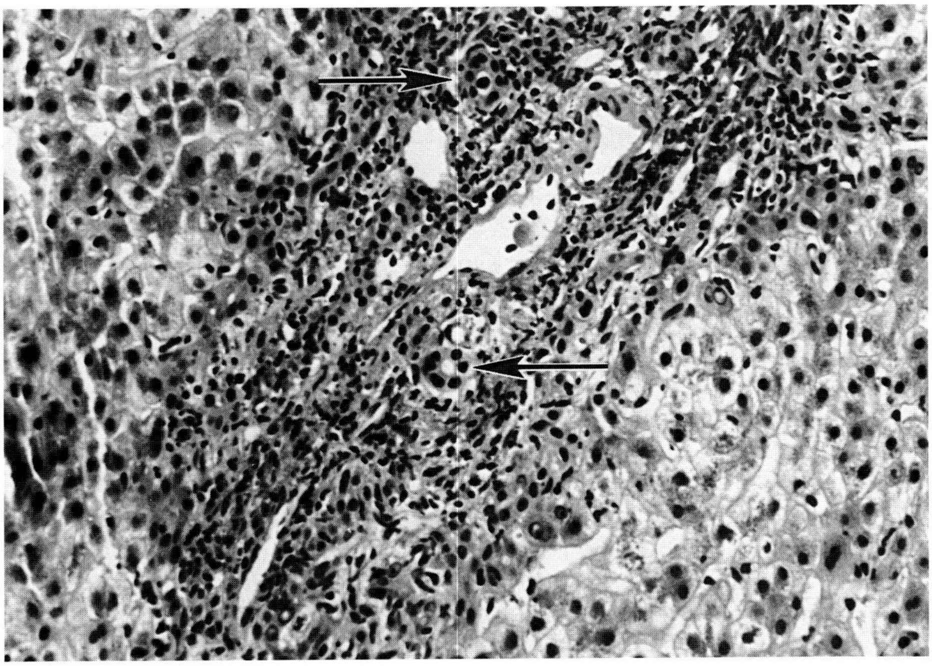

Figure 17-18. Portal fibrosis and inflammation with piecemeal necrosis. The inflammatory infiltrate consists predominantly of lymphocytes. The bile ducts are intact (arrows). This chronic hepatitis with significant activities is seen in a patient with recurrent hepatitis C 15 months after OLT (H&E, ×100).

disease(s) being treated with these agents may affect the allograft itself, and (3) hepatotoxicity of drugs commonly used in allograft recipients such as cyclosporine A and FK506 have not been defined.

Hepatotoxicity secondary to cyclosporine A therapy has been reported in transplant recipients. The frequency has ranged from 6–100% in renal allograft recipients and up to 86% in bone marrow transplant recipients.[88-90] The most frequent abnormality is elevation of the serum bilirubin level, which is dose-dependent and may be reversible if the dosage of cyclosporine A is lowered. Elevation of serum bilirubin level has also been observed in heart transplant recipients[91] and in patients receiving cyclosporine A for endogenous uveitis.[92] This mild cholestatic liver injury is usually self-limited and asymptomatic but may cause diagnostic difficulty if a preexisting liver disease is present. Obviously the most difficult group of patients to study cyclosprine A hepatotoxicity is liver transplant recipients in whom many factors may contribute to the elevation of serum bilirubin or the activities of liver enzymes. The role of cyclosporine A in "functional cholestasis," which is observed early after liver transplantation, for example, is not known. Documentation of the histopathologic findings in cyclosporine A hepatotoxicity is limited to individual case reports and animal studies.[93] These findings include cholestasis and occasional acidophilic degeneration of hepatocytes.[94] Centrolobular steatosis, in addition to the above findings, has been reported in animal studies.[93]

The other known hepatotoxic drugs are thought to cause liver damage in allografts, similar to that in native livers. We have seen acute drug-induced hepatitis in a patient who continued to take prophylactic isoniazide after OLT. The serum aminotransferase levels started to rise 9 days after transplantation. The liver biopsy specimen at that time revealed acute hepatitis, which persisted in the subsequent biopsy 14 days later. The serum aminotransferase levels normalized with cessation of the drug.

Hyperalimentation

Prolonged total parenteral nutrition (TPN) is sometimes necessary in liver allograft recipients. The histopathologic alterations produced by TPN are similar to those described in nongrafted livers.[95-98] These changes include hepatocellular and canalicular cholestasis, steatosis, portal inflammation, and fibrosis with proliferation of bile ductules. It is important to recognize the changes due to TPN, so that they are not imputed to other causes such as mechanical biliary obstruction.

Recurrent Diseases

Hepatic malignancies,[99,100] viral hepatitis type B and C,[82,86,101-103] and Budd-Chiari syndrome[104] are known to recur after liver transplantation.

Tumor Recurrence

Tumor recurrence is the most common cause of death in patients who underwent liver transplantation for hepatocellular carcinoma, cholangiocarcinoma, or metastatic tumors.[99] Recurrent or metastatic neoplasms may occur either in the transplanted liver or at extrahepatic sites. Longer survival, however, is seen in patients who have low-grade malignant tumors, such as fibrolamellar hepatocellular carcinoma, epithelioid hemangioendothelioma, and metastatic neuroendocrine tumors.

Recurrence of Viral Hepatitis

Hepatitis B. Recurrence of hepatitis B in the allografts has been well documented. The histopathologic findings are identical to those described in intercurrent hepatitis B (see above). Because of the high recurrence rate of this infection, liver transplantation for hepatitis B patients should be considered only when HBV DNA is undetectable in the serum. The native livers removed during transplantation in our cases revealed cytoplasmic HBsAg and no or rare nuclear HBcAg, as demonstrated by immunohistochemical studies. This pattern of HBV antigen expression is consistent with an inactive phase of HBV replication.[83,84,105] In one case, in addition to cytoplasmic HBsAg, rare cytoplasmic HBcAg was noted. HBV infection recurred in this patient 8 months after transplantation. The liver biopsy specimen contained scattered ground-glass hepatocytes and mild lobular necroinflammatory lesions. Unfortunately, three other patients died early (7, 14, and 34 days) after transplantation from other causes. One patient is still free from HBV infection (serum HBV DNA is negative) 3 months posttransplantation.

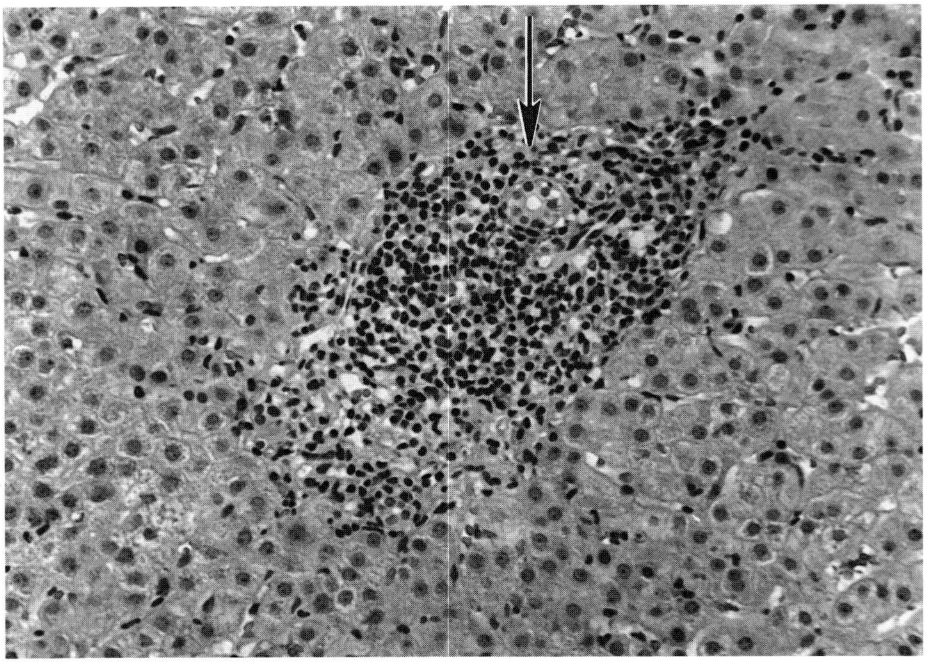

Figure 17-19. Recurrent hepatitis C in patient 2 years after OLT. The portal tract is infiltrated predominantly by lymphocytes which spare the bile duct (arrow). Piecemeal necrosis is minimal (H&E, ×100).

Hepatitis C. With the availability of specific markers for HCV, such as the detection of HCV-RNA following PCR, recurrent HCV infection in liver allografts has been documented.[87] The histopathologic findings range from acute hepatitis to chronic hepatitis with or without piecemeal necrosis (Figs. 17-18, 17-19).

Budd-Chiari Syndrome

Budd-Chiari syndrome may recur.[105] The incidence of recurrence is lower when the underlying disease, such as myeloproliferative disorder, is being treated.

Recurrence of other chronic diseases of the liver such as primary biliary cirrhosis, primary sclerosing cholangitis, and autoimmune chronic active hepatitis have been reported.[106,107] The lack of unequivocal markers of these diseases and specific or pathognomonic biopsy findings, however, make it difficult or impossible to confirm the diagnosis.

REFERENCES

1. Kakizoe S, Yanaga K, Starzl TE, et al: Evaluation of protocol before transplantation and after reperfusion biopsies from human orthotopic liver allografts: Considerations of preservation and early immunological injury. *Hepatology* 11:932–941, 1990.
2. Todo S, Demetris AJ, Makowka L, et al: Primary nonfunction of hepatic allografts with preexisting fatty infiltration. *Transplantation* 47:903–905, 1989.

3. Thung SN, Bach N, Miller CM, Schaffner F: Antibody-mediated liver allograft rejection is associated with poor prognosis. *Hepatology* 10:673, 1989.
4. Evrard H, Miller C, Schwartz M, et al: Resistant hepatic allograft rejection successfully treated with cyclophosphamide and plasmapheresis. *Transplantation* 50:702–704, 1990.
5. Shieh YSC, Shim KS, Lampertico P, et al: Detection of hepatitis C sequences in liver tissue by the polymerase chain reaction. *Lab Invest* 65:408–411, 1991.
6. Thung SN, Gerber MA, Sarno E, Popper H: Distribution of 5 antigens in hepatocellular carcinoma. *Lab Invest* 41:101–105, 1979.
7. Lai Y-S, Thung SN, Gerber MA, et al: Expression of cytokeratin in normal and diseased livers and in primary liver carcinomas. *Arch Pathol Lab Med* 113:134–138, 1989.
8. Theise ND, Schwartz M, Miller C, Thung SN: Macroregenerative nodules and hepatocellular carcinoma in forty-four sequential adult liver explants with cirrhosis. *Hepatology* 14:49A, 1991.
9. Demetris AJ, Jaffe R, Starzl TE: A review of adult and pediatric post-transplant liver pathology. *Pathol Annu* 11:347–386, 1987.
10. Ludwig J: Histopathology of the liver following transplantation. In Maddrey WC: *Transplantation of the Liver,* p 191, New York, Elsevier, 1988.
11. Gerber MA, Thung SN: Normal histology of the liver. *Am J Surg Pathol* 11:709–722, 1987.
12. Christoffersen P, Poulsen H, Skeie E: Focal liver cell necrosis accompanied by infiltration of granulocytes arising during operation. *Acta Hepato-Splenologia (Stuttgart)* 17:240–245, 1970.
13. Gall EA, Dobrogorski O: Hepatic alterations in obstructive jaundice. *Am J Clin Pathol* 41:126–130, 1964.
14. Review by an International Group: Histopathology of the intrahepatic biliary tree. *Liver* 3:161–175, 1983.
15. Male AJ: The minute structure of the liver: a review. *Glasgow Med J* 32:283–301, 1951.
16. Mitra SK: The terminal distribution of the hepatic artery with special reference to arterio-portal anastomosis. *J Anat* 100:651–663, 1966.
17. Masuko K, Rubin E, Popper H: Proliferation of bile ducts in cirrhosis. *Arch Pathol* 78:421–431, 1964.
18. Thung SN: The development of proliferating ductular structures in liver disease. An immunohistochemical study. *Arch Pathol Lab Med* 114:407–411, 1990.
19. Wight DGD: Differential diagnosis of cholestasis in liver allografts. *Transplant Proc* 18:152–156, 1986.
20. Loeffler L: Factors determining necrosis or survival of liver tissue after ligation of hepatic artery. *Arch Pathol* 21:496–503, 1936.
21. McMaster P, Walton RM, White DGD, et al: The influence of ischaemia on the biliary tract. *Br J Surg* 67:321–324, 1980.
22. Seeley TT, Blumenfeld CM, Ikeda R, et al: Hepatic infarction. *Human Pathol* 3:265–276, 1972.
23. Rappaport AM: Physioanatomic considerations. In Schiff L, Schiff ER: *Diseases of the Liver,* 5th ed, pp 1–57, Philadelphia, Lippincott, 1982.
24. Tzakis AG, Gordon RD, Shaw BW, Jr, et al: Clinical presentation of hepatic artery thrombosis after liver transplantation in the cyclosporine era. *Transplantation* 40:667–671, 1985.

25. Russo PA, Yunis EJ: Subcapsular hepatic necrosis in orthotopic liver allografts. *Hepatology* 6:708–713, 1986.
26. Lerut JP, Iwatsuki S, Starzl TE: Human orthotopic liver transplantation: surgical aspects in 393 consecutive grafts. *Transplant Proc* 20:603–606, 1988.
27. Hubscher SG, Adams DH, Buckels JAC, et al: Massive haemorrhagic necrosis of the liver after liver transplantation. *J Clin Pathol* 42:360–370, 1989.
28. Demetris AJ, Lasky S, Van Thiel DH: Pathology of hepatic transplantation. A review of 62 adult allograft recipients immunosuppressed with a cyclosporine/steroid regimen. *Am J Pathol* 118:151–161, 1985.
29. Snover DC, Freese DK, Sharp HL, et al: Liver allograft rejection. An analysis of the use of biopsy in determining outcome of rejection. *Am J Surg Pathol* 11:1–10, 1987.
30. Vierling JM, Fennell RH, Jr: Histopathology of early and late human hepatic allograft rejection: evidence of progressive destruction of interlobular bile ducts. *Hepatology* 5:1076–1082, 1985.
31. Gouw ASH, Snover DC, Grond J, et al: Acute rejection in human liver grafts: a comparative histologic study of cases maintained on azathioprine and prednisone versus cyclosporine A and low-dose steroids. *Hum Pathol* 19:1036–1042, 1988.
32. Kemnitz J, Ringe B, Cohnert TR, et al. Bile duct injury as a part of diagnostic criteria for liver allograft rejection. *Hum Pathol* 20:132–143, 1989.
33. Eggink HF, Hofsteen N, Gips CH, et al. Histopathology of serial graft biopsies from liver transplant recipients. *Am J Pathol* 114:18–31, 1984.
34. Ludwig J, Wiesner RH, Batts KP, et al. The acute vanishing bile duct syndrome (acute irreversible rejection) after orthotopic liver transplantation. *Hepatology* 7: 476–483, 1987.
35. Portmann B, Neuberger JM, William R: Intrahepatic bile duct lesions. In Calne RY: *Liver Transplantation: The Cambridge–Kings's College Hospital Experience*, pp 279–287, New York, Grune & Stratton, 1983.
36. Cuervas-Mons V, Martinez AJ, Dekker A, et al: Adult liver transplantation: an analysis of the early causes of death in 40 consecutive cases. *Hepatology* 6:495–501, 1986.
37. Ludwig J, Batts KP, Ploch M, et al: Endotheliitis in hepatic allografts. *Mayo Clin Proc* 64:545–554, 1989.
38. Ludwig J. Classifications and terminology of hepatic allograft rejection: Whither bound? *Mayo Clin Proc* 64:676–679, 1989.
39. Hubscher SG, Clements D, Elias E, et al: Biopsy findings in cases of rejection of liver allograft. *J Clin Pathol* 38:1366–1373, 1985.
40. Snover DC, Sibley RK, Freese DK, et al: Orthotopic liver transplantation. A pathological study of 63 serial liver biopsies from 17 patients with specific reference to the diagnostic features and natural history of rejection. *Hepatology* 4:1212–1222, 1984.
41. Busch GJ, Reynolds ES, Galvanek EG, et al: Human renal allografts. The role of vascular injury in early graft failure. *Medicine* 50:29–83, 1971.
42. Weil R, Clarke DR, Iwaki, et al: Hyperacute rejection of a transplanted human heart. *Transplantation* 32:71–72, 1981.
43. Williams GM, DePlangue B, Graham WR, et al: Participation of antibodies in acute cardiac-allograft rejection in man. *New Engl J Med* 281:1145–1150, 1969.
44. Williams GM, Hume DM, Hudson RP, Jr, et al: "Hyperacute" renal-homograft rejection in man. *New Engl J Med* 279:611–618, 1968.

45. Duquesnoy RJ: Is there hyperacute rejection of the liver? *Transplant Proc* 21:3506–3507, 1989.

46. Demetris AJ, Jaffe R, Tzakis A, et al: Antibody mediated rejection of human orthotopic liver allografts: a study of liver transplantation across ABO blood group barriers. *Am J Pathol* 132:489–502, 1988.

47. Starzl TE, Demetris AJ, Todo S, et al: Evidence for hyperacute rejection of human liver grafts: the case of the canary kidneys. *Clin Transplant* 3:37–45, 1989.

48. Brasile L, Zebre T, Rabin B: Identification of the antibody to vascular endothelial cells in patients undergoing cardiac transplantation. *Transplantation* 40:672–675, 1985.

49. Claas FHJ, Paul LC, VanEs LA, et al: Antibodies against donor antigens on endothelial cells and monocytes in eluates of rejected kidney allografts. *Tissue Antigens* 15(Suppl):19–24, 1980.

50. Stastny P: Endothelial-monocyte antigens. *Transplant Proc* 12(Suppl):32–36, 1980.

51. Knechtle SJ, Kolbeck PC, Tsuchimoto S, et al: Hepatic transplantation into sensitized recipients. *Transplantation* 43:8–12, 1987.

52. Houssin D, Bellon B, Brunaud MD, et al: Interactions between liver allografts and lymphocytotoxic alloantibodies in inbred rats. *Hepatology* 6:994–998, 1986.

53. Demetris AJ, Lasky S, Van Thiel DH, et al: Induction of Dr/Ia antigens in human liver allografts. *Transplantation* 40:504–509, 1985.

54. Perkins JD, Rakela J, Sterioff S, et al: Immunohistologic pattern of the portal T-lymphocyte infiltration in hepatic allograft rejection. *Mayo Clin Proc* 64:565–569, 1989.

55. Gouw ASH, Huitema S, Grond J, et al: Early induction of MHC antigens in human liver grafts. An immunohistologic study. *Am J Pathol* 133:82–94, 1988.

56. Wight DCD: Pathology of rejection. In Calne RY: *Liver Transplantation: The Cambridge–King's College Hospital Experience,* pp 247–277, New York, Grune & Stratton, 1983.

57. Fennel RH, Jr, Vierling JM: Electron microscopy of rejected human liver allografts. *Hepatology* 5:1083–1087, 1985.

58. Ludwig J, Gross JB, Jr, Perkins JD, et al: Persistent centrilobular necroses in hepatic allografts. *Hum Pathol* 21:656–661, 1990.

59. Oguma S, Banner B, Zerbe T, et al: Participation of dendritic cells in vascular lesions of chronic rejection of human allografts. *Lancet* 2:933–936, 1988.

60. Oguma S, Belle S, Starzl TE, et al: A histometric analysis of chronically rejected human liver allografts: insights into the mechanisms of bile duct loss: direct immunologic and ischemic factors. *Hepatology* 9:204–209, 1989.

61. Grond J, Gouw ASH, Poppema S, et al: Chronic rejection in liver transplants: a histopathologic analysis of failed grafts and antecedent serial biopsies. *Transplant Proc* 18:128–135, 1986.

62. Nakkleh RE, Schwarzenberg SJ, Bloomer J, et al: The pathology of liver allografts surviving longer than one year. *Hepatology* 11:465–470, 1990.

63. Markin RS, Hollins S, Wood RP, et al: Main autopsy findings in liver transplant patients. *Modern Pathol* 2:339–342, 1989.

64. Paya CV, Hermans PE: Bacterial infections after liver transplantation. *Eur J Clin Microbiol Infect Dis* 8:499–504, 1989.

65. Cuervas-Mons V, Martinez AJ, Dekker A, et al: Adult liver transplantation: An analysis of the early causes of death in 40 consecutive cases. *Hepatology* 6:495–501, 1986.

66. Gorensek MJ, Carey WD, Vogt D, et al: A multivariate analysis of risk factors for cytomegalovirus infection in liver transplant recipients. *Gastroenterology* 98:1326–1332, 1990.

67. Salt A, Sutehall G, Sargaison M, et al: Viral and *Toxoplasma gondii* infections in children after liver transplantation. *J Clin Pathol* 43:63–67, 1990.

68. Bach N, Thung SN, Berk PD: The liver in acquired immunodeficiency syndrome (AIDS). In Bianchi L, Gerok W, Maier KP: *Infectious Diseases of the Liver,* p 333, Boston, Kluwer Academic Publishers, 1990.

69. Sieratzki J, Thung SN, Gerber MA, et al: Major histocompatibility antigen expression in the liver in acquired immunodeficiency syndrome. *Arch Pathol Lab Med* 111:1045–1049, 1987.

70. Paya CV, Holley KE, Wiesner RH: Early diagnosis of cytomegalovirus hepatitis in liver transplant recipients: role of immunostaining, DNA hybridization and culture of hepatic tissue. *Hepatology* 12:119–126, 1990.

71. Erice A, Jordan MC, Chace BA, et al: Ganciclovir treatment of cytomegalovirus disease in transplant recipients and other immunocompromised hosts. *JAMA* 257:3082–3087, 1987.

72. Gerber MA, Thung SN: Viral hepatitis: Pathology. In Berk JE, Haubrich WS, Kalser MH, Roth JLA, Schaffner F: *Bockus Gastroenterology,* Vol V, *The Liver,* p 2825, Philadelphia, Saunders, 1985.

73. Randhawa PS, Markin RS, Starzl TE, et al: Epstein-Barr virus associated syndromes in immunosuppressed liver transplant recipients. Clinical profile and recognition on routine allograft biopsy. *Am J Surg Pathol* 14:538–547, 1990.

74. Ho M, Jaffe R, Miller G, et al: The frequency of EBV infection and associate lymphoproliferative syndrome after transplantation and its manifestations in children. *Transplantation* 45:719–727, 1988.

75. Nalesnik MA, Jaffe R, Starzl TE, et al: The pathology of posttransplant lymphoproliferative disorders occurring in the setting of cyclosporine A- prednisone immunosuppression. *Am J Pathol* 133:173–192, 1988.

76. Hanto DW, Frizzera G, Gajl-Peczalska KJ, et al: Epstein-Barr virus, immunodeficiency, and B-cell lymphoproliferation. *Transplantation* 39:461–472, 1985.

77. Purtilo DT, Tatsumi E, Manolov G, et al: Epstein-Barr virus as an etiological agent in the pathogenesis of lymphoproliferative and aproliferative diseases in immune deficient patients. *Int Rev Exp Pathol* 27:113–181, 1985.

78. Starzl TE, Nalesnik MA, Porter KA, et al: Reversibility of lymphomas and lymphoproliferative lesions developing under Cyclosporine-steroid therapy. *Lancet* 2:584–587, 1984.

79. Carmichael GP, Jr, Zahradnik JM, Mayer GF, et al: Adenovirus hepatitis in an immunosuppressed adult. *Am J Clin Pathol* 71:352–355, 1979.

80. Zuckerman AJ: *Virus Diseases of the Liver,* p 98, London, Butterworths, 1970.

81. Leevy CM, Popper H, Sherlock S (criteria committee): Diseases of the liver and biliary tract: standardization of nomenclature, diagnostic criteria and diagnostic methodology. *Fogarty International Center Proceedings No 22, DHEW Publication No (NIH) 76-725.* Washington, DC, US Government Printing Office, 1976.

82. Demetris AJ, Jaffee R, Sheahan DG, et al: Hepatitis B in liver allograft recipients. Differentiation between viral hepatitis B and rejection. *Am J Pathol* 125:161–172.

83. Gerber MA, Thung SN: The localization of hepatitis virus in tissues. *Int Rev Exp Pathol* 29:49–76, 1979.

84. Gerber MA, Thung SN: The diagnostic value of immunohistochemical demonstration for hepatitis viral antigens in the liver. *Hum Pathol* 18:771–774, 1987.

85. Hoofnagle JH, Dusheiko GM, Seeff LB, et al: Seroconversion from hepatitis B antigen to antibody in chronic type B hepatitis. *Ann Int Med* 94:744–748, 1981.

86. Ming W, Todo S, Fung JJ, et al: Analysis of hepatitis B viral antigen expression in liver allografts: correlation with HBV serology and histopathology. *Hepatology* (in press).

87. Shim K-S, Thung SN, Shieh YSC, et al: Hepatitis C in liver transplants. *Gastroenterology* 100:795, 1991

88. Starzl TE, Klintmalm GBG, Weil R, et al: Cyclosporine A and steroid therapy in 66 cadaver kidney recipients. *Surg Gynecol Obstet* 153:486–494, 1981.

89. European Multicentre Trial Group: Cyclosporine in cadaveric renal transplantation: One year follow-up of a multicentre trial. *Lancet* 2:986–987, 1983.

90. Klintmalm GB, Iwatsuki S, Starzl TE: Cyclosporin A hepatotoxicity in 66 renal allograft recipients. *Transplantation* 32:488–496, 1981.

91. Schade RR, Gugliemi DH, Van Thiel DH, et al: Cholestasis in heart transplant recipients treated with cyclosporine. *Transplant Proc* 15:2757–2760, 1983.

92. Kassianides C, Nussenblatt R, Palestine AG, et al: Liver injury from Cyclosporine A. *Dig Dis Sci* 35:693–697, 1990.

93. Farthing MJG, Clark ML: Nature of the toxicity of cyclosporin A in the rat. *Biochem Pharmacol* 30:3311–3316, 1981.

94. Hamilton DV, Evans DB, Thiru S: Toxicity of cyclosporin A in organ grafting. In White DJG: *Cyclosporin A: Proceedings of an International Conference on Cyclosporin A,* p 393, Amsterdam, Elsevier, 1982.

95. Hodes JE, Grosfeld JL, Weber TR, et al: Hepatic failure in infants on total parenteral nutrition (TPN): clinical and histopathologic observations. *J Ped Surg* 17:463–468, 1982.

96. Cohen C, Olsen MM: Pediatric total parenteral nutrition. Liver histopathology. *Arch Pathol Lab Med* 105:152–156, 1980.

97. Fouin-Fortunet H, LeQuernec L, Erlinger S, et al: Hepatic alterations during total parenteral nutrition in patients with inflammatory bowel disease. A possible consequence of lithocholate toxicity. *Gastroenterology* 82:932–937, 1982.

98. Barrett Dahms B, Halpin TC Jr: Serial liver biopsies in parenteral nutrition—associated cholestasis of early infancy. *Gastroenterology* 81:136–144, 1981.

99. Portmann B, O'Grady J, Williams R: Disease recurrence following orthotopic liver transplantation. *Transplant Proc* 13:136–143, 1986.

100. Iwatsuki S, Gordon RD, Shaw B, Starzl TE: Role of liver transplantation in cancer therapy. *Ann Surg* 202:401–406, 1985.

101. Wight DGD: Pathology of liver transplantation (other than rejection). In Calne RY: *Liver Transplantation: The Cambridge–King's College Hospital Experience,* p 289, New York, Grune & Stratton, 1983.

102. Corman JL, Putman CW, Iwatsuki S, et al: Liver allograft. Its uses in chronic active hepatitis with macronodular cirrhosis, hepatitis B surface antigen. *Arch Surg* 114:75–78, 1979.

103. Todo S, Demetris AJ, Van Thiel DH, et al: Orthotopic liver B transplantation for patients with hepatitis B virus related liver disease: *Hepatology* 13:619–626, 1991

104. Seltman HJ, Dekker A, Van Thiel DH, et al: Budd-Chiari syndrome recurring in a transplanted liver. *Gastroenterology* 84:640–643, 1983.

105. Gerber MA, Thung SN: Biology of disease: molecular and cellular pathology of hepatitis B. *Lab Invest* 52:572–590, 1985.

106. Neuberger J, Portmann B, Macdougall BRD, et al: Recurrence of primary biliary cirrhosis after liver transplantation. *New Engl J Med* 306:1–4, 1982.

107. Neuberger J, Portmann B, Calne R, et al: Recurrence of autoimmune chronic active hepatitis following orthotopic liver grafting. *Transplantation* 37:363–365, 1983.

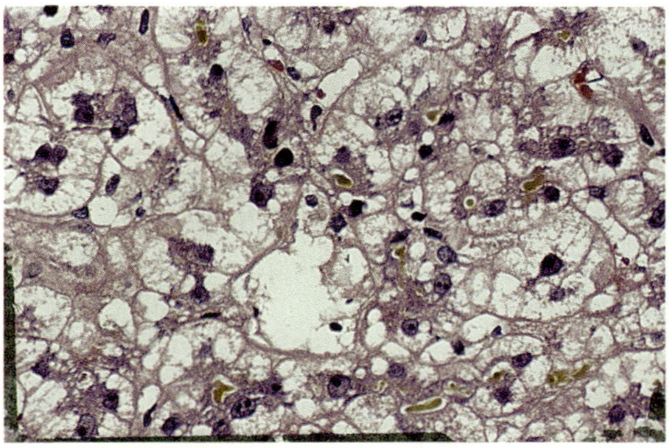

Plate 1: Functional cholestasis. Centrolobular cholestasis and feathery degeneration of hepatocytes observed 7 days after OLT (H&E, ×400).

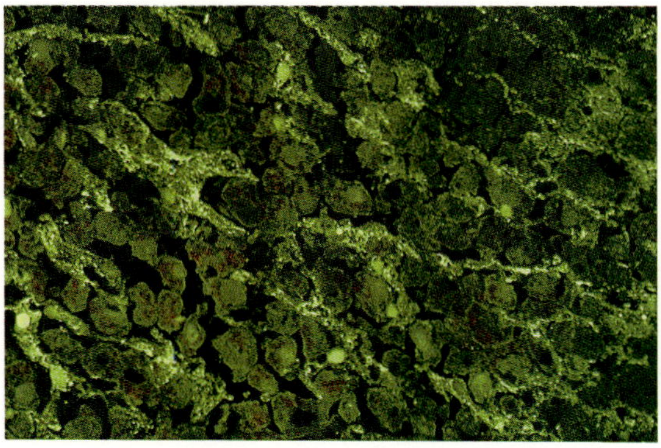

Plate 2: Hyperacute allograft rejection. Granular deposition of IgG within the sinusoids in a 2 hours postperfusion liver biopsy specimen. (Direct immunofluorescence, ×250).

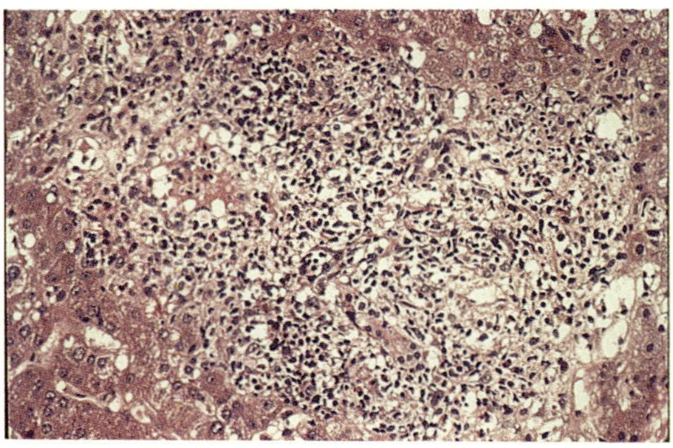

Plate 3: Acute cellular rejection. Edema and mixed cellular inflammatory infiltration of the portal tract. Endothelitis of the portal vein and rejection cholangitis are noted. (H&E, ×100).

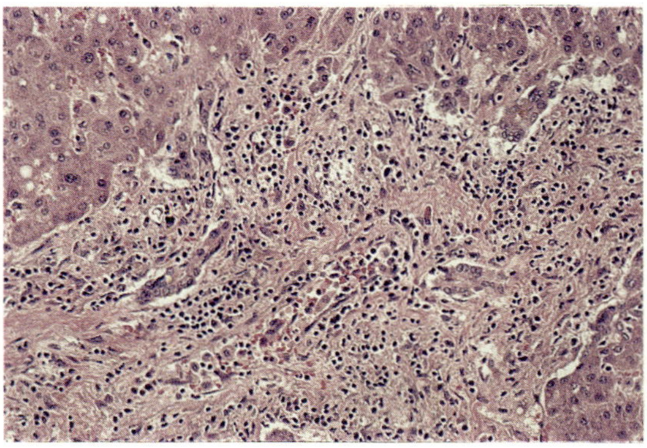

Plate 4: Partially treated rejection. Portal tract is still enlarged, but contains less inflammatory cells. There is mild proliferation of bile ductules. (Same patient as Color plate 3 after 1 week of antirejection treatment; H&E, ×100).

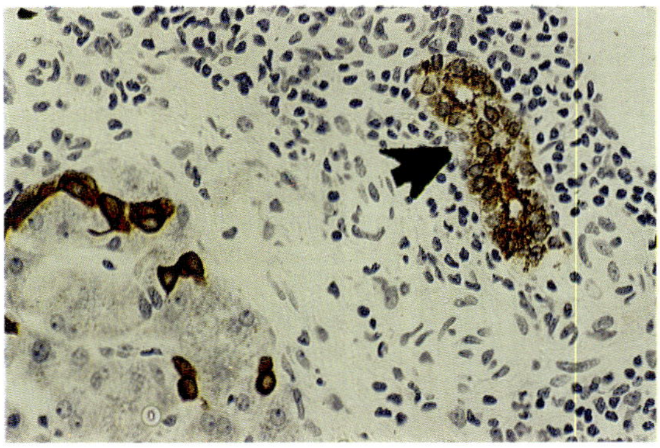

Plate 5: Partially treated rejection. The bile duct remains abnormal (arrow). (Same biopsy specimen as in color plate 4; immunoperoxidase stain using anti-cytokeratin antibodies, ×100).

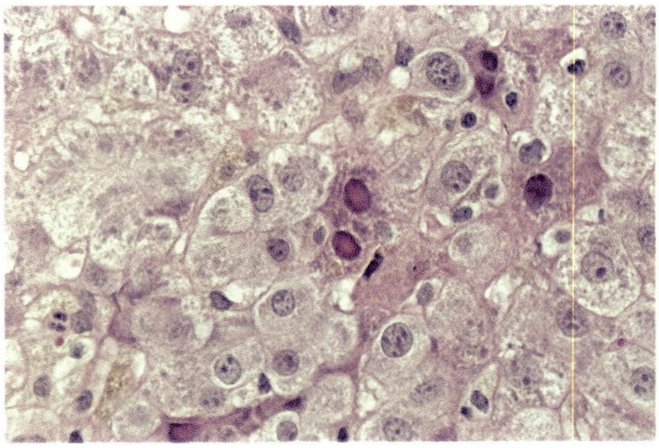

Plate 6: Herpes hepatitis. Many hepatocytes undergoing eosinophilic degeneration. Two of them have ground glass nuclei. (H&E, ×100).

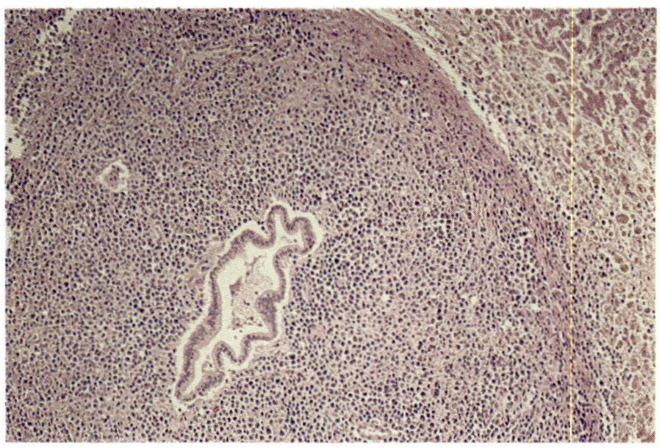

Plate 7: Posttransplantation lymphoproliferative disease. Portal tract enlargement by "monomorphic" immunoblasts in liver biopsy specimen 7 weeks after OLT. The bile duct (center) is intact (H&E, ×100).

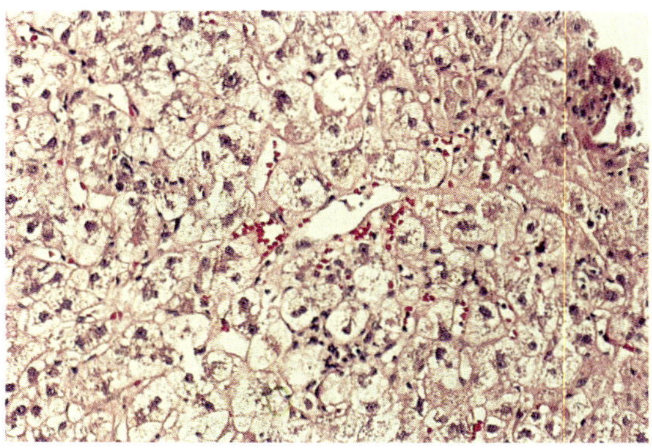

Plate 8: Acute hepatitis B. Ballooning of hepatocytes in a patient who acquired hepatitis B infection after OLT. Liver biopsy specimen taken two and a half months after OLT (H&E, ×250).

— Appendix A —
SOCIAL SUPPORT FOR LIVER TRANSPLANTATION

Barbara Klion and Erica Miller

Liver transplantation marks a monumental event in the lives of all transplant recipients and their families. This potential gift of life imposes an entirely new and unique set of rules and guidelines for daily activity and has a profound impact on patients, families, and friends.

Beginning with evaluation and acceptance for transplantation, entire families must face the enormity of this medical crisis. They are immediately confronted with the possibility that the patient may actually die while awaiting transplantation, thus creating a very strong desire to be with their loved one in order to provide both physical and emotional assistance during this pretransplant period. Transplantation is not only the patient's problem, but the problem of the entire family. They all need to be supported in order to be supportive.

Entire families may be uprooted from their homes and jobs. They can experience an abrupt change in their social and/or economic status resulting in an acute dependence on others. They may also face problems of separation, role reversal, and loneliness. Some patients experience feelings of guilt, as a manifestation of their illness, because of the burden that their illness imposes on their family and friends.

FAMILY CENTERS

One nonmedical solution to this extraordinary medical crisis has been the establishment of guest houses to accommodate the transplant family. Whether known as "family houses," "hospitality houses," or "Ronald McDonald houses," the effect that these alternative shelters have on the total recovery of the patients along with the well-being of their families has proved to be invaluable. Families need a caring environment where they can share their feelings. They need to know they are never quite alone and that there are others who also share their hopes, expectations, fears, trepidations, sorrows, and joys. They need to know that some normalcy of life can go on during an otherwise less than normal time. The complete transplant experience is not just the patient's problem, but it is the problem of the entire family. The family centers provide a temporary, economic, and safe haven where private sleeping accommodations, combined with communal living, cooking, and dining spaces become their own form of support group. The natural networking that takes place between displaced persons is enormously important and is a major force in their recuperation because it allows them to dispell their anxieties and fears.

A family care facility can benefit many people in the transplant program, and the effects are currently being examined across the country. In many cities, such as Pittsburgh, Pennsylvania and Rochester, Minnesota, these centers are already an integral part of the entire transplantation program. The initial benefits are to the family members who are provided with a housing alternative that is considerably less costly than that of a standard hotel. Transplant patients benefit simultaneously as they are now relieved of their concerns for their families' safety and comfort and can direct all their energy into their recovery. Physicians know that patients with good family support mend and heal better. Recovery is further hastened by early hospital discharge, which is made possible when the family center is used as a stepdown unit. Logistically, coordinators and medical personnel benefit because they can now work in concert with the entire family.

Family centers provide the climate for both patients and their families to overcome the challenges of a life-threatening illness and provide a helping hand to those who need it. They offer the arena where new personal relationships can be formed and act as the surrogate family. Most families, when questioned, admitted that the midday hour and after visiting hours are the most difficult. In the shelter of a family house, families are able to draw strength from others who are experiencing similar emotions. Family centers also enable children to be with their parents while enabling parents to be with their children. Tender loving care needs to be administered to allay the anxieties, depression, and withdrawal experienced by all. The family center provides the physical space for cooking, eating, and cleaning, and participating together in these daily routines helps prevent the separation that frequently occurs in a medical crisis.

When a loved one is admitted to a hospital far from home, the accompanying family member is left completely alone. New York City is scary to the out-of-towner and carries with it its own brand of apprehension. Plans are currently under way to establish a family care facility in New York City, named the Transplant Living Center (TLC). Here, liver transplant patients and their families will find a caring staff in a supportive environment where they can interact with each other. The Transplant Living Center will provide the supportive atmosphere where sharing the challenges of a life-threatening illness can help convert strangers into friends and ultimately result in extended families.

SUPPORT GROUPS

There are several independent support groups functioning outside the environs of the hospital that are also invaluable to the total rehabilitation of the transplant patient. The American Liver Foundation, with more than 25 chapters throughout the United States, is a national, voluntary health agency that supports research and education and provides a referral service for support groups for all liver patients and their families. One of the local American Liver Foundation chapters has initiated their own "buddy system" where patients are matched with those experiencing similar ailments, needs, and crises. Their "liver line" is open daily and available to answer any and all questions. Monthly meetings feature a guest lecturer with special expertise in the field. They publish a monthly newsletter that not only informs but also supports. There are various social functions, including a dinner dance auction as well as a golf tournament taking place throughout the year which further the comraderie between the members and helps to diminish any feelings of isolation.

Adhering to the basic principle that the patient who feels cared for is more likely to comply with a medical regimen, independent support groups are establishing chapters in many towns and cities throughout the United States. The National Transplant Support Network is currently being established. The purpose of this organization is to centralize information and assistance on a national basis. They refer for legal assistance, offer social work services and financial counseling, and advocate lobbying for legislation for transplant patients' rights.

Transplant Recipients International Organization (TRIO), meeting monthly, has chapters in many locations. TRIO is a nonprofit, international organization whose main concern is to improve the quality of life for the transplant family. Understanding that the major obstacle in providing transplants to patients is obtaining a transplantable organ, TRIO is very involved in donor awareness and public education programs. Local chapters of TRIO hold monthly meetings and publish a supportive and informative newsletter.

There is a specialty pharmacy program, servicing the national transplant community, which provides support through group meetings every other week on Long Island. They also host specialty meetings for spouses and children. This organization offers a teleconference support group that can accommodate groups of up to 20, thus enabling the homebound or newly relocated to participate. They have their own toll-free (800), 24-hr, hotline and publish a quarterly newsletter.

There are also in-hospital-based support groups at all transplant centers that meet weekly under the guidance of social workers and specially trained personnel. In the New York, metropolitan area, the Mt. Sinai Medical Center offers a support and bereavement group that meets weekly.

The Well Spouse Foundation, located in San Diego, California, is an organization that aids millions of well spouses across the country through support groups and newsletters. This organization acknowledges and supports the role of the well partner.

The timely scheduling of the various support group meetings within a metropolitan area makes it possible for a patient to seek a different group almost every day. These various groups play an integral role in preparing the patient who is waiting as well as the patient who is posttransplant and healing. Continuing public education programs are a very important part of all support group activities, and recognizing that legislative issues are very therapeutic, most support groups are generally involved in lobbying and campaigning.

The International Transplant games, held every other year, offer another form of support system. Here transplanted patients meet, compete in athletic activities, and exchange experiences while keeping fit. More than 55 competitors from over 30 countries met and competed in Budapest, Hungary in 1991.

Encore: Another Chance for Life is a quartely publication that provides a broad look at the many issues facing the transplant community. The main focus of this magazine, which is distributed as a service to the transplant community, is to share information and provide encouragement to its readers.

Support groups demonstrate that transplant works help to restore the recipients' self-image and encourage them to make the most of the gift of life. Following surgery, the entire transplant family faces a lifelong challenge and it is the support groups and family centers that help them begin to "manage" and enjoy their "rebirth" following transplantation.

RESOURCES

The American Liver Foundation
1425 Pompton Avenue, Cedar Grove, NJ 07009
1-800-223-0179

The American Liver Foundation, Long Island Chapter
101 Shinebone Lane, Commack, NY 11725
516-453-2700

Encore Magazine
Cronimed Publishing
13911 Ridgedale Drive, Minnetonka, MN 55343
1-800-444-5951

MHI Social Work Services and Support Groups
80 Air Park Drive, Ronkonkomo, NY 11779
1-800-637-5633

The Mount Sinai Medical Center
Liver Transplant Support–Bereavement Group
1 Gustave Levy Place, New York, NY 10029
Joan Pietro, MSW
(212) 241-1693
Emily Vaill Pfaff, MSW
(212) 241-1764

National Transplant Support Network
New York City
Information source: 516-981-0034

TRIO
PO Box 922
Huntington, NY 11743-0922
516-421-3258
244 North Bellefield Ave.
Pittsburgh, PA 15213
412-687-2210

Well Spouse Foundation
PO Box 28876, San Diego, CA 92189

World Transplant Games
Contact: Wayne Clark
207-871-2196

— Appendix B —

COMPUTER DATABASE SYSTEMS IN LIVER TRANSPLANT

Myron E. Schwartz and Wayne Dewell

Liver transplantation is an endeavor of great complexity that requires a large commitment of personal, institutional, and societal resources. It is the responsibility of transplant centers to review their results critically, to conduct active research, and to present this work to the medical community and to the public. The generation, collection, and storage of meaningful data in a manner that facilitates analysis are paramount to the successful development and evaluation of a liver transplant program.

Current computer technology provides the tools for the creation of systems to maintain this information, so-called computer databases. Quite simply, a computer database is an electronic record-keeping system the overall purpose of which is to maintain information that has traditionally been kept in voluminous paper files. The components of such a computer system are illustrated below (Fig. A.1); they include: data, hardware, software, and users.

Data. The data constitute all information stored in the database. Items such as patient names, background demographics, diagnoses, and laboratory results are examples of data elements.

Hardware. The hardware of a computer system includes all of its physical components, such as the keyboard, monitor, central processing unit (CPU), hard-disk drives, and cables.

Software. The software is the interface between the hardware components and the users of the database. Software, or "computer programs," include all the necessary executable commands required to run a computer system.

Users. The users of a computer system are the administrator(s) and the end users. The database administrator is the one who is responsible for the writing of the applications (computer programs) that access information from the database. The end users of the database are those

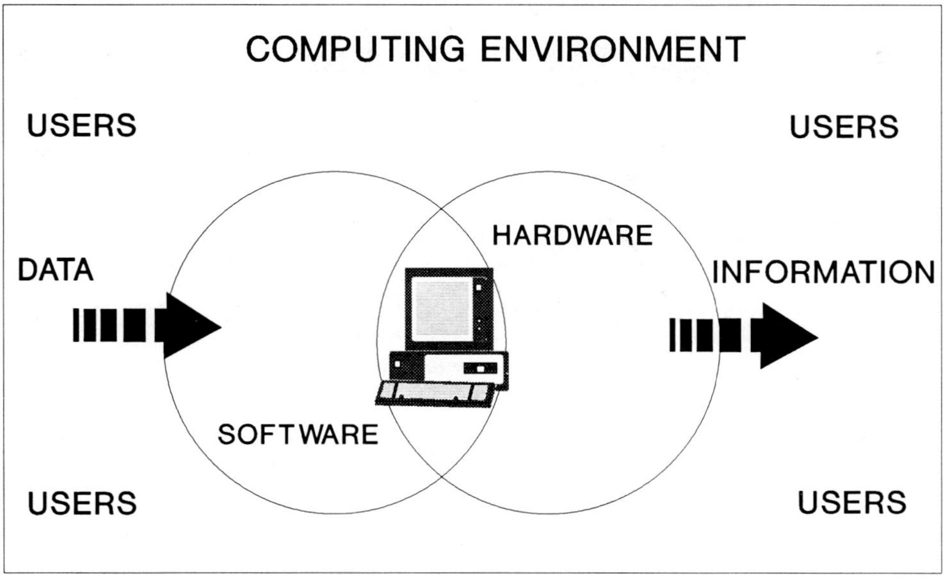

Figure B-1. Components of a computer database system.

individuals who interact with the system from an online terminal using the application.

Advantages of a computer database include the speed with which vital information can be made available, as well as the elimination of much of the tedium of maintaining paper files by hand. In addition to enabling research, such systems can help to maximize the efficiency of a busy clinical service.

The implementation of a computer system involves a well-thought-out eight-stage process.

1. *Evaluation.* The first and often the most important step is the *evaluation* phase. During this stage, a transplant program must form an evaluation team that will follow and monitor the implementation of the computer system to its completion. This group must include experts from administrative, operational, and technological backgrounds. This group can evaluate the informational needs of a transplant program and dovetail it with existing hardware and software technologies available in the marketplace.
2. *Planning.* Second, and equally important, is the *planning* phase. This is actually a continuation of the evaluation phase. The hardware and software components of the system are now purchased. Long-term program objectives and direction need to be discussed at this point. The team will begin to define the timing of the following steps 3–8.
3. *Installation.* Once a plan is in place, technical personnel install and test the hardware and software components of the computer system. It may be necessary to purchase additional hardware and software at this point.
4. *Customization.* When the computer system has been installed and tested, the database administrator can begin to custom tailor the software applications to meet the needs of the transplant program. Screen appearance and

database structure are created during this interval. It is helpful to examine the informational needs of the various end users to assist in identifying the data elements to be recorded. A balance must be struck between the complexity and comprehensiveness of the database and the resources available to gather and enter data. The database administrator defines user access and security levels during this phase based on the operational structure of the transplant program. Adequate backup facilities are installed.

5. *Conversion.* The fifth phase of computerization entails replacing the previous paper filing system with an electronic system. During this phase, forms should be customized to allow easy data collection. The forms should be complete and should eliminate any ambiguity in interpretation. Once the preexisting forms have been converted to data-entry forms, virtually any clerical staff member should be able to enter data.
6. *Migration and/or evolution.* This is often the most difficult and labor-intensive stage in the computerization process. New technologies are often met with apprehension by staff who are used to doing things "the old way." Computer training can help to ease this anxiety and to eliminate the mystique that often surrounds computers. The original evaluation and planning team must keep abreast of the issues that arise during the implementation of a new computer system.
7. *Operation.* Before abandoning the preexisting files, it is wise to operate both systems in parallel for a period of time during which the reliability of the new database may be validated and any wrinkles in the standard operating procedures may be ironed out. A glossary of important terms and their definitions must be maintained, and any changes in procedures should be recorded.
8. *Maturation.* The final stage is an ongoing process. Criteria for the classification of data in all cases cannot be adequately predefined. Clarification will be required as new situations are encountered. Evolving informational needs are continually woven into the structure of the database. Technological advances in computer hardware and software are evaluated critically, and appropriate enhancements are incorporated into the system. When considering the replacement of an existing computer system, care should be taken to evaluate alternative hardware and software products so as to decide which best fit the needs of the office environment.

THE MOUNT SINAI LIVER TRANSPLANT DATABASE

Prior to the initiation of the clinical Liver Transplant Program at Mount Sinai, a decision was made to create a computer database and to prospectively enter data on our transplant patients for purposes of clinical research and quality assurance. Program directors at other centers were contacted in an attempt to acquire suitable computer software for this purpose, but none was found suitable, so we have initiated the development of a database. After examining several of the available relational database applications development systems, we have implemented our database on MS-DOS using DataEase. This software package has a number of attributes, including ease of application development, full data security, the simple creation of predefined "choice fields" that eliminate error in the data entry process, a user-friendly report-generating system, and network support.

Planning the Database Design

Logical database design begins with the development of critical protocols for the major aspects of patient care. Protocols ensure high-quality clinical care and facilitate data collection. Such protocols, for example, have been developed for medical, nutritional, psychosocial candidate evaluation, donor evaluation and procurement, recipient prophylaxis against infection, intraoperative monitoring of coagulation, initial immunosuppression, surveillance for infection, liver biopsies, cholangiograms, duplex Doppler ultrasound studies, and the treatment of rejection and infection in posttransplant patients. Definition of the problems to be answered is a critical element of successful database design. Before structuring our database, a wide-ranging list of questions dealing with many of the controversial issues in liver transplantation was developed by a team, including members of the surgery, hepatology, pathology, immunology, pediatrics, and infectious diseases services. Definition of the data items was then begun.

Eighteen data files have been created. Patients are assigned a unique identification number (ID#) at the time of initial entry into the system; information contained within the files is related to a particular patient through this number. Additional relationships between files have been constructed in situations where recurring events (retransplantation, rejection, etc.) must maintain linkage with the appropriate data in other files (e.g., transplant and donor files, transplant and rejection files).

A full-time data coordinator and a data-entry clerk have been hired to gather and enter the data, to maintain the database, and to generate reports as required. Data collection forms were created and have been used successfully for prospective data collection. Errors in the data entry process are minimized by assigning this task to one individual. Following data entry, data forms are marked as entered and filed for permanent storage. Regular backup of the database is performed.

The data forms are listed below, with the number of data items required in each:

FORM	DATA ITEMS	FORM	DATA ITEMS
REFERRALS	51	BIOPSIES	84
CONTROL	35	COMPLICATIONS	20
CANDIDATES	170	LABORATORY PANEL	58
PRE-TX COMPLICATIONS	11	REJECTIONS	67
UNOS LISTING FILE	35	INFECTIONS	22
DEMOGRAPHICS	30	NONTRANSPLANT	
MD ADDRESS	16	OPERATIONS	23
TRANSPLANTS	90	FOLLOW-UP	45
DONORS	74	DEATH SUMMARY	20
ADMISSIONS	31		

TOTAL ITEMS = 882

Data Collection Protocol

For the database to be effective data must be entered as soon as possible after generation. For this reason, the data coordinator must be integrated into the clinical team, both in the hospital and in the outpatient clinic. The cooperation of key team members including the hepatologist, pathologist, and surgeon is essential. Following are the specifics of our data-gathering procedures:

Candidate evaluation data. Baseline data is collected for all patients evaluated for transplantation. A log is maintained of all new patients seen, and a chart containing the referral information, previous test results, and the findings on history and physical is created for each new patient. For all patients who enter the evaluation protocol, a flow sheet is begun (Fig. A.2) which is used to record the results of the various tests and to assure the completion of all elements of the CANDIDATES form (Fig. A.3). This phase of the data-entry process must be done retrospectively and there is thus some risk for loss of data. We have found the flow sheets to be helpful in avoiding data loss.

Transplant-related data. The DONORS form (Fig. A.4) is taken along to the donor hospital to be completed by the surgical team. TRANSPLANTS forms (Fig. A.5) are stored in the transplant operating room; the immediate preoperative laboratory values and patient status are recorded as well as the operative details. The surgeon performing the transplant completes this form, thus minimizing error.

Pathology data. The BIOPSIES form (Fig. A.6) is completed by the pathologist. Information about the pathology of the native liver is entered into the CANDIDATES file.

In-hospital postoperative data. The data coordinator accompanies the transplant team on daily rounds. INFECTIONS, COMPLICATIONS, and REJECTIONS forms (Figs. A.7–A.9) are completed, or the data gathered to ensure their completion, in a prospective fashion. The requisite lab values for the periodic completion of the LAB PANELS form are gathered independently by the database personnel.

Postdischarge follow-up data. The data coordinator joins the surgeon and transplant physician in the outpatient clinic, where the requisite data for the completion of the FOLLOW-UP form are captured. Complications are noted as they arise, and the appropriate forms are completed.

Databases as management tools. Apart from its use in clinical research, the database is a useful tool in managing the day-to-day operation of a transplant service. Databases are used in the scheduling and billing of a transplant program's services. Quality assurance is another feature that can be built into a program's design. Figures on a program's patient and graft survival, hospitalized average daily population (ADP), average hospital length of stay (LOS), and complication rates are a few of the indicators that can be reported and monitored on a routine basis. These data provide the framework for which a program can evaluate itself as well as plan for future patient care.

LIVER TRANSPLANT RECIPIENT EVALUATION

Name: ______________________________

DOB: ______________ Age: ______________

Address: ______________________________

____

Ph #: ______________________________

S.S. #: ______________________________

Insurance: ______________________________

NOK: ______________________________

Backup Number: ______________________________

Beeper: ______________________________

Referring M.D.: ______________________________

Address: ______________________________

____

Ph #: ______________________________

THE MOUNT SINAI MEDICAL CENTER
LIVER TRANSPLANTATION EVALUATION

CANDIDATE NAME ____________ AGE ______ HOSPITAL NUMBER ____________

ABO ________ Ht ________ IBW ________ CC ________ LV/ELL ________

DATE			TEMP	WEIGHT	BLOOD PRESSURE			BLOOD GASES			HEMATOLOGY												BLOOD CHEMISTRIES																
			High in 24 hr.				24 Hour Volume								Differential																								
YEAR	MONTH	DAY	C°	Kg	Sys	Dias	Urine	PO_2	PCO_2	PH	Fibrinogen	Hgb / HCT	WBC	Platelets	Seg	Bands	Lymph	Atyp Lymph	Mono	Eos	PT	PTT	Na	K	Cl	CO_2	BUN	Creat	T.P.	Alb	Mg	Ca	P	Amy	Glu	LDH	GGTP / Alk Phos	Bili / T/D	(ALT) SGPT	(AST) SGOT

DIAGNOSIS ____________ INDICATIONS FOR TX ____________ REFERRING M.D. ____________

Hbs Ag ________ CMV ________ Re Op ________

COMMENTS

SPECIALTY LAB RESULTS

DAY 1:	Date Sent	Results
Type & Screen #1		
HIV		
Hepatitis Profile		
PPD		
Mumps		
Candida		
Creatine Clearance		

DAY 2: VIRAL STUDIES	Date Sent	Results
CMV		
HSV		
EBV		
Varicella		
VDRL		
AFP		
CEA		
Type & Screen #2		

DAY 3:	Date
Vaccines	
Flu	
Pnemorax	
Heptorax	

OPTIONAL	Date Sent	Results
IPEP		
SPEP		
AMA		
ANA		
TOXO		
ASHA		
HLA/PRA		

CONSULTATIONS

Consultant / Comments

Surgery ________
Hepatology ________
Tx. Coordinator ________
Social Work ________
Nutrition ________
Anesthesia ________
Pulmonary ________
Dental ________
Administrator ________

Additional Consults

PROCEDURES (Date & Results)

CT Scan ________
USG - Duplex ________
PFT's ________
EKG ________
Liver Biopsy ________

LIVER TRANSPLANT DATABASE

CANDIDATES

NAME: ________ MS-OLTX# ________ DOB: ________

SEX: ________ RACE: ________ NATIONALITY: ________

DIAGNOSIS 1 ________ SOC SEC #: ________

2 ________ CATEGORY: ________

VERICEAL BLEED: ESOPH ____ GASTRIC ____ # BLEEDS ____ FATIGUE ____
(WHEN)

SCLEROTHERAPY ____ # SESSIONS ____ ENCEPHALOPATHY ____ ITCHING ____
(WHEN)

HYPERSPLENISM ____ WASTING ____ ASCITES ____ SBP ____ # EPISODES ____
(WHEN)

PAST MEDICAL HISTORY

HEART DISEASE ____ DIABETES ____ HYPERTENSION ____ RENAL DISEASE ____

MALIGNANCY ____ PULMONARY DISEASE ____ INFLAM BOWEL DIS ____ IVDA ____

PRIOR ABD SURGERY: 1 ________

2 ________

BLOOD TX ____ SMOKING ____

COMMENT: ________

____

PHYSICAL EXAMINATION

HEIGHT: ____IN WEIGHT: ____LB

RADIOLOGIC STUDIES

CT SCAN: LIVER VOLUME ____ CC/EXPECTED ____ CC DUPLEX: ____

TUMOR MARKERS

CEA: _______ AFP: _______

BLOOD GROUP: ABO _______ RH _______

IMMUNOLOGIC MARKERS

IgA _______ IgG _______ IgM _______ ANA: _______ AMA: _______ ASMA: _______

VIRAL STUDIES

HIV: ELISA _____________ WESTERN BLOT _____________ PCR _____________

HEPATITIS B: HBsAg _______ HBsAb _______ HBcAb _______ HBcAb (IgM) _______

HBeAg _______ HBeAb _______ HDAb: _______ HAAb: TOTAL _______ IgM _______

CMV: _______ HSV: _______ EBV: _______

FTA-ABS: _____________

PATIENT
ADDRESS: ____________________ CITY: ____________________ STATE: _______

TEL: ____________________________

MD #1 LAST NAME __________ FIRST NAME __________ SPECIALTY __________

ADDRESS: ____________________ CITY: ____________________ STATE: _______

TEL: ____________________________

MD #2 LAST NAME __________ FIRST NAME __________ SPECIALTY __________

ADDRESS: ____________________ CITY: ____________________ STATE: _______

TEL: ____________________________

LIVER TRANSPLANT DATABASE

DONORS

RECIPIENT NAME: __________ MS-OLTX#: __________ FOR GRAFT # ______

DATE: ____________ DONOR NAME: ______________________________

INSTITUTION: ________________ CITY: ________________ STATE: ______

DONOR AGE: ____ SEX: ____ RACE: __________ HGT: ____IN WGT: ____LBS

DAYS IN HOSPITAL: ____ CAUSE OF DEATH: _______ CARDIAC ARREST? ____

BLOOD GROUP: ______ RH ______ DONOR SURGEON: ________________

SGOT: PEAK ___ LAST ___ SGPT: PEAK ___ LAST ___ BILI: PEAK ___ LAST ___

CMV STATUS: ______ VDRL/FTA: ______

SURGEON'S ASSESSMENT OF LIVER

BILE PRODUCTION: ______________ LIVER CONSISTENCY: ______________

TECHNIQUE: _____________ FLUSH: _____________ OKT3: _____________

ORGANS PROCURED:

HEART ____ LUNG ____ HEART-LUNG ____ KIDNEYS ____ PANCREAS ____

CROSS-CLAMP TIME: __________________________

LIVER TRANSPLANT DATABASE

TRANSPLANTS

NAME: ______________________________ MS-OLTX#: __________

DATA OF TX: ______________ GRAFT # ______________

PRETRANSPLANT PATIENT STATUS

____

WEIGHT: ______ LBS MENTAL STATUS: ______________________

PRETRANSPLANT LABORATORY EVALUATION

CBC: HB ____ HCT ____ WBC ____ PLT ____ PRO TIME: ____ FIBRINOGEN: ____

BUN: ____ CREAT: ____ T. PROT: ____ ALBUMIN: ____ ALK PHOS: ____ GGTP: ____

BILI: TOT ______ DIR ______ SGPT: ______ SGOT: ______

INDICATION: ____________________

HEPATIC ALLOGRAFT

ISCHEMIA: TOTAL ____HR WARM ____MIN ARTERY ANATOMY: __________

BACK TABLE RECONSTRUCTION REQUIRED? ______

PRIMARY SURGEON: ______________ DURATION OF SURGERY: ______ HR

ASCITES REMOVED: __L TRANSFUSION: PRBC __U FFP __U CRYO __U PLT __U

VENO-VENOUS BYPASS: ______ PLACEMENT OF LIVER: ______________

PORTAL VEIN: STATUS ______________ TECHNIQUE ______________

HEPATIC ARTERY: INFLOW __________ ANASTOMOTIC TECHNIQUE __________

FLOW: RESTING ____ CC/MIN AUGMENTED ____ CC/MIN PORTAL ____L/MIN

CARDIC OUTPUT: ______L/MIN DUCT RECONSTRUCTION: __________

INITIAL IMMNOSUPPRESSION PROPHYLAXIS

STEROIDS ______ CYCLOSPORINE ______ AZATHIOPRINE ______

OKT3 ______ CYTOXAN ______ ALG ______

LIVER TRANSPLANT DATABASE

BIOPSIES

NAME: ______________________________ MS-OLTX#: ________

DATE OF BIOPSY: ___________ GREATER THAN 4 PORTAL TRACTS? __________

PORTAL TRACTS

INFLAMMATION: ______________________________

COMPOSITION OF INFLAMMATION: ___________ EOSINOPHILS: ___________

PORTAL FIBROSIS: ______________ PORTAL TRACT EDEMA: ______________

BILE DUCTS

SEVERITY OF BILE DUCT DAMAGE: ________ INFILTRATION BY PMN: ________

INFILTRATION BY LYMPHOCYTES: _____ VACUOLIZATION OF BILE DUCT: _____

DETACHMENT OF BILE DUCT EPITHELIUM FROM BASEMENT MEMBRANE: _____

EOSINOPHILIC DEGENERATION OF BILE DUCT EPITHELIUM: ___________

IF >0 THEN % OF DUCTS DAMAGED: __________ BILE DUCT LOSS: __________

BILE DUCTULAR CHOLESTASIS: _______

HEPATIC ARTERY

ENDOPHLEBITIS: ________ HYPERTROPHY: ________ FOAMY CELLS: ________

THROMBUS FORMATION: _______

OTHER: ______________________________

PORTAL VEIN

ENDOPHLEBITIS: ________________ FOAMY CELLS: ________________

OTHER: ______________________________

TERMINAL HEPATIC VENULE

NECROSIS: _____ ENDOPHLEBITIS: _____ CELL TYPE _____ THROMBUS: _____

NARROWING OF THE LUMEN: ______________ FIBROSIS: ______________

CONGESTION: _______

HEPATIC PARENCHYMA

DISTRIBUTION OF INFLAMMATION: ______________ DEGREE: ______________

COMPOSITION OF INFLAMMATION: ______________________________

DEGREE OF NECROSIS: ______________ TYPE OF CELLS: ______________

DISTRIBUTION OF NECROSIS: __________ PIECEMEAL NECROSIS: __________

EOSINOPHILIC DEGENERATION: ______ INFARCT: ______ STEATOSIS: ______

SINUSOIDAL CELL ACTIVATION: ______ BALLOONING DEGENERATION: ______

MISCELLANEOUS

CHOLESTASIS: __________ GRANULOMAS: __________ MITOSIS: __________

PSEUDODUCTULAR FORMATION: __________ BINUCLEATED CELLS: __________

OTHER: ______________________________

DIAGNOSIS ______________________________

____

LIVER TRANSPLANT DATABASE

INFECTIONS

NAME: ______________ MS-OLTX#: ______________

DATE OF DIAGNOSIS: ______________ AFTER TRANSPLANT # ______________

TYPE/SITE OF INFECTION: ______________________________

ORGANISM #1: ______________ ORGANISM #2: ______________

TREATMENT ______________________________

SURGICAL INTERVENTION REQUIRED? ______________ DATE: ______________

LIVER TRANSPLANT DATABASE

COMPLICATIONS

NAME: ______________________ MS-OLTX# ______________________

DATE: ______________________

COMPLICATION: ______________________

COMMENT: ______________________

SURGERY REQUIRED? ______________ DATE: ______________

LIVER TRANSPLANT DATABASE

REJECTIONS

NAME: ______________________ MS-OLTX#: ________

DATE OF REJECTION: ____________

	BILI	SGPT	SGOT	ALK PHOS
PRE-REJECTION:	______	______	______	______
PEAK:	______	______	______	______

BIOPSY? __________ GRADE: __________ IMMUNOFLUORESCENCE: __________

IMMUNOSUPPRESSION PREREJECTION:

STEROID __________ DOSE __________ CsA __________ LEVEL __________

IMURAN ______ DOSE ______

THERAPY:

STEROID RECYCLE ______ RESPONSE ______ REPEAT? ___ RESPONSE ___

OKT3 ______ RESPONSE ______

AGL ______ RESPONSE ______

CYTOXAN ______ RESPONSE ______

PLASMAPHERESIS ______ RESPONSE ______

IMMUNOSUPPRESSION POSTREJECTION:

STEROID ____________ DOSE ____________ CsA ____________ LEVEL ____________

IMURAN ____________ DOSE ____________ CYTOXAN ____________ DOSE ____________

REPEAT CROSSMATCH: ____________________ DATE: ____________________

ADMISSIONS

NAME: ____________________ MS-OLTX#: ____________________

DATE OF ADMISSION: ____________ DATE OF DISCHARGE: ____________

REASON FOR ADMISSION: ______________________________

COMMENT: ______________________________

____

NONTRANSPLANT OPERATIONS

NAME: ____________________ MS-OLTX#: ____________________

DATE OF OPERATION: ______________________________

SURGEON: ____________ INDICATION FOR SURGERY: ____________

PROCEDURE: ______________________________

COMMENT: ______________________________

____

— Appendix C —

TRANSPLANTATION OF FOREIGN NATIONALS

Lynn Rogut

During the early 1980s, the provision of transplant services to foreign nationals (nonresident aliens permitted to enter the United States temporarily) became extremely controversial. This was partly attributable to the practice of some transplant centers giving foreign nationals waiting list priority due to their willingness to pay higher fees for medical care. A second element of the controversy was related to the provision of scarce donor organs to foreign nationals when there were American candidates in need of transplants. In its report to Congress in 1986, the Task Force on Organ Transplantation recommended limiting the proportion of foreign nationals transplanted at each transplant center to 10%. This recommendation along with other limitations have been incorporated into the policies of the OPTN.

Transplant centers that accept nonresident aliens must adhere to the following guidelines:

- Organs must be allocated to foreigners on the waiting list in accordance with UNOS policies without favoritism or discrimination.
- Nonresident aliens must be charged the same fees as domestic patients.
- No contractual arrangements can be made with foreign governments for transplantation of nonresident aliens.
- The provision of training programs in organ transplantation that include physicians from underserved nations is desirable.
- A mechanism for community participation and review of the candidate selection process should be established.

In addition, transplant centers must allow the UNOS Foreign Relations Committee to review and audit all activities related to the transplantation of nonresident aliens. A center that exceeds the 10% limitation triggers a review by the Committee.

BIBLIOGRAPHY

1. Task Force on Organ Transplantation, *Organ Transplantation, Issues and Recommendations, Report of the Task Force on Organ Transplantation,* Washington, DC, US Government Printing Office, 1986, p 95.
2. UNOS, *UNOS Policies,* pp 18–19, Richmond, VA, June 1989.

— Appendix D —

DIET FOR PATIENTS WITH END-STAGE LIVER DISEASE

Franklin M. Klion and Thomas L. Fabry

A. FOODS PERMITTED IN UNLIMITED QUANTITIES;

Marshmallows
Saltfree hard candies
Honey, Jams and Jellies
Molasses and maple syrup
Non-dairy toppings
Jelly
Popcorn (plain)
Fats such as sweet butter and sour cream
Sugar
Chewing gum
Jelly Beans, Gum Drops

B. SAMPLE MENU FOR ONE DAY:

40 gm. protein/day
32 oz. liquid/day
500 mg. sodium/day

Breakfast—total 14 gm. protein, 150 mg. sodium, 12 oz. liquid
1 egg
1 slice toast or 1 pancake (plain, homemade)
Oatmeal
butter (sweet)
Jelly or Jam
Coffee or tea—8 oz.
Orange juice—4 oz.

Lunch—total 9.9 gm. protein, 240 mg. sodium, 8 oz. liquid
Fresh fruit—1 cup
Fresh vegetables—1 cup
Pasta—1 cup cooked
Bread—1 slice
Butter
Coffee or Tea—8 oz.

Dinner—total 16 gm. protein, 85 mg. sodium, 12 oz. liquid
Chicken or hamburger—2 1/2 oz.

Baked Potato w/o skin
Sweet butter
Sour cream
Beets—1/2 cup
Spinach—1/2 cup or salad greens with fresh lemon dressing
Tea or Coffee—8 oz.

C. FOOD EXCHANGE LISTS

1. DAIRY PRODUCTS—

MILK—1 oz. = 1 gr. protein, unless fortified.

	CALORIES	PROTEIN grm.	SODIUM mg.
Whole Milk 8 oz. =	150	8	122
CHEESE—			
Cream—1 oz. =	99	2.1	8
Swiss—1 oz. = (Imported)	107	8.1	74
CREAMS—			
1/2 & 1/2 1 T =	20	0.4	6
Sour—1 T =	26	0.4	6
Whipping—1 T =	52	0.3	6
BUTTER—1 t =	36	0	41
EGGS—			
One raw egg = approximately	80	6.5	70

2. GRAINS—

	CALORIES	PROTEIN grm.	SODIUM mg.
CEREALS—			
Oatmeal—3/4 c =	108	4.5	0
Wheatena—3/4 c =	101	3.7	0
Farina—3/4 c =	87	2.5	0
Grits—1 c =	146	3.0	0
Cream of Rice—3/4 c =	95	1.6	1
Puffed Rice—1 cup =	57	.9	0
Puffed Wheat—1 cup =	52	2.1	1
Shredded Wheat—1 =	83	2.6	0
BREADS—			
Boston Brown	95	2.5	113
Cracked Wheat	66	2.3	108
Bread Sticks—2	77	2.4	140
Wheat—1 slice	66	2.3	108
Raisin—1 slice	70	2.1	94
White—1 slice	64	2.0	123
CRACKERS—			
Cracker Meal—2 T	50	1.0	0
Holland Rusk—1	60	1.0	35
Rice Cakes—1	35	0.4	0
Royal Lunch—1	60	1.0	80
Zweiback—1 piece	30	0.7	18
PANCAKES—			
Plain—1 4″	62	1.9	115

	CALORIES	PROTEIN gm.	SODIUM mg.
PASTA—			
Macaroni—1 cup ckd.	159	5.2	1
Noodles—enr. ckd. 1 cup	200	6.6	3
Spaghetti—enr. ckd. 1 cup	159	5.2	1
TORTILLAS—			
Corn—enr.	67	2.1	53
Taco-tostado shell	50	1.0	72
3. MEATS & POULTRY—			
Brisket—3.5 oz. lean	241	29.4	72
Chuck Pot Rst.—3.5 oz.	231	33.0	66
Ground ext. lean—3.5 oz.	250	24.5	49
Lamb—1 rib chop	273	13.5	33
Pork—ctr. loin 3.5 oz.	354	29.4	51
Rib—shortribs 3.5 oz.	471	21.6	50
Round—bottom 3.5 oz.	261	29.8	51
Veal—loin 3 oz.	199	22.4	55
Eel—smoked 3.5 oz.	330	18.6	0
Frogs Legs—3.5 oz.	73	16.4	18
Snail—3.5 oz.	90	16.1	0
Chicken—dark meat 3.5 oz.	192	26.0	74
light meat 3.5. oz.	230	29.0	75
Duck 3.5 oz.	337	19.0	59
4. FISH—			
Bass, striped—3 oz. raw	82	15.1	59
Bluefish—3 oz.	105	17.0	51
Butterfish—3 oz. raw	124	14.7	75
Carp—3 oz. raw	108	15.2	42
Clams—3 oz. raw	63	10.9	47
Cod—3 oz. raw	70	15.1	46
Crayfish—3 oz.	76	15.9	45
Flounder/Sole—3.5 oz.	68	14.9	56
Grouper—3 oz.	78	16.5	45
Haddock—3 oz.	74	16.1	58
Halibut—3 oz.	93	17.7	46
Lobster—3 oz.	77	16.0	0
Mackerel—3 oz.	174	15.8	76
Monkfish—3 oz.	64	12.3	16
Perch—3 oz.	77	16.5	52
Pike—3 oz.	75	16.4	33
Pompano—3 oz.	140	15.7	55
Salmon—3 oz. raw	121	16.9	3
Snapper—3 oz.	85	17.4	54
Sole—3.5 oz.	68	14.9	56
Shad—3 oz.	167	14.4	44
Smelt—4–5	98	18.6	0
Swordfish—3 oz.	103	16.8	76
Tuna in water canned no salt—lt. chunk 2 oz.	60	13.0	43
Tuna, raw—3 oz.	122	19.8	33

	CALORIES	PROTEIN gm.	SODIUM mg.
5. VEGETABLES—			
Alfalfa Sprouts—1 cup	10	1.3	2
Artichoke—1 med.	53	2.8	79
Asparagus—6 spears	22	2.3	4
Avacado—1 med.	306	3.6	21
Bean Green—4 oz. boiled	22	1.2	2
Beets—1/2 cup boiled	26	0.9	42
Broccoli—1/2 cup boiled	12	1.3	12
Brussel Spr.—4 sprts. boiled	30	2.0	17
Cabbage—1/2 cup raw	8	0.4	6
Carrots—1 med. raw	31	0.7	25
Cauliflower—1/2 cup	12	1.0	7
Celery—1 stalk	6	0.3	35
Corn—1/2 cup boiled	89	2.7	14
Eggplant—1/2 cup raw	11	0.5	1
Mushrooms—1/2 cup raw	9	0.7	1
Onions—1/2 cup	27	0.9	2
Parsnips—1/2 cup	63	1.0	8
Peas—1/2 cup	63	4.2	4
Peppers—1	12	0.4	2
Potato w/o skin	88	2.3	7
w skin	220	4.7	16
Pumpkin—1/2 cup boiled	24	9	2
Rhubarb—1 cup	29	0.8	2
Rice—white, enr. 1 cup	223	4.1	0
Soybeans—1/2 cup boiled	127	11.0	0
Spinach—1/2 cup raw	6	0.8	22
Squash—1/2 cup raw	13	0.8	1
Tomato—1	30	1.5	16
6. FRUITS—			
Apple—1	81	0.3	1
Apricot—3	51	1.5	1
Banana—1	105	1.2	1
Blackberries—1/2 cup	37	0.5	0
Blueberries—1 cup	82	1.0	9
Raspberries—1 cup	61	1.1	0
Strawberries—1 cup	45	0.9	2
Cantaloupe—1 cup	57	1.4	14
Cranberry—1 cup raw	46	0.4	1
Figs—1 med.	37	0.4	1
Citrus–1	35	0.7	0
Grapes—1 cup	58	0.6	2
Pear—1 med.	98	0.7	1
Pineapple—1 cup raw	77	0.6	1
Prunes—10 dried	201	2.2	3
Raisins—2/3 cup seedless	300	3.2	12
Watermelon—1 cup	50	1.1	3
7. DRESSINGS & CONDIMENTS—			
Oil & vinegar—1 T	72	0	0
Horseradish—1 T	6	2	14
Vinegar & Oil Homemade—	72	0	0

INDEX

D